Diagnosis and Management *of* Fetal Arrhythmias

EDITORS

Bettina F. Cuneo, MD
Professor, Pediatrics (Cardiology) and Obstetrics
Director of Perinatal Cardiology and
Fetal Cardiac Telemedicine
University of Colorado School of Medicine
Aurora, Colorado

Julia A. Drose, BA, RDMS, RDCS, RVT
Associate Professor, Radiology
Chief Sonographer, Divisions of Diagnostic
Ultrasound and Prenatal Diagnosis & Genetics
University of Colorado School of Medicine
Aurora, Colorado

D. Woodrow Benson, MD, PhD
Professor of Pediatrics (Cardiology)
Medical College of Wisconsin
Milwaukee, Wisconsin

Wolters Kluwer

Philadelphia • Baltimore • New York • London
Buenos Aires • Hong Kong • Sydney • Tokyo

Acquisitions Editor: Chris Teja
Development Editor: Thomas Celona
Editorial Coordinator: Ashley Pfeiffer
Editorial Assistant: Brian Convery
Marketing Manager: Phyllis Hitner
Production Project Manager: Kim Cox
Design Coordinator: Teresa Mallon
Manufacturing Coordinator: Beth Welsh
Prepress Vendor: TNQ Technologies

9 8 7 6 5 4 3 2 1

Printed in China

Library of Congress Cataloging-in-Publication Data

ISBN: 978-1-9751-2286-7

Cataloging in Publication data available on request from publisher.

shop.lww.com

CCS0720

FOREWORD

Huge progress has been made in the diagnosis and treatment of various fetal conditions. Ultrasound has provided the essential information regarding the nature of abnormalities of structure, growth, and function and has allowed the understanding of how the fetus adapts to these conditions. It is now clear that the fetal heart, while centrally involved in structural anomalies, can also play a major secondary functional role in other conditions involving the placenta and fetal brain. On the maternal side of the placenta, diabetes, obesity, autoimmune diseases, hemoglobinopathies, and even medications can have a major effect on the fetal heart, which is the epicenter of fetal response to these challenges.

Ultrasound has been the major diagnostic vehicle for identifying congenital heart disease. Interestingly, the technology has undergone an exponential expansion, evolving from 2D and M-mode ultrasound, through pulsed and color Doppler real-time advances to the new speckle tracking techniques used to assess fetal ventricular contractility. However, the current technology has arrived before many clinicians in the field have had a chance to understand, or even exploit, its potential. This book should fill the knowledge gap that has arisen from one set of particularly thorny problems: fetal cardiac arrhythmias. A novel challenge for healthcare providers managing fetal arrhythmias is the care of two patients—the fetus and the mother. This book, a compilation of topics written by multidisciplinary experts in the field and edited by Cuneo, Drose, and Benson, is the first textbook to exclusively address fetal cardiac arrhythmias. In this book, the approach to fetal cardiac arrhythmias is comprehensive and includes diagnosis, treatment of the fetus, maternal management, and etiology including genetic origins.

The editors represent an ideal coalition of professionals, each representing a separate component in the collaborative delivery of care to fetuses suspected of having cardiac arrhythmias. Julia Drose is a sonographer who has been immersed in fetal echocardiography almost from its inception. D. Woodrow Benson is a well-known and prolific electrophysiologist and cardiovascular geneticist, and Bettina Cuneo is a widely published fetal cardiologist who has made numerous contributions to our understanding of fetal cardiac arrhythmias.

Each chapter is well laid out by selected contributors from pediatric cardiology and maternal-fetal medicine and embellished with beautiful images to illustrate the accompanying text. Every aspect of the diagnosis, treatment, and surveillance of arrythmias is addressed in the book, as well as future approaches to dealing with problem arrhythmias, that will become standard of care in the coming years.

This book beautifully arms the clinician with the most up-to-date knowledge to deal with some of our greatest challenges.

John Hobbins, MD
Professor Emeritus of Obstetrics and Gynecology
Division of Maternal Fetal Medicine
University of Colorado School of Medicine
Aurora, Colorado

PREFACE

The birth of fetal arrhythmology, the diagnosis and treatment of arrhythmias, occurred in the early 1980s. Using a 3.5-MHz nonfocused transducer with a strip chart recorder, teams of maternal fetal medicine (MFM) specialists and pediatric cardiologists from Yale University and the Cardiothoracic Unit in Guy's Hospital successfully diagnosed various fetal arrhythmias. The first transplacental treatment of "fetal paroxysmal atrial tachycardia" with digoxin was reported in the *New England Journal of Medicine* in 1983 by the team of Charlie Kleinman, Greg DeVore, John Hobbins, and others at Yale University. Across the pond at Guy's Hospital in London, Lindsey Allan was publishing her results of transplacental treatment of fetal arrhythmias with digoxin and verapamil. The fortitude and "disruptive thinking" of these early investigators can be summed up in the dedication to Dr. Allan's *Manual of Fetal Echocardiography*: "To all those people....who have inspired me by telling me my proposed next step was impossible." We think it is important to acknowledge the bravery, determination, and vision of the "founders of fetal arrhythmology."

Over the next 25 years, the field of fetal arrhythmology will advance to a state where the electrophysiology mechanisms of complex arrhythmias will be incorporated into clinical practice. Currently, the precise diagnosis and treatment of fetal tachycardia is the standard of care, and the genetics of fetal arrhythmias are making their way to the bedside. It was time for a book about fetal arrhythmias, written in the spirit of the multidisciplinary collaboration, so essential for a successful fetal cardiology program.

The diagnosis and treatment of fetal arrhythmias are intended for a broad audience. There are many illustrations and a chapter on how to obtain the Doppler and M-mode images that allow for accurate diagnosis. Parts 1 and 2 focus on the basics of fetal rhythm analysis. Parts 3 to 5 cover arrhythmias in greater detail and include suggestions for fetal management, maternal arrhythmia treatment, and care of the mother at risk for fetal arrhythmia. Part 6 is intended to spark interest in newer techniques that we believe will further advance the field.

Compiling a book of this type requires a village, and we wish to acknowledge those who made the undertaking possible. First, we are forever humbled by the mothers and families who have entrusted the care of their children to us. Their bravery and resilience are inspirational. Second, we are grateful for what we have learned from our mentors, students, and colleagues. This acknowledgment includes the obstetricians, maternal fetal medicine specialists, pediatric cardiologists, radiologists, electrophysiologists, cardiovascular geneticists, and sonographers with whom we collaborate everyday. We are so fortunate that they have shared our passion for excellent patient care and advancement of the field.

Lastly, we wish to thank our families for their continued support and encouragement, which provide the inspiration for us to "dream things that never were" for other families.

Bettina F. Cuneo Denver, CO

Julia A. Drose Denver, CO

D. Woodrow Benson Milwaukee, WI

Alfred Abuhamad, MD
Mason C. Andrews Professor of Obstetrics & Gynecology
Chairman Department of Obstetrics & Gynecology
Eastern Virginia Medical School
Norfolk, Virginia

Fayeza Alrais, MBSS, FRCSC
Consultant
Maternal-Fetal-Medicine (MFM)
Department of Obstetrics and Gynecology
Tawam Hospital in Affiliation with Johns Hopkins Medicine
SEHA Abu Dhabi Health Services, Co.
Al Ain, United Arab Emirates

Yaniv Bar-Cohen, MD
Professor of Clinical Pediatrics and Medicine
Department of Pediatrics
Keck School of Medicine
University of Southern California
Los Angeles, California

Nico A. Blom, MD, PhD
Head Pediatric Cardiology
Department of Pediatrics
AUMC
Amsterdam, The Netherlands

Ramen H. Chmait, MD
Associate Professor
Department of Obstetrics and Gynecology
University of Southern California
Los Angeles, California

Sally-Ann Barker Clur, MBBCh, MSc(Med), FCP(Paed)SA, PhD
Paediatric Cardiologist and Head of Fetal Cardiology Center for Congenital Heart Defects Amsterdam-Leiden (CAHAL)
Department of Paediatric Cardiology
Amsterdam UMC
University of Amsterdam, Heart Center
Amsterdam, The Netherlands

Bettina F. Cuneo, MD
Professor
Pediatrics (Cardiology) and Obstetrics
Director of Perinatal Cardiology and Fetal Cardiac Telemedicine
University of Colorado School of Medicine
Aurora, Colorado

Mary T. Donofrio, MD
Professor of Pediatrics
George Washington University
Washington, District of Columbia

Julia A. Drose, BA, RDMS, RDCS, RVT
Associate Professor, Radiology
Chief Sonographer, Divisions of Diagnostic Ultrasound and Prenatal Diagnosis & Genetics
University of Colorado School of Medicine
Aurora, Colorado

Susan Etheridge, MD
Professor
Department of Pediatrics
University of Utah
Salt Lake City, Utah

Frank A. Fish, MD
Professor
Departments of Pediatrics and Medicine
Vanderbilt University Medical Center
Nashville, Tennessee

Gerard Frunzi, MBA
Telehealth Services Manager
Telehealth
Children's Hospital Colorado
Aurora, Colorado

Henry L. Galan, MD
Professor
Department of Obstetrics and Gynecology
Division of Maternal-Fetal Medicine
University of Colorado School of Medicine
Colorado Fetal Care Center
Children's Hospital of Colorado
Aurura, Colorado

Helena M. Gardiner, MD, PhD
Professor
The Fetal Center
UT Health
Houston, Texas

John Hobbins, MD
Professor Emeritus of Obstetrics and Gynecology
Division of Maternal Fetal Medicine
University of Colorado School of Medicine
Aurora, Colorado

Hitoshi Horigome, MD, PhD
Professor
University of Tsukuba
Department of Pediatrics
Tsukuba, Ibarkai, Japan

Lisa K. Hornberger, MD
Professor of Pediatrics/Adjunct Professor
Department of Pediatrics/Obstetrics & Gynecology
University of Alberta
Edmonton, Alberta

Lisa Willis Howley, MD
Director
Fetal Cardiology
The Children's Heart Clinic
Children's Hospital Minnesota
Minneapolis, Minnesota

Stacy Ann Stratemann Killen, MD, MSCI
Assistant Professor
Department of Pediatrics, Division of Pediatric Cardiology
Vanderbilt University School of Medicine
Nashville, Tennessee

Katherine Anne Kosiv, MD
Assistant Professor of Clinical Pediatrics
Department of Pediatrics
Yale University School of Medicine
New Haven, Connecticut

Gerald E. Loeb, MD
Professor
Biomedical Engineering
University of Southern California
Los Angeles, California

Lindsay Meyers, MS, LCGC
Adjunct Faculty
Department of Pediatrics
University of Utah
Salt Lake City, Utah

Anita J. Moon-Grady, MD
Professor of Clinical Pediatrics
Department of Pediatrics
University of California San Francisco
San Francisco, California

Christina A. Olson, MD
Assistant Professor
Department of Pediatrics
University of Colorado
Aurora, Colorado

Jay D. Pruetz, MD
Associate Professor of Clinical Pediatrics and Obstetrics and Gynecology
Department of Pediatrics
Keck School of Medicine
University of Southern California
Los Angeles, California

Rachel L. Rodel, MD
Clinical Assistant Professor
Department of Obstetrics and Gynecology
University of South Dakota Sanford School of Medicine
Vermillion, South Dakota

Michael J. Silka, MD
Professor of Pediatrics
Keck School of Medicine
University of Southern California
Los Angeles, California

Danna Spears, MSc, MD, FRCP(C)
Division of Cardiology - Electrophysiology
Medical Director - UHN Cartwright Inherited Cardiomyopathy and Arrhythmia Program
U of T Pregnancy and Heart Disease Program - Arrhythmia Clinic
University Health Network - Toronto General Hospital
Toronto, Ontario, Canada

Janette F. Strasburger, MD
Professor of Pediatrics
Department of Pediatrics and Cardiology Medical College of Wisconsin
Milwaukee, Wisconsin

J. Fred Thomas, PhD
Associate Professor
Department of Medicine, Public Health and Nursing
School of Medicine and School of Public Health
University of Colorado Anschutz Medical Campus
Aurora, Colorado

Arja Suzanne Vink, MD, MSc (EBP)
Department of Clinical and Experimental Cardiology
Amsterdam UMC
University of Amsterdam, Heart Center
Amsterdam, The Netherlands

Ronald Wakai, PhD
Professor
Department of Medical Physics
University of Wisconsin
Madison, Wisconsin

CONTENTS

PART 1 Background

PART 2 Techniques to Analyze Fetal Rhythm

PART 3 Presentation and Diagnosis of Fetal Arrhythmias

PART 6 Fetal Arrhythmias: Future Directions

PART

1

Background

Overview of Fetal Arrhythmias

Julia A. Drose • Bettina F. Cuneo

THE NORMAL CARDIAC CONDUCTION SYSTEM

An understanding of the normal cardiac conduction system is necessary to understand fetal arrhythmia **(FIG. 1.1.1)**. Electrical conduction begins in the sinoatrial (SA) node located in the right atrium (RA). The SA node fires, sending electrical impulses to the left and right atria, causing them to contract. These impulses are then conducted to the atrioventricular (AV) node.

From the AV node, electrical impulses are conducted to the right and left bundle branches, via the bundle of His, then to the Purkinje fibers within the myocardium, resulting in ventricular contraction. If the impulses from the AV node are delayed, 1° block occurs. If the impulses are not conducted due to a structural or functional anomaly of the AV node, 2° or 3° block results and the ventricles beat at an independent and slower rate than the atria. The more distal the damage to the conduction system, the slower the ventricular rate. On the other hand, if electrical impulses from the bundle of His to the Purkinje fibers are accelerated, ventricular or junctional tachycardia occurs.

Atrial depolarization corresponds to the P-wave on the ECG **(FIG. 1.1.2)**, the A-wave on the mitral inflow/aortic outflow spectral Doppler **(FIG. 1.1.3A)**, retrograde flow during atrial systole on the spectral Doppler tracing of a systemic or pulmonary vein **(FIG. 1.1.3B** and **C)**, and the atrial deflections on simultaneous M-mode tracing of atria and ventricles **(FIG. 1.1.3D)**. Atrial deflections are unusually sharp and clear when the M-mode cursor is positioned simultaneously through the RA and LA in the longitudinal view of the aortic arch **(FIG. 1.1.4)**.

The QRS complex on an ECG **(FIG. 1.1.2)** corresponds to excitation of the ventricles as seen by the antegrade flow on the spectral Doppler tracing of aorta or pulmonary artery **(FIG. 1.1.3A-C)** and the ventricular deflections on simultaneous M-Mode tracing of atria and ventricles **(FIG. 1.1.3D)**.

(text continued on page 6)

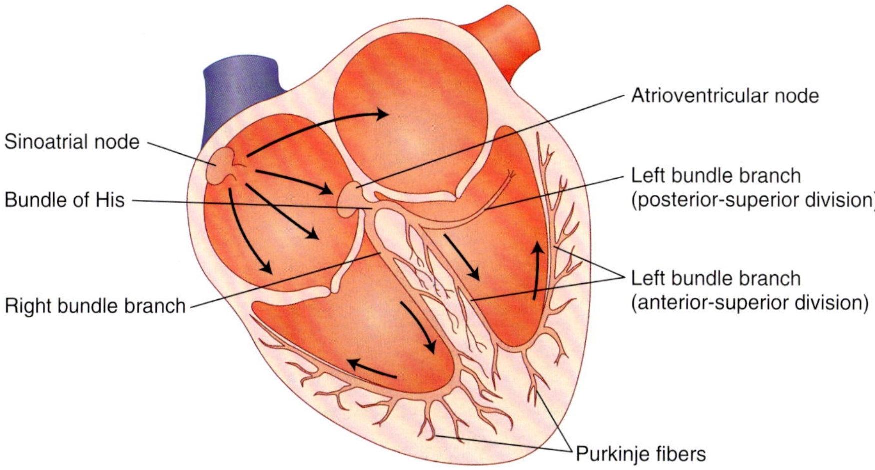

FIGURE 1.1.1 Normal cardiac conduction system. (Modified from Jones RM. *Patient Assessment in Pharmacy Practice*. 3rd ed. Philadelphia, PA: Wolters Kluwer; 2015.)

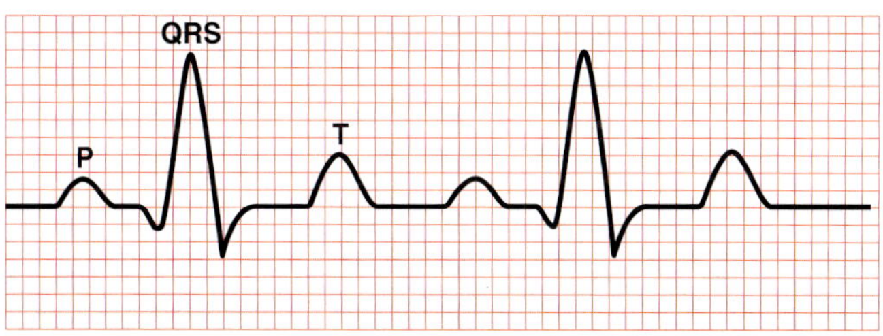

FIGURE 1.1.2 Diagram of a normal electrocardiogram (ECG) tracing. The P-wave represents the onset of atrial contraction. The QRS complex represents ventricular contraction. The T-wave represents ventricular repolarization. The distance between the P-wave and the R-wave represents the time interval from atrial to ventricular contraction of the heart (the PR interval).

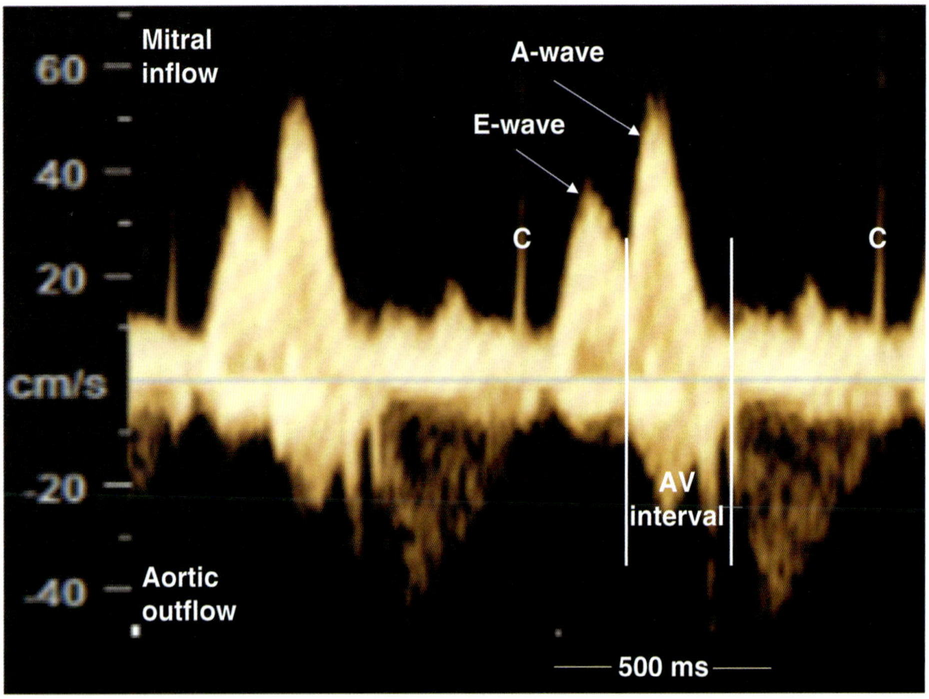

A.

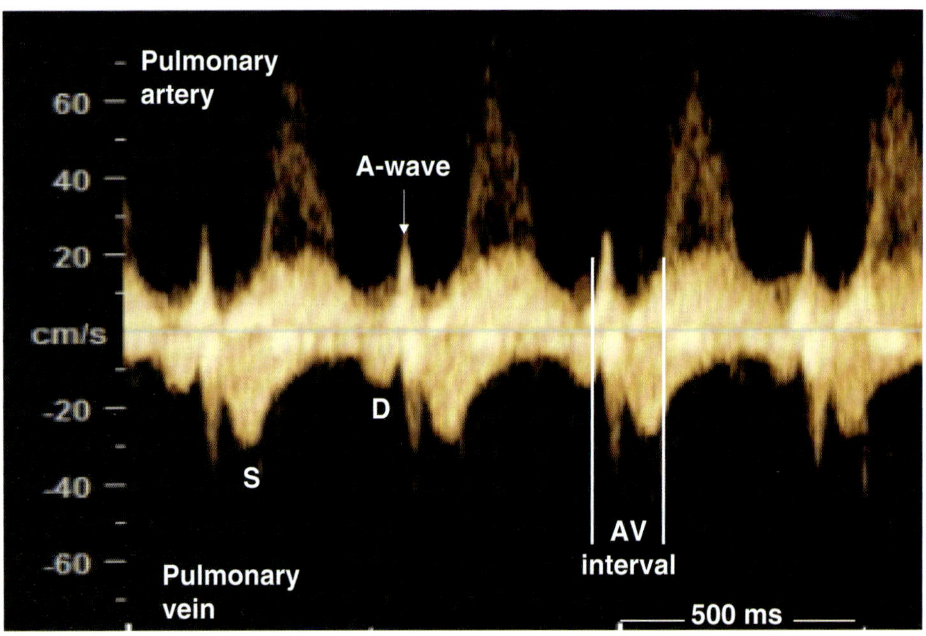

B.

FIGURE 1.1.3 **A:** Spectral Doppler tracing of mitral valve inflow (top tracing) and aortic valve outflow (bottom tracing). The A-wave of the mitral valve corresponds to the P-wave on an ECG and represents atrial contraction. The aortic outflow waveform represents ventricular contraction and corresponds to the ECG QRS. **B:** Pulmonary artery and pulmonary vein spectral Doppler showing atrial contraction represented by reverse flow (the A-wave) in the pulmonary vein. The pulmonary artery waveform (arrow) represents ventricular contraction. The time between the two is the AV interval. D, diastole; S, systole. **C:** Wave forms of the aorta and innominate vein from the three-vessel tracheal view. Atrial contraction is noted as retrograde flow in the innominate vein (IV), and antegrade flow in the transverse aortic arch (Ao) represents ventricular contraction. White circle highlight A-wave of innominate vein. **D:** Tracing with the M-mode cursor placed simultaneously through the left ventricle and the right atrium to show atrial contractions (a) and ventricular contractions (V). AV, atrioventricular; C, aortic valve clicks; LA, left atrium; LV, left ventricle; RA, right atrium; RV, right ventricle.

C.
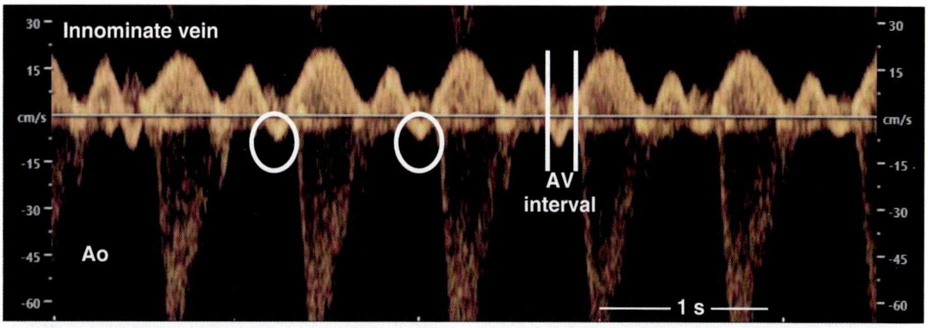

D.
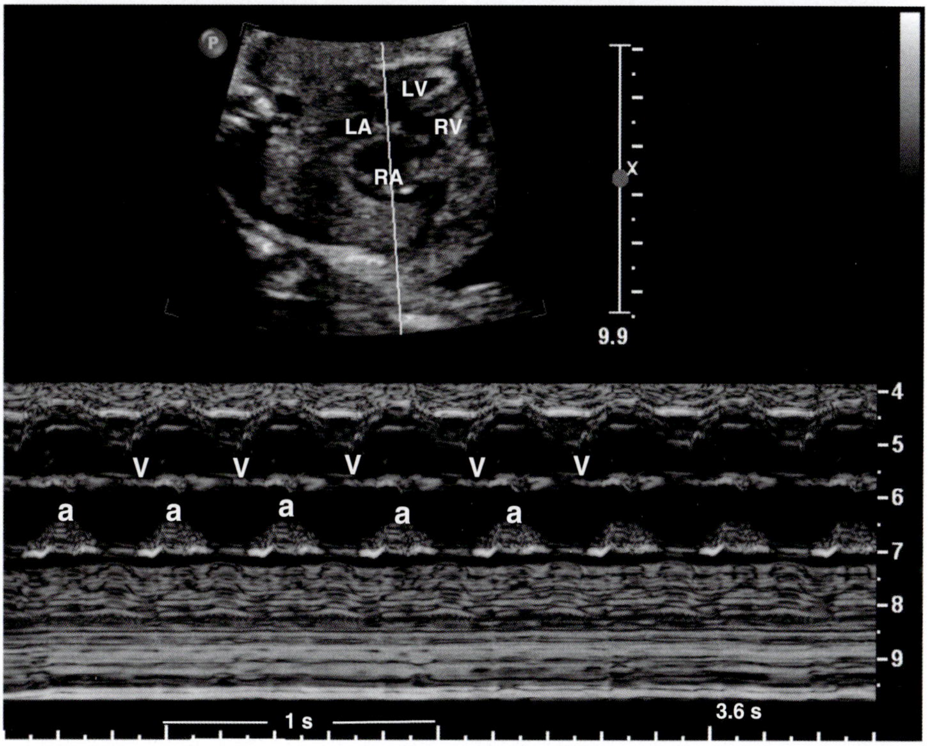

FIGURE 1.1.3 Cont'd

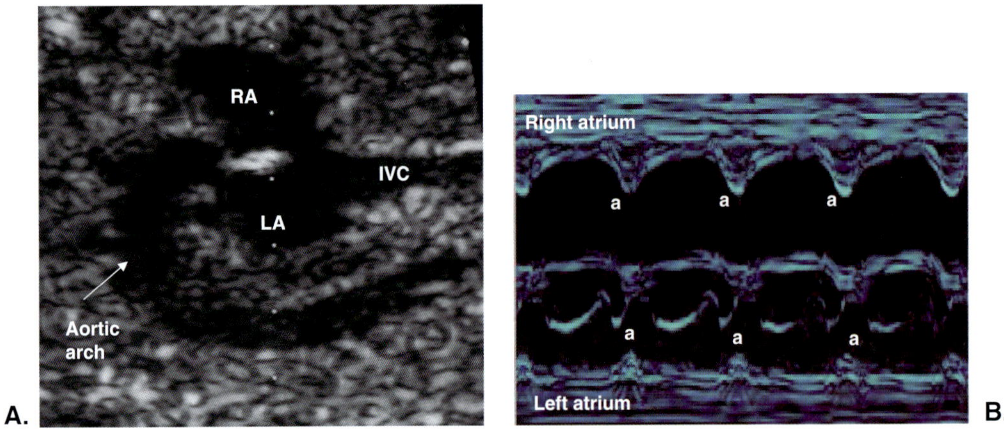

FIGURE 1.1.4 **A:** Positioning the M-mode cursor through the right atrium (RA) and left atrium (LA) simultaneously in longitudinal view of the aortic arch (arrow) to obtain **(B)** a sharp M-mode tracing of atrial contractions (a).

OCCURRENCE OF ARRHYTHMIAS

Fetal arrhythmias are common, occurring in approximately 1% to 3% of all pregnancies.[1,2] The most common arrhythmias occurring in utero are isolated ectopic premature atrial contractions (PACs). Although benign, atrial ectopic beats carry a small risk of developing into sustained supraventricular tachyarrhythmias (SVTs) (Part 3, Chapter 2). Approximately 10% of fetal rhythm abnormalities are significant and may require treatment either in utero or immediately following delivery. Of these, tachyarrhythmias (fetal heart rate [FHR] >180 beats/min [bpm]) are more prevalent, accounting for about 7% of cases, while bradyarrhythmias (FHR <the third percentile for gestational age [GA]) occur in around 3%.[3] Arrhythmias can occur both with structural or functional cardiac defects and in the normal heart.[4,5]

EVALUATION OF FETAL HEART RATE AND RHYTHM

Echocardiographic evaluation of FHR and rhythm should follow a systematic approach to include the following (FIG 1.1.5), as well as an assessment of cardiac structure:

1. What is the fetal heart rate (the ventricular rate) and what is the atrial rate?

The ventricular rate can be measured from one ventricular deflection to the next on M-mode or, for more precise measurements, spectral Doppler of the aortic or pulmonary valve clicks (FIG. 1.1.3A). Likewise, the atrial rate can be measured between two atrial contractions on M-mode, the A-waves of tricuspid or mitral inflow spectral Doppler, or reverse flow during atrial contraction in the pulmonary, systemic, hepatic vein, or ductus venosus (FIGS. 1.1.4 and 1.1.6).[6]

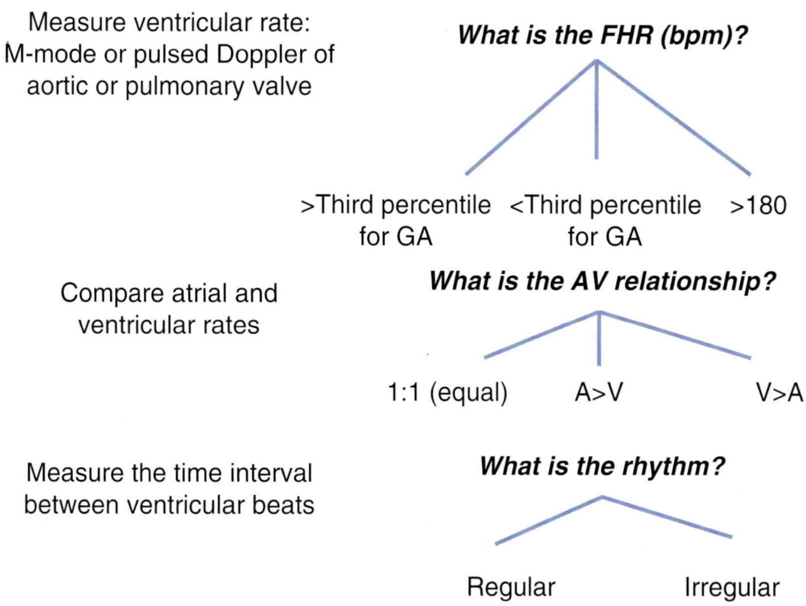

FIGURE 1.1.5 Step-by-step evaluation of fetal heart rate and rhythm. A, atrial; AV, atrioventricular; BPM, beats per minute; FHR, fetal heart rate; V, ventricular.

2. What is the atrioventricular (AV) relationship?

The AV relationship is normally 1:1 and can be assessed by simultaneous atrial and ventricular M-mode or color M-mode or spectral Doppler of mitral inflow and aortic outflow or any vein and artery simultaneously.[7-9] Doppler interrogation is advantageous because the exact time between atrial and ventricular contraction, that is the AV interval (also known as the mechanical PR interval), can be measured. The normal AV interval varies by gestational age but, in general, should be <160 ms.[10-12] The E- and A-waves are not normally fused; however, if the FHR is >150 bpm or there is severe ventricular dysfunction and the isovolumic contraction time is prolonged, ventricular filling may be monophasic **(FIG. 1.1.7)**. In these situations, an accurate AV interval can be measured by sampling a pulmonary or systemic vein and the pulmonary artery or aorta **(FIG. 1.1.3B** and **C)**. The normal values for the AV interval differ based on the sampling location and are longer when measured between mitral inflow and aortic outflow tracings.[11,12]

Quantifying the FHR and the AV relationship is diagnostic in many arrhythmias. Bradycardia can have a 1:1 **(FIG. 1.1.8)** or ≥1:1 AV relationship **(FIGS. 1.1.9** and **1.1.10)**. Likewise, tachycardia can have a 1:1 **(FIG. 1.1.11)**, >1:1 **(FIG. 1.1.12)**, or <1:1 **(FIG. 1.1.13)** AV relationship.

3. Is the rhythm regular or irregular?

Normally the fetal heart rhythm is regular, that is the V-V intervals do not vary by more than about 10 ms. The differential diagnosis of an irregular rhythm is atrial or ventricular ectopy (premature atrial or ventricular contractions) **(FIG. 1.1.14)** and intermittent

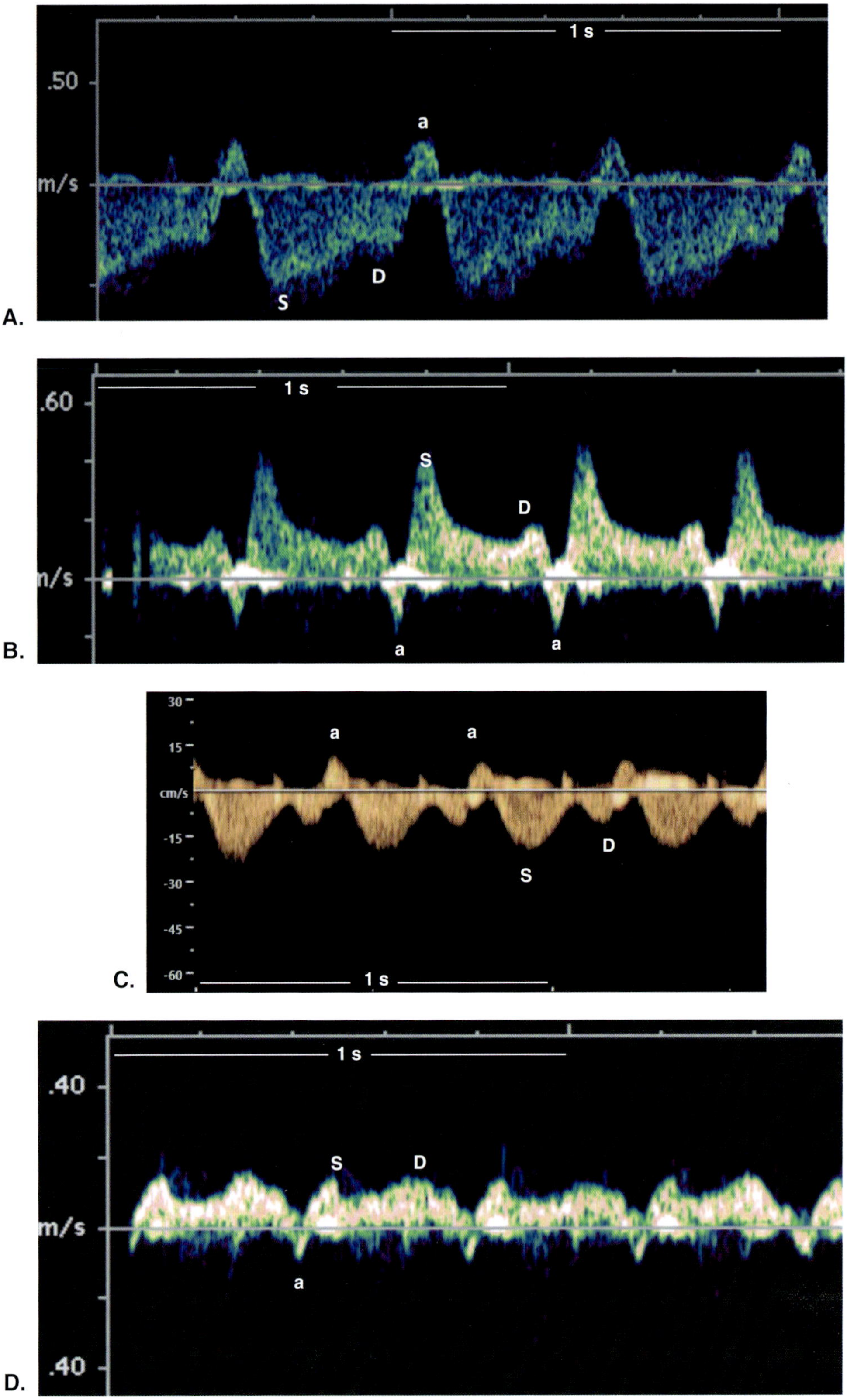

FIGURE 1.1.6 Atrial contractions as seen as reverse flow in the **(A)** ductus venosus; **(B)** pulmonary vein; **(C)** systemic vein; **(D)** hepatic vein. A, atrial contractions; D, diastole; S, systole.

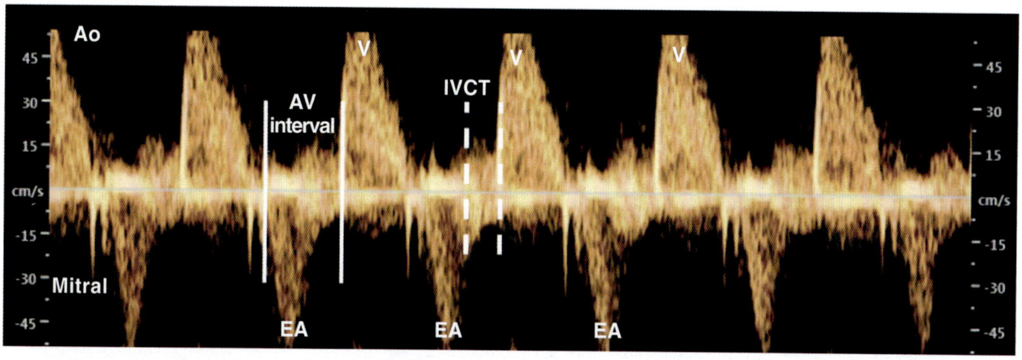

FIGURE 1.1.7 Spectral Doppler of monophasic (fused E- and A-waves) of mitral inflow (below baseline). The atrioventricular (AV) interval is marked by the solid lines. Comprising part of the AV interval is the isovolumic contraction time (IVCT) which occurs from the end of atrial contraction to the beginning of ventricular contraction and is marked on the figure by the dotted lines. Aortic outflow (Ao) is seen above baseline.

AV block **(FIG. 1.1.15)**. One approach to the fetus with an irregular rhythm is to first obtain an atrial M-mode from the aortic arch view **(FIG. 1.1.4)**. If the atrial rate is regular and all atrial deflections appear the same, the diagnosis is most likely AV block. If the atrial rate is regular, but the atrial beats do not all have the same morphology, or if the atrial rate is regular and there are periods of atrial silence, premature ventricular contractions (PVCs) with retrograde conduction to the atrium **(FIG. 1.1.16A** and **B)** or PVCs with no retrograde conduction **(FIG. 1.1.16C)** can be diagnosed.

4. Is the heart structurally normal?

Any structural heart defect that causes an anatomical disruption in the normal conduction system can be associated with an arrhythmia. Therefore, a thorough evaluation of all cardiac structures is always warranted with a fetal arrhythmia diagnosis. For

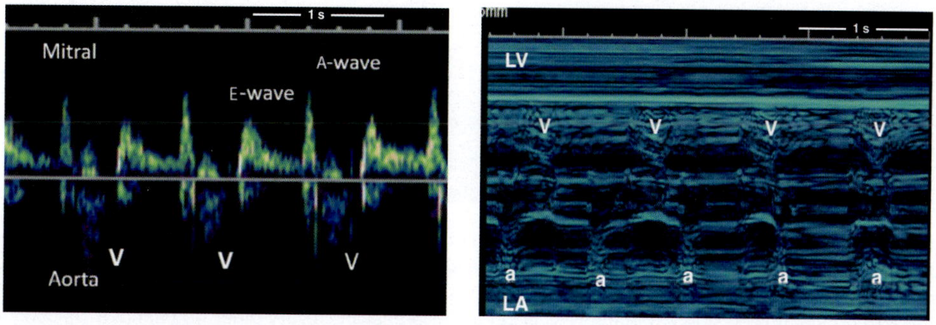

FIGURE 1.1.8 Bradycardia with 1:1 atrioventricular (AV) conduction. **A:** Spectral Doppler tracing showing simultaneous mitral valve inflow and aortic valve outflow. The mitral E-waves and A-waves are well separated (above baseline), and there is 1:1 AV conduction as every A-wave (above baseline) is followed by a V (below baseline). **B:** Left atrial (LA) and left ventricular (LV) M-mode demonstrating a 1:1 A-wave and V-wave relationship at a fetal heart rate of 90 bpm.

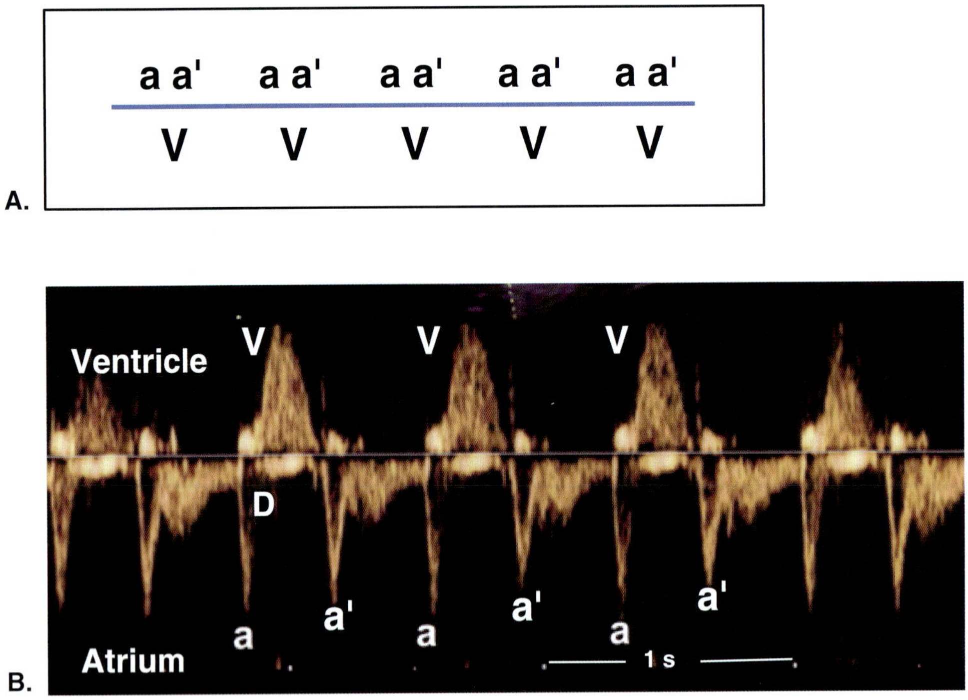

FIGURE 1.1.9 Blocked atrial bigeminy. **A:** Diagram showing the pattern of conducted (a) and nonconducted (a′) atrial beats in relation to ventricular (V) beats seen with blocked atrial bigeminy. **B:** Spectral Doppler of mitral inflow (below baseline). Note a-a′ interval is longer than a′-a interval, where a is the conducted beat and a′ is premature and not conducted. Aortic outflow (V) is above baseline.

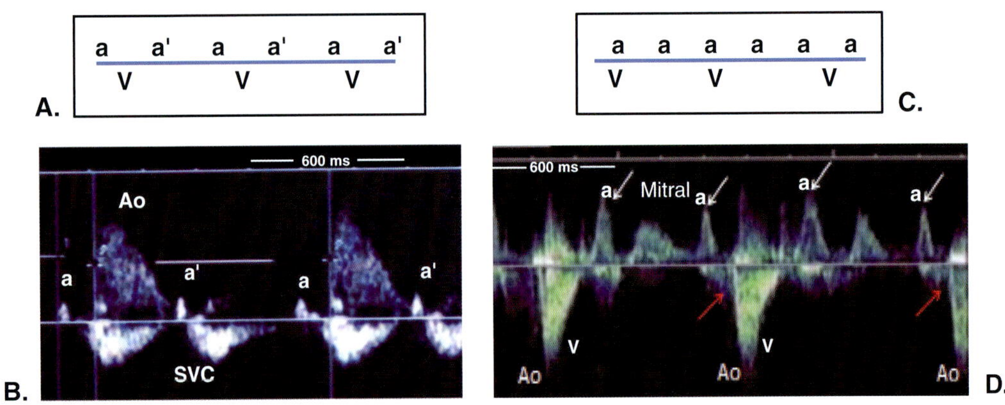

FIGURE 1.1.10 2° AV block and 3° AV block. **A:** Cartoon of 2° AV block. The a-a′ interval and a′-a intervals (atrial beats) are consistent, but every other beat (a, not a′) is conducted to the ventricles (V). **B:** Spectral Doppler of simultaneous interrogation of the superior vena cava (SVC, below baseline) and aorta (Ao, above baseline). Retrograde flow during atrial systole (a) in the SVC is seen above baseline: every other (a) but not a′, is conducted to the aorta (V). **C:** Cartoon of 3° AV block. There is no relationship between atrial contractions (a) and ventricular contractions (V). The atrial rate is faster than the ventricular rate. **D:** Spectral Doppler of simultaneous mitral inflow (above baseline) and aortic outflow (below baseline) of a fetus with 3° AV block. The mitral A-waves are shown by white arrows. Note that the AV intervals (red arrows) are different, indicating no AV relationship. AV, atrioventricular.

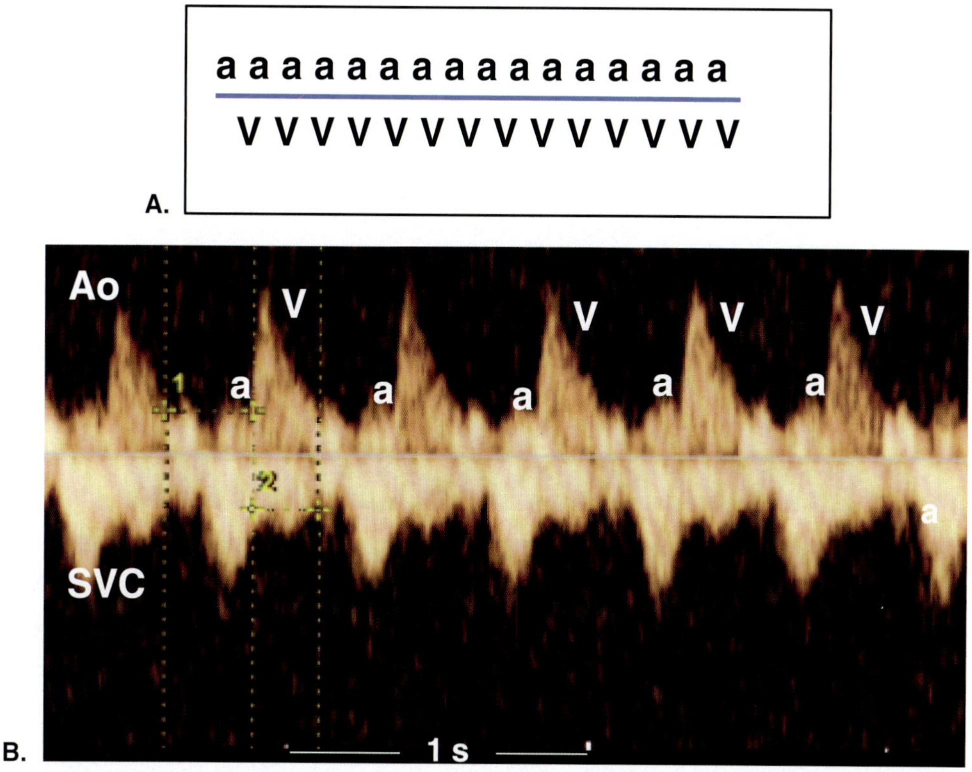

FIGURE 1.1.11 Supraventricular and ventricular tachycardia. **A:** Cartoon of supraventricular tachycardia (SVT) with 1:1 atrioventricular (AV) conduction. a, atrial contractions; V, ventricular contractions. **B:** Spectral Doppler of superior vena cava (SVC) (below baseline) and aorta (Ao) (above baseline) demonstrating SVT with 1:1 AV conduction. The lines indicate the AV and the ventriculoatrial (VA) intervals (see below).

example, arrhythmias are common in the heterotaxy syndromes and in congenitally corrected transposition of the great vessels (CC-TGV), due to morphological aberrations of the conduction system.[13-20] Approximately, 17% to 20% of patients with Ebstein anomaly will have SVT secondary to enlargement of the right atrium and the prevalence of accessory pathways.[21] Cardiac tumors, such as a rhabdomyoma or teratoma, may also result in intermittent ectopy or sustained arrhythmias, depending on the size and location.[22-24]

(text continued on page 16)

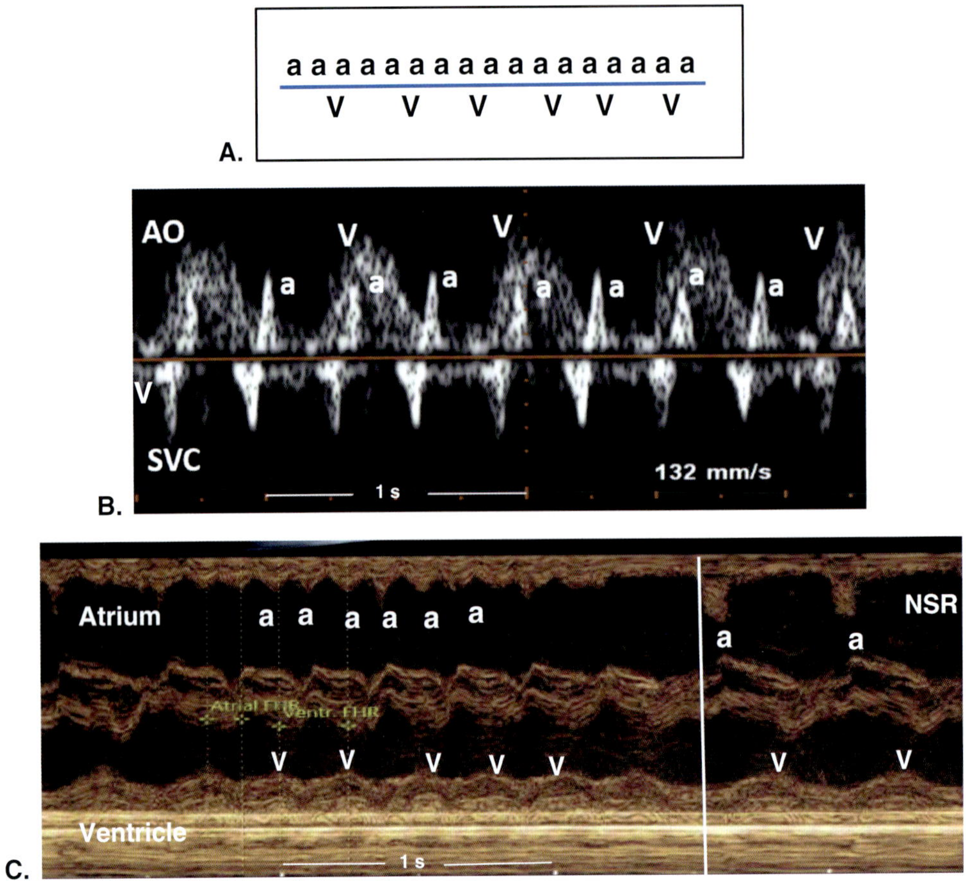

FIGURE 1.1.12 Atrial flutter. **A:** Diagram of atrial flutter (a) showing 2:1 and 3:1 block with slower ventricular (V) rate. **B:** Simultaneous spectral Doppler tracing of the aorta (Ao) above baseline and superior vena cava (SVC) below baseline. Reverse flow in the SVC during atrial contraction (a) demonstrates two atrial beats for every ventricular beat (V) (both above baseline). **C:** Simultaneous M-mode tracing through the right atrium (RA) and left ventricle (LV) during atrial flutter (left of white line). The a-a interval is about 300 ms, with ventricular response of about 200 bpm. To the right of the white line, there is spontaneous conversion to normal sinus rhythm (NSR) with 1:1 AV conduction and normal atrial (a) and ventricular (V) rates.

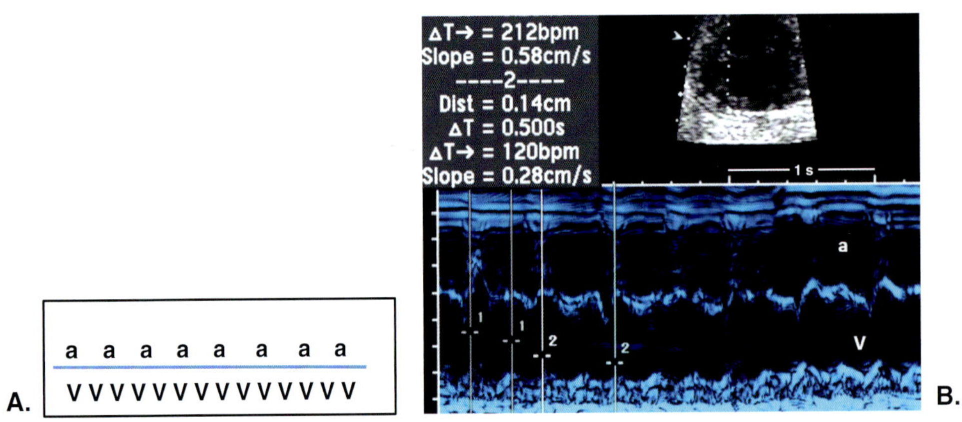

FIGURE 1.1.13 Ventricular tachycardia **A:** Cartoon of ventricular tachycardia (VT) showing faster ventricular beat rates (V) with slower and normal atrial beat rates (a). There is also atrioventricular (AV) dissociation. **B:** M-mode of a fetus in VT demonstrating the faster ventricular rates (V) compared to the atrial rates (a).

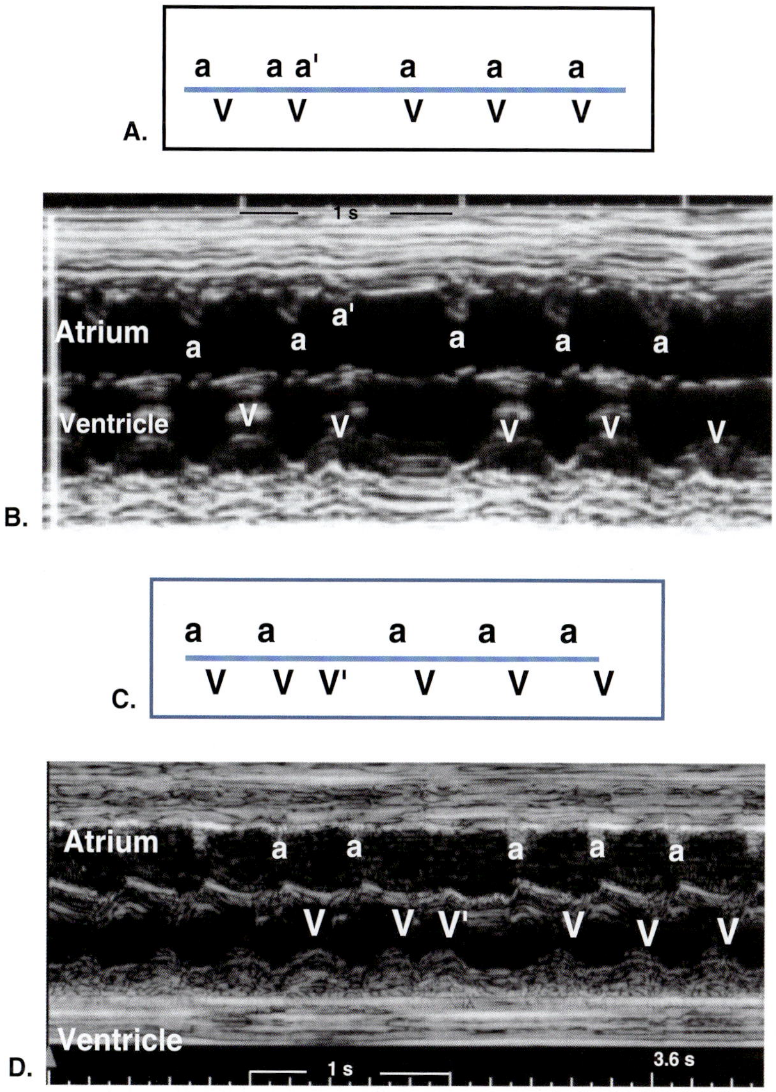

FIGURE 1.1.14 Atrial and ventricular ectopy **A:** Diagram showing the pattern of atrial (a) to ventricular (V) contractions seen with premature atrial contractions (PACs). The premature beat is marked as a′. Note the irregular ventricular rhythm. **B:** Atrial (a, top) and ventricular (V, bottom) M-mode. Regular atrial contractions (a's,) are interrupted by a premature atrial beat (a′) which results in a ventricular pause (V) and a "dropped beat." **C:** Diagram of premature ventricular contractions (PVCs). The regular ventricular rhythm (V's) is interrupted by a premature ventricular beat (V′). There is no retrograde conduction to the atrium in this example, thus the atrial rate (a) is also irregular. **D:** Simultaneous atrial (a's) and ventricular (V's) M-mode tracing showing a PVC (V′). The diagnosis of a PVC can be made because the premature beat seen in the ventricles is not preceded by a premature beat in the atria (a).

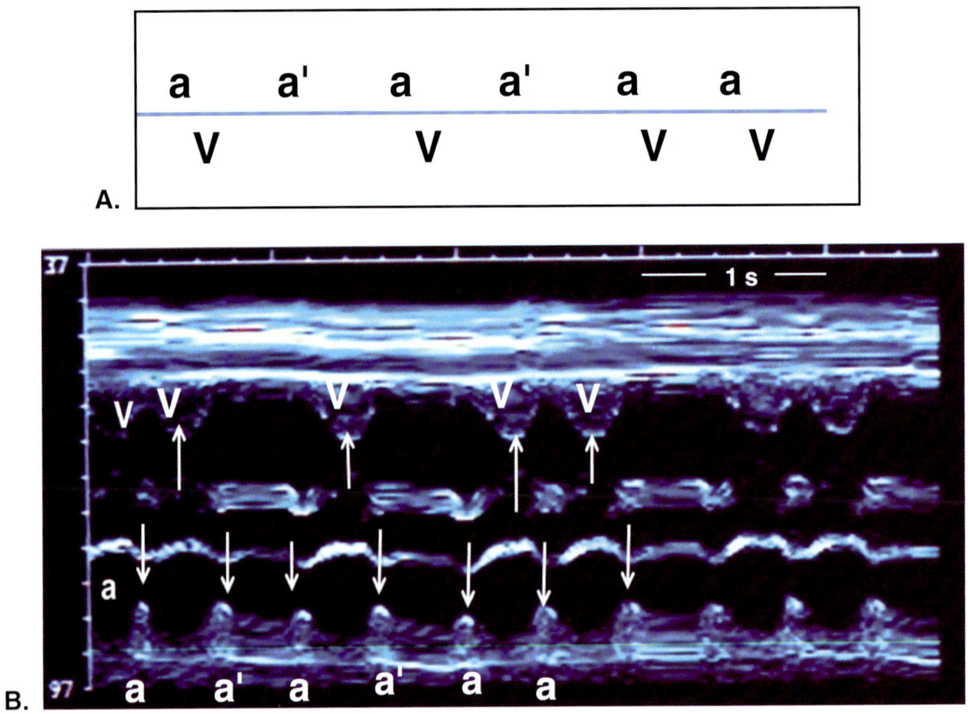

FIGURE 1.1.15 Evolving fetal 2° AV block in an anti-Ro/SSA–positive pregnancy. **A and B:** Diagram and simultaneous atrial and ventricular M-mode showing the relationship between the atrium (a) and the ventricles (V). Some of the beats appear to be conducted (a), while others are blocked (a′). In the absence of a spectral Doppler to measure the atrioventricular (AV) times, it is not clear if this is type 1 or type 2 of 2° AV block. SSA, Sjögren syndrome–related antigen A.

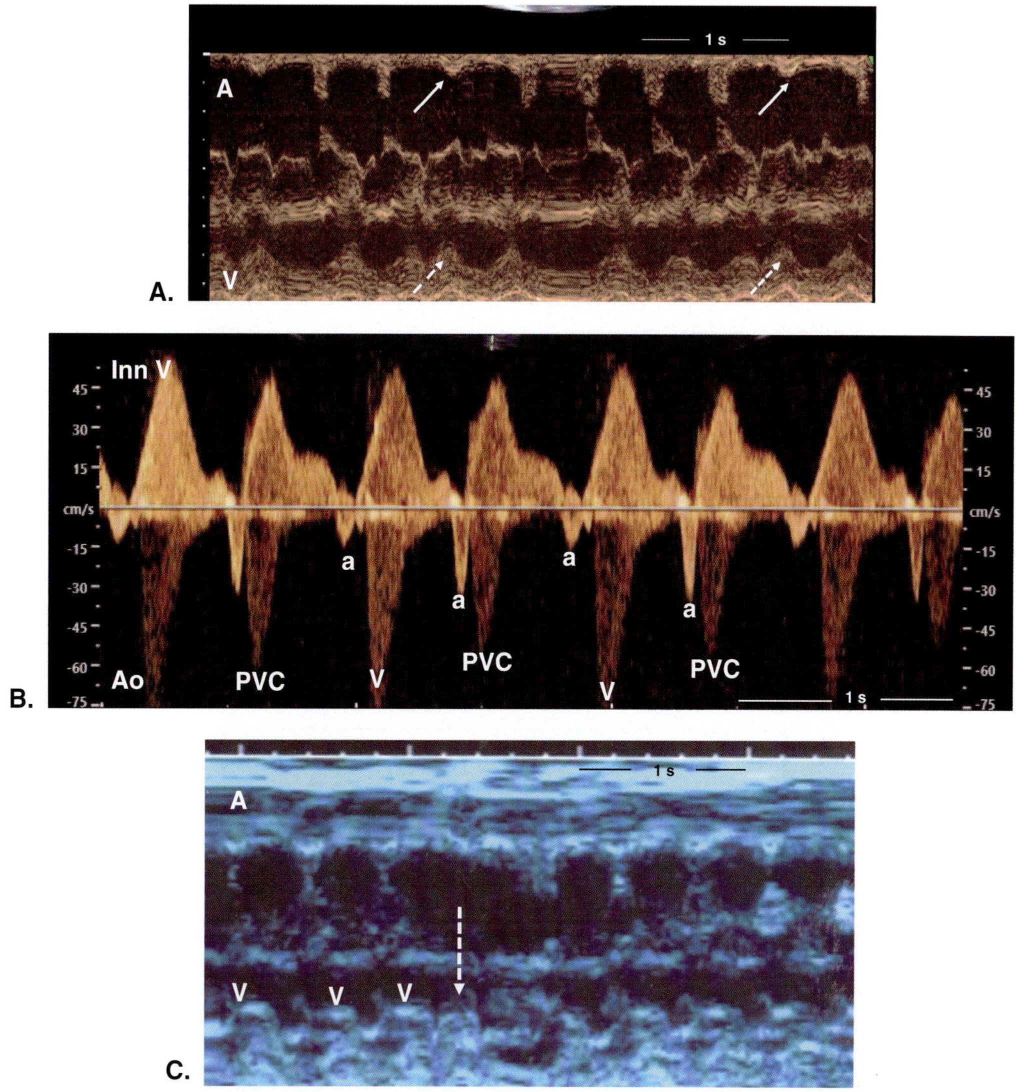

FIGURE 1.1.16 Premature ventricular contractions. **A:** M-mode of atrial (A at top of m-mode) and ventricular (V at bottom of m-mode) contractions. The premature ventricular beat (dotted arrow) occurs with retrograde conduction to the atrium, but the atrial beat, while coming on time, has a different morphology than the normal atrial beats. **B:** Spectral Doppler of innominate vein (Inn V above baseline) and aorta (A below baseline) from the three-vessel view. **C:** M-mode showing the premature ventricular beat (dotted arrow) with no retrograde conduction; hence no atrial contraction.

CLASSIFICATION OF ARRHYTHMIAS

Ectopy

An ectopic rhythm is defined as an irregular heart rhythm due to a premature or "extra" beat that originates in the atria or ventricle.

Premature Atrial Contractions (PAC)

The most common type of fetal ectopy is PACs, which can occur secondary to maternal stimulants, a redundant aneurysm of the fossa ovalis, or for no apparent reason. A PAC can be "conducted," that is followed by an early ventricular contraction, or it can be "nonconducted" or "blocked," meaning it is not followed by a ventricular contraction (FIGS. 1.1.14A, B and 1.1.17). Although most fetal irregular rhythms are benign and self-limited atrial ectopy, it is not possible to distinguish by auscultation between atrial ectopy, ventricular ectopy and pathologic and progressive intermittent AV block (FIG. 1.1.15). This is especially of concern between 18 and 25 weeks of gestation, when fetal AV block due to maternal anti-Ro/SSA (Sjögren syndrome–related antigen A) antibodies presents. Finally, in a coexisting structural cardiac defect, intracardiac tumors,

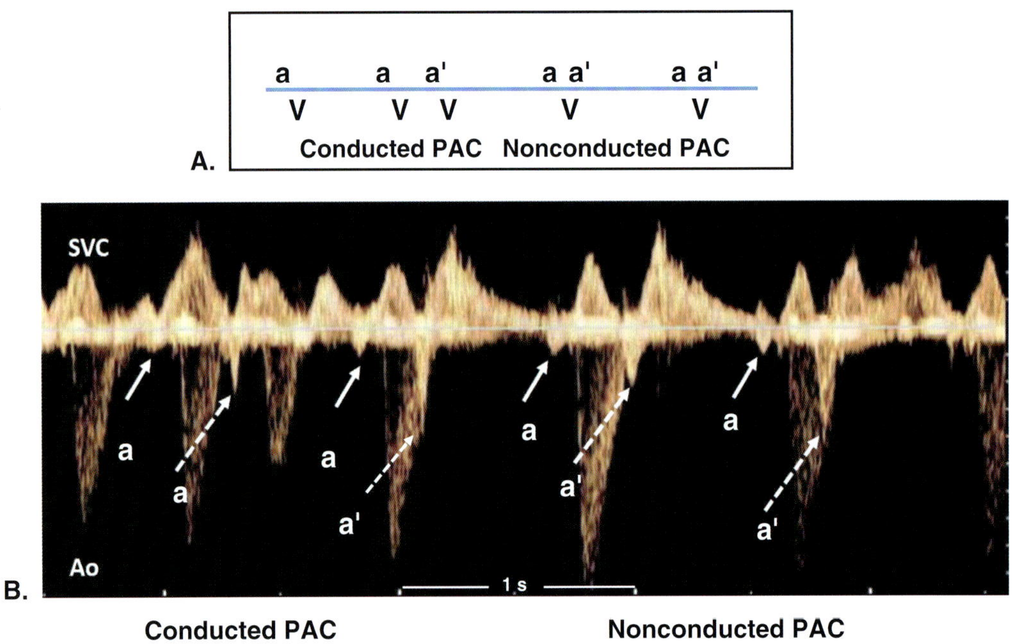

FIGURE 1.1.17 Conducted and nonconducted premature atrial contractions. **A:** Cartoon of the spectral Doppler shown in **(B)**. **B:** Simultaneous superior vena cava (SVC, above baseline) and aortic (Ao, below baseline) spectral Doppler. There is normal atrioventricular (AV) conduction (solid arrows, below baseline) and premature atrial contractions (dotted arrows, below baseline). When the atrial contraction comes just after the ventricular beat (a, with dotted arrow), it is conducted, and the subsequent ventricular beat comes early (third ventricular beat from the right) and has a lower velocity, thus the rhythm is irregular. If the atrial beat comes too early (see A-waves buried in ventricular beats below baseline, a′ and dotted arrow), the atrial contraction is blocked, and the ventricular rhythm becomes regular, but the rate is slow.

diverticulum, and aneurysm are found in a small percentage of fetuses with ectopy.[22-24] In general, isolated atrial ectopic beats of the fetal heart are harmless and self-limiting, but at least, weekly fetal heart rhythm auscultation is suggested since 2% to 3% of fetuses with atrial ectopy will develop SVT.[25] Atrial bigeminy and trigeminy occur if every other or every third atrial beat is premature but still conducted to the ventricles.

Premature Ventricular Contractions (PVC)

The other type of ectopy is PVCs (**FIGS. 1.1.14C, D** and **1.1.15**). Like PACs, PVCs present with an irregular rhythm; however, they are much less common. The two types of ectopy can only be distinguished by simultaneous interrogation of atrial and ventricular contractions with M-mode or spectral Doppler. Ventricular wall defects, such as congenital ventricular aneurysms or ventricular diverticula, and cardiac tumors can also be associated with PVCs.[22-24] PVCs can also be associated with cardiac channelopathies.

Blocked Atrial Bigeminy

Blocked atrial bigeminy (BAB) is another pattern of atrial ectopy which manifests as a slow heart rate and regular rhythm, in contrast to isolated PACs, which result in an irregular rhythm (see above). Lasting from hours to months, BAB occurs when a conducted atrial beat is followed by a PAC that is not conducted to the ventricle; thus, only every other atrial beat is conducted, resulting in ventricular bradycardia (**FIG. 1.1.9**). BAB is not considered a significant arrhythmia unless it is present at the time of delivery, as the obstetrician cannot distinguish fetal distress when the baseline heart rate is 60 to 70 bpm as it is during BAB. In addition, BAB can be mistaken for AV block, resulting in unnecessary concern for the family. The differentiating feature between AV block and BAB is that in AV block, all atrial beats should occur at evenly spaced intervals (**FIG. 1.1.10**), while in BAB, every other atrial beat will be premature (**FIG. 1.1.9**). Ironically, the fetus with BAB has the same risk of developing sustained SVT as the fetus with isolated atrial ectopy.[25]

Tachyarrhythmias

A sustained FHR of >180 bpm is diagnostic of tachycardia. Sustained fetal tachyarrhythmias can be associated with significant sequalae, including fetal and neonatal death. Specifically, in hydropic fetuses with sustained tachycardia, a mortality rate of 17% has been reported.[26-29] Therefore, sustained fetal tachyarrhythmias require in utero drug management. All efforts should be made to avoid an early operative delivery as the outcome of a preterm hydropic infant is poor. Tachycardia is classified based on the atrial rate and correlation of the ventricular response (**TABLE 1.1.1**).

Supraventricular Tachyarrhythmias (SVT)

SVT, defined as an increased heart rate of >180 to 300 bpm, with a 1:1 AV conduction (equal ventricular and atrial rates) accounts for the majority of fetal tachyarrhythmias, occurring in up to 66% to 90% of cases.[26-29] Most fetal SVT is due to atrioventricular reentry using an accessory connection,[30,31] and in utero treatment is based on slowing

TABLE 1.1.1 DIFFERENTIAL DIAGNOSIS OF FETAL ARRHYTHMIAS BASED ON AV CONDUCTION AND FETAL HEART RATES (FHRS)

Finding	Normal	Bradycardia	Tachycardia
1:1 AV conduction and structurally normal heart; sinus rhythm	1. Normal	1. Viral or anti-Ro antibody damage to normal SA node 2. Ectopic atrial rhythm 3. Inherited channelopathy	1. SVT 2. PJRT 3. AET 4. JET
>1:1 AV conduction	Atrial flutter	1. AV block 2. BAB	Atrial flutter
<1:1 AV conduction	–	–	1. VT 2. JT
Irregular rhythm	PACs or PVCs	Type 1, 2° AV block Intermittent type 2, 2° AV block	Intermittent tachycardias (see above)

AET, atrial ectopic tachycardia; AV, atrioventricular; BAB, blocked atrial bigeminy; GA, gestational age; JET, junctional ectopic tachycardia; JT, junctional tachycardia; LQTS, long QT syndrome; PAC, premature atrial contraction; PJRT, permanent junctional reciprocating tachycardia; PVC, premature ventricular contraction; SVT, supraventricular tachycardia; VT, ventricular tachycardia.

conduction in the AV node and/or the accessory connection to interrupt the tachycardia cycle. Accessory connections are associated with Wolff-Parkinson-White (WPW) and cannot be diagnosed by fetal echocardiography, but the electrocardiographic manifestation of WPW as "pre-excitation" can be seen by fetal magnetocardiography.[32]

Fetal SVT (FIG. 1.1.12A and B) can be divided into two categories based on length of the ventriculoatrial (VA) interval and distinguished by Doppler echocardiography or M-mode (FIG. 1.1.18).[33] Short VA tachycardias, defined when the VA interval is <½ the RR interval (cardiac cycle length), initiate with reentry and comprise the "typical" SVT and some cases of atrial flutter (FIG. 1.1.18A). The mechanism of the long VA tachycardias can be either reentrant (permanent junctional ectopic tachycardia, junctional ectopic tachycardia, and some types of ventricular tachycardia) or automatic (sinus tachycardia, atrial ectopic tachycardia, and other types of ventricular tachycardia). The long VA tachycardias (FIG. 1.1.18B) are notoriously difficult to successfully treat, and at times, only the ventricular rate can be slowed sufficiently to prevent hydrops. The short VA tachycardias respond very well to digoxin, flecainide, and sotalol. A large randomized control trial is currently underway to define the most efficacious treatment for fetal reentrant supraventricular arrhythmias. Detailed information about SVT and treatment is found in later chapters in this book.

Atrial Flutter

Atrial flutter occurs with an atrial rate usually between 300 and 500 bpm, with varying degrees of AV block, which presents as a ventricular rate often between 160 and 240 bpm (FIG. 1.1.12).[26-29] Up to 30% of fetuses diagnosed with atrial flutter will also have a structural heart defect, usually Ebstein malformation of the tricuspid valve.[21] It is important to distinguish atrial flutter from SVT as prognosis and in utero antiarrhythmic treatment differ.

A.

B.

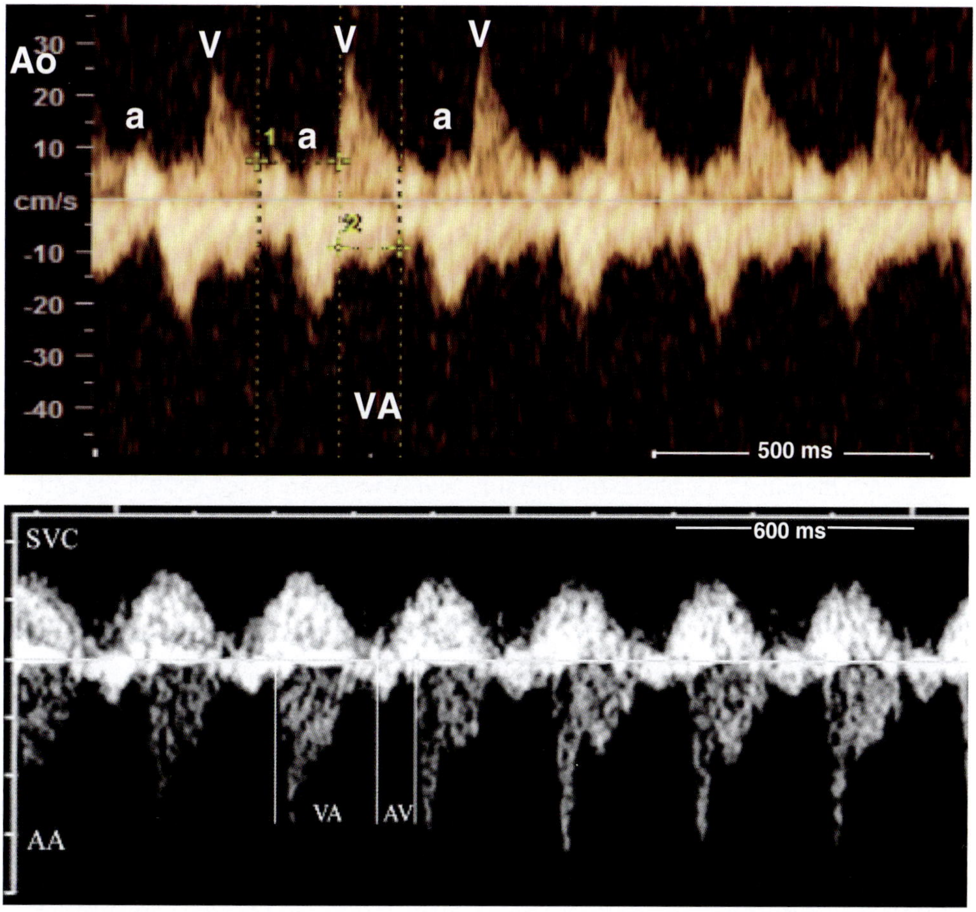

FIGURE 1.1.18 Short ventriculoatrial (VA) and long VA supraventricular tachycardia. **A:** Short VA tachycardia. Simultaneous superior vena cava (SVC, below baseline) and aortic (Ao, above baseline) spectral Doppler. The time from onset of Ao ejection to A-wave reversal in the SVC is shorter than the time from A-wave reversal in the SVC to the onset of Ao ejection. **B:** Long RP tachycardia. Simultaneous spectral Doppler of the SVC (above baseline) and ascending aorta (AA, below baseline). Note, the VA interval is significantly longer than the atrioventricular (AV) interval. (B, Reprinted from Fouron JC. Fetal arrhythmias: the Saint-Justine hospital experience. *Prenat Diagn*. 2004;24(13):1068-1080.)

Ventricular Tachycardia

Ventricular tachycardia is very rare and should be considered when the ventricular rate is >180 bpm and exceeds the atrial rate, which is usually normal **(FIG. 1.1.13)**. Ventricular tachycardia has been reported to be associated with long QT syndrome and cardiac tumors.[23,27,34]

Bradyarrhythmias

Fetal bradycardia has been defined as a sustained FHR < 110 bpm, but a more accurate definition is a FHR < third percentile for GA.[35,36] Transient fetal bradycardia is usually benign, occurring from increased vagal stimulation due to transducer pressure during the ultrasound examination or a nuchal cord.

Sustained sinus bradycardias (bradycardia with 1:1 AV conduction) (FIG. 1.1.8) can be seen with the heterotaxy syndromes (right atrial or left atrial isomerism, secondary to abnormal or multiple sinus nodes), viral or anti-Ro/SSA antibody–mediated damage to normal sinus node, genetic variants, maternal medications, and long QT syndrome (LQTS). Bradycardia with >1:1 AV conduction indicates AV block or BAB.

AV Block

The most common cause of fetal AV block in the structurally normal heart is inflammation and fibrosis of the AV node caused by maternal anti-Ro/SSA antibodies.[37] As previously noted, AV block can also complicate CC-TGV and left atrial (LA) isomerism due to morphologic abnormalities of the AV node. 1° AV block in the fetus is not a bradyarrhythmia but occurs with a prolonged AV interval (>160 ms) and may be a harbinger of more advanced fetal block in the anti-Ro/SSA antibody–positive pregnancy. Often in 1° AV block, the mitral E- and A-waves are fused (FIGS. 1.1.19 and 1.1.20). The findings of 1° AV block with a structurally normal heart should prompt maternal testing for anti-Ro/SSA antibodies, and, if antibodies are present, the fetus should be followed closely for progression to 2° or 3° AV block.

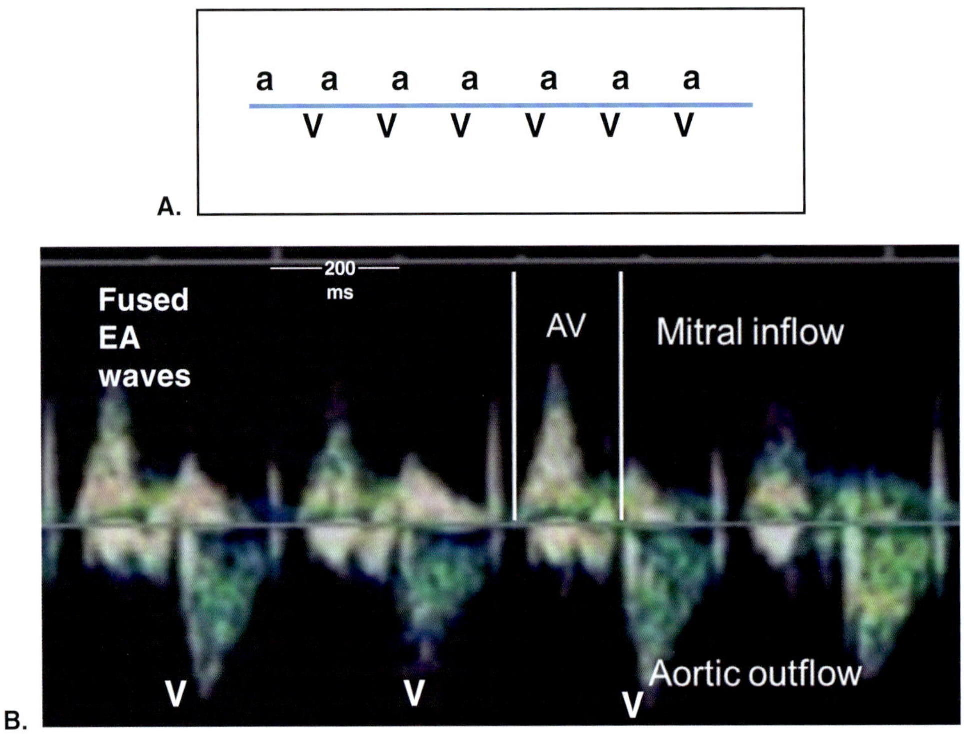

FIGURE 1.1.19 1° AV block. **A:** Diagram showing the pattern of atrial (a) to ventricular (V) contractions seen in 1° AV block. There is 1:1 AV conduction, but the AV interval is prolonged. Atrial contractions occur at evenly spaced intervals. **B:** Simultaneous mitral inflow and aortic outflow showing monophasic mitral inflow (fused EA waves above baseline) and a prolonged AV interval (~200 ms). There is still 1:1 AV conduction with a normal atrial and ventricular rate. One week later, this fetus was in 3° AV block (not shown). AV, atrioventricular.

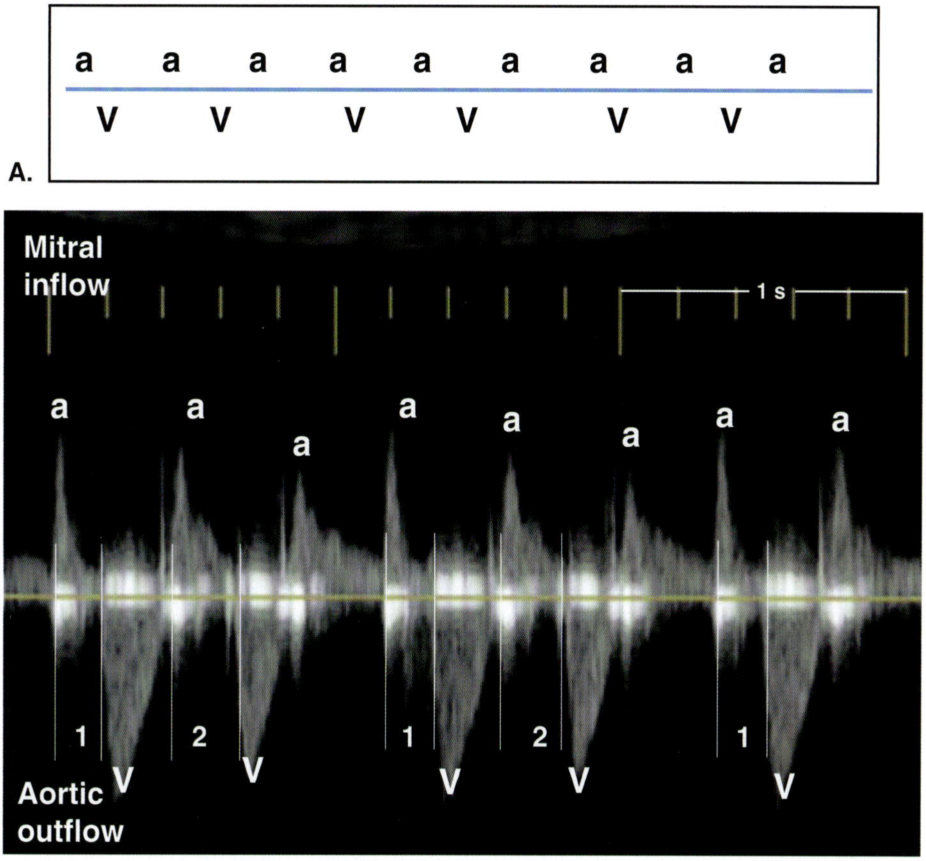

FIGURE 1.1.20 Type 1, 2° AV block (Wenckebach periodicity). **A:** Cartoon. The first AV interval is normal, the second is longer, and the third A-wave does not conduct. This pattern is repeated and results in an irregular rhythm. **B:** Simultaneous mitral inflow (top) and aortic outflow (bottom). The AV interval #1 is shorter than AV interval #2, and the ventricular rate (V) is irregular. Note that the mitral E-wave and A-waves are fused and thus monophasic. AV, atrioventricular.

There are two types of 2° AV block: type 1 (**FIG. 1.1.20**) and type 2 (**FIG. 1.1.10A** and **B**). Type 1 2° AV block is diagnosed when the AV interval prolongs until the atrial beat is not conducted to the ventricles (**FIG. 1.1.20**). Type 2 2° AV block is diagnosed when every other atrial beat is conducted to the ventricles in a 2:1 fashion (**FIG. 1.1.10A** and **B**). If only M-mode is used, it can be difficult to distinguish between type 1 and type 2 2° AV block. In both type 1 and type 2, 2° AV block, the atrial rhythm and rates are normal, but the ventricular rhythm can be irregular or regular with a slow rate. A "functional" or "pseudo" type 2 2° AV block occurs in LQTS: the AV node conducts perfectly, but repolarization is so prolonged that atrial contraction initiates before ventricular repolarization ends (**FIG. 1.1.21**).

Complete or 3° AV block implies complete disassociation between the atria and the ventricles (**FIG. 1.1.10C** and **D**).[34] The atrial rate is typically normal, while the ventricular rate is <80 bpm. The fetus with 3° AV block is at high risk for hydrops, in utero demise, or very premature delivery, especially in the setting of left atrial isomerism.[38,39]

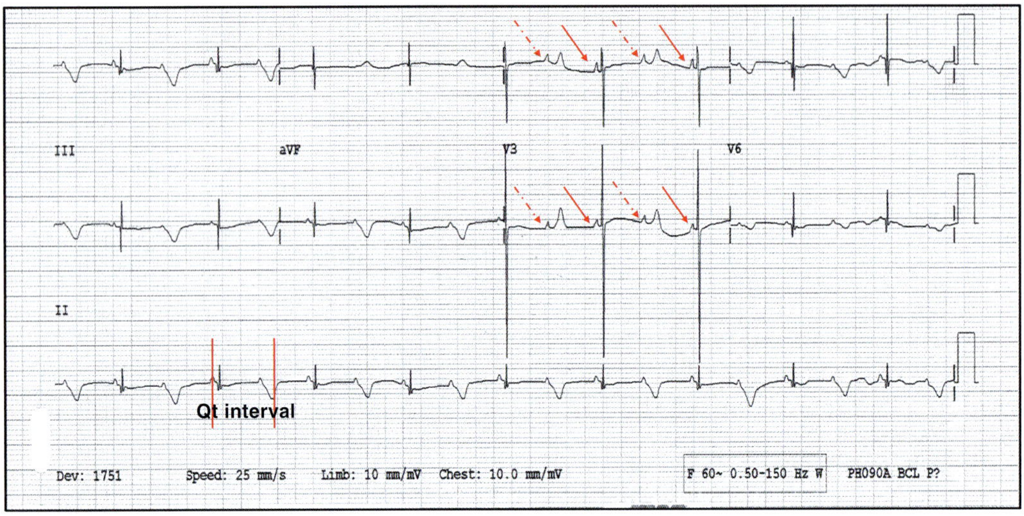

FIGURE 1.1.21 12-Lead electrocardiogram of an infant with long QT syndrome due to a pathogenic calmodulin variant. The rhythm is functional 2° AV block with 2:1 AV conduction. The QT interval (red lines) is so long that atrial depolarization (dotted arrows) occurs before ventricular repolarization is complete, thus it is functional. The "conducted" P-waves are marked by solid arrows. AV, atrioventricular.

SUMMARY

Understanding the type and significance of a particular fetal arrhythmia is important in determining prognosis, need for in utero treatment, and the risk of associated structural cardiac or extracardiac abnormalities. Although initially daunting, diagnosis of fetal arrhythmias becomes more straightforward with practice and a step-by-step analysis of atrial and ventricular rates, AV relationship, type of rhythm, and the presence or absence of morphological cardiac anomalies.

References

1. Strasburger JF. Fetal arrhythmias. *Prog Pediatr Cardiol.* 2000;11(1):1-17.
2. Strasburger JF, Cheulkar B, Wichman HJ. Perinatal arrhythmias: diagnosis and management. *Clin Perinatol.* 2007;34(4):627-652.
3. ACOG Committee on Practice Bulletins. Intrapartum fetal heart rate monitoring: nomenclature, interpretation and general management principals. *Obstet Gynecol.* 2009;114:192-202.
4. Cuneo BF. Outcome of fetal cardiac defects. *Curr Opin Pediatr.* 2006;18(5):490-496.
5. Cuneo BF, Strasburger JF, Wakai RT, Ovadia M. Conduction system disease in fetuses evaluated for irregular cardiac rhythm. *Fetal Diagn Ther.* 2006;21(3):307-313.
6. Saemundsson Y, Johansson C, Wenling S, Gudmundsson S. Hepatic venous Doppler in the evaluation of fetal extrasystoles. *Ultrasound Obstet Gynecol.* 2011;37(2):179-183.
7. Carvalho JS, Prefumo F, Ciardelli V, Sairam S, Bhide A, Shinebourne EA. Evaluation of fetal arrhythmias from simultaneous pulsed wave Doppler in pulmonary artery and vein. *Heart.* 2007;93(11):1448-1453.
8. Fouron JC, Fournier A, Proulx F, et al. Management of fetal tachyarrhythmia based on superior vena cava/aorta Doppler flow recordings. *Heart.* 2003;89(10):1211-1216.
9. Howley LW, Schuchardt E, Park D, Gilbert L, Gruenwald J, Cuneo BF. Simultaneous recording of pulsed-wave Doppler signals in innominate vein and transverse aortic arch: new technique to evaluate atrioventricular conduction and fetal heart rhythm. *Ultrasound Obstet Gynecol.* 2018;52(4):544-545.

10. Cuneo BF, Bitant S, Strasburger JF, Kaizer AM, Wakai RT. Assessment and outcome of AV conduction in normal and anti-Ro/SSA antibody positive pregnancies evaluated by echocardiography and magnetocardiography. *Ultrasound Obstet Gynecol.* 2019;54(5):625-633.
11. Adelfinger G, Fouron JC, Sonesson S-E, Proulx F. Reference values for time intervals between atrial and ventricular contractions for the fetal heart measured by two Doppler techniques. *Am J Cardiol.* 2001;88:1433-1436.
12. Ni M, Hamilton RM, Fenwick L, Kingdom JCP, Roman KS, Jaeggi ET. Assessment of fetal atrioventricular time intervals by tissue Doppler and pulsed Doppler echocardiography: normal values and correlation with fetal electrocardiography. *Heart.* 2006;92:1831-1837.
13. Berg C, Geipel A, Kamil D, et al. The syndrome of left isomerism: sonographic findings and outcome in prenatally diagnosed cases. *J Ultrasound Med.* 2005;24:921-931.
14. Dickinson DF, Wilkinson JL, Anderson KR, Smith A, Ho SY, Anderson RH. The cardiac conduction system in situs ambiguous. *Circulation.* 1979;59:879-885.
15. Ho SY, Fagg N, Anderson RH, Cook A, Allan L. Disposition of the atrioventricular conduction tissues in the heart with isomerism of the atrial appendages: its relation to congenital complete heart block. *J Am Coll Cardiol.* 1992;20:904-910.
16. Bharati S, Lev M. The course of the conduction system in dextrocardia. *Circulation.* 1978;57:163-171.
17. Moorman AF, Christoffels VM, Anderson RH. Anatomic substrates for cardiac conduction. *Heart Rhythm.* 2005;2(8):875-886.
18. Hernandez-Madrid A, Paul T, Abrams D, et al. Arrhythmias in congenial heart disease: a position paper of the European Heart Rhythm Association (EHRA), Association for European Paediatric and Congenital Cardiology (AEPC), and the European Society of Cardiology (ESC) Working Group on Grown-up Congenital heart disease, endorsed by HRS, PACES, APHRS, and SOLAECE. *Europace.* 2018;20(11):1719-1753.
19. Cheung Y, Cheng VY, Yung T, Chau AK. Cardiac rhythm and symptomatic arrhythmia in right atrial isomerism. *Am Heart J.* 2002;144:159-164.
20. Paladini D, Volpe P, Marasini M, et al. Diagnosis, characterization and outcome of congenitally corrected transposition of the great arteries in the fetus: a multicenter series of 30 cases. *Ultrasound Obstet Gynecol.* 2006;27(3):281-285.
21. Delhaas T, Sarvaas GJ, Rijlaarsdam ME, et al. A multicenter, long-term study on arrhythmias in children with Ebstein anomaly. *Pediatr Cardiol.* 2010;31:229-233.
22. Holley DG, Martin GR, Brenner JI, et al. Diagnosis and management of fetal cardiac tumors: a multicenter experience and review of published reports. *J Am Coll Cardiol.* 1995;26:516-520.
23. Wacker-Gussmann A, Strasburger JF, Cuneo BF, Wiggins D, Gotteiner N, Wakai R. Fetal arrhythmias associated with fetal rhabdomyomas. *Heart Rhythm.* 2014;11(4):677-683.
24. Peters C, Wacker-Gussman A, Strasburger JF, et al. Electrophysiologic features of fetal ventricular aneurysms and diverticula. *Prenat Diagn.* 2015;35(2):129-136.
25. Srinivasan S, Strasburger J. Overview of fetal arrhythmias. *Curr Opin Pediatr.* 2008;20(5):522-531.
26. Hinkle KA, Peyvandi S, Stiver C, et al. Postnatal outcomes of fetal supraventricular tachycardia: a multicenter study. *Pediatr Cardiol.* 2017;38(7):1317-1323.
27. Jaeggi ET, Carvalho JS, De Groot E, et al. Comparison of transplacental treatment of fetal supraventricular tachyarrhythmias with digoxin, flecainide, and sotalol: results of a nonrandomized multicenter study. *Circulation.* 2011;124(16):1747-1754.
28. Alsaied T, Baskar S, Fares M, et al. First-line antiarrhythmic transplacental treatment for fetal tachyarrhythmia: a systematic review and meta-analysis. *J Am Heart Assoc.* 2017;6(12):e007164.
29. Donofrio MT, Moon-Grady AJ, Hornberger LK, et al. Diagnosis and treatment of fetal cardiac disease: a scientific statement from the American Heart Association. *Circulation.* 2014;129(21):2183-2242.
30. Kannankeril PJ, Gotteiner NL, Deal BJ, Johnsrude CL, Strasburger JF. Location of accessory connection in infants presenting with supraventricular tachycardia in utero: clinical correlations. *Am J Perinatol.* 2003;20(3):115-119.
31. Naheed ZJ, Strasburger JF, Deal BJ, Benson DW Jr, Gidding SS. Fetal tachycardia: mechanisms and predictors of hydrops fetalis. *J Am Coll Cardiol.* 1996;27(7):1736-1740.
32. Wakai RT, Strasburger JF, Li Z, Deal BJ, Gotteiner NL. Magnetocardiographic rhythm patterns at initiation and termination of fetal supraventricular tachycardia. *Circulation.* 2003;107:307-312.
33. Jaeggi E, Fouron JC, Fournier A, van Doesburg N, Drblik SP, Proulx F. Ventriculo-atrial time interval measured on M mode echocardiography: a determining element in diagnosis, treatment, and prognosis of fetal supraventricular tachycardia. *Heart.* 1998;79(6):582-587.
34. Cuneo BF, Etheridge SP, Horigome H, et al. Arrhythmia phenotype during fetal life suggests long-QT syndrome genotype: risk stratification of perinatal long-QT syndrome. *Circ Arrhythm Electrophysiol.* 2013;6(5):946-951.

35. Mitchell JL, Cuneo BF, Etheridge SP, Horigome H, Weng HY, Benson DW. Fetal heart rate predictors of long QT syndrome. *Circulation.* 2012;126(23):2688-2695.
36. Winbo A, Fosdal I, Lindh M, et al. Third trimester fetal heart rate predicts phenotype and mutation burden in the type 1 long QT syndrome. *Circ Arrhythm Electrophysiol.* 2015;8(4):806-814.
37. Buyon JP, Friedman DM. Autoantibody-associated congenital heart block: the clinical perspective. *Curr Rheumatol Rep.* 2003;5(5):374-378.
38. Izmirly PM, Saxena A, Kim MY, et al. Maternal and fetal factors associated with mortality and morbidity in a multi-racial/ethnic registry of anti-SSA/Ro-associated cardiac neonatal lupus. *Circulation.* 2011;124(18):1927-1935.
39. Jaeggi ET, Hornberger LK, Smallhorn JF, Fouron JC. Prenatal diagnosis of complete atrioventricular block associated with structural heart disease: combined experience of two tertiary care centers and review of the literature. *Ultrasound Obstet Gynecol.* 2005;26(1):16-21.

Before Diagnosis: Initial Evaluation of the Pregnancy With Fetal Arrhythmia

Julia A. Drose • Bettina F. Cuneo

INTRODUCTION

The assessment of fetal arrhythmias begins not with the echocardiogram, but with a detailed history of the current pregnancy. Obstetrical, past medical, and family histories may give additional important clues to both the diagnosis and the severity of the arrhythmia. For example, a fetus with a normal rhythm a few days prior to presenting with a sustained tachycardia is less likely to be in heart failure than a fetus who was last evaluated weeks before and whose mother reports decreased fetal movement. A mother with a history of multiple fetal losses and a current pregnancy with a fetal heart rate (FHR) <3rd percentile for gestational age may be the proband of a family with undiagnosed mosaic or heterozygous long QT syndrome (LQTS) **(FIG. 1.2.1)**.[1-3] Alternatively, a mother with a history of Sjogren syndrome or a family history of autoimmune disease with FHR of 60 beats per minute may have anti-Ro/SSA antibodies and fetal atrioventricular (AV) block.[4] The objective of this chapter is to review assessment of the pregnancy when a fetal arrhythmia is suspected.

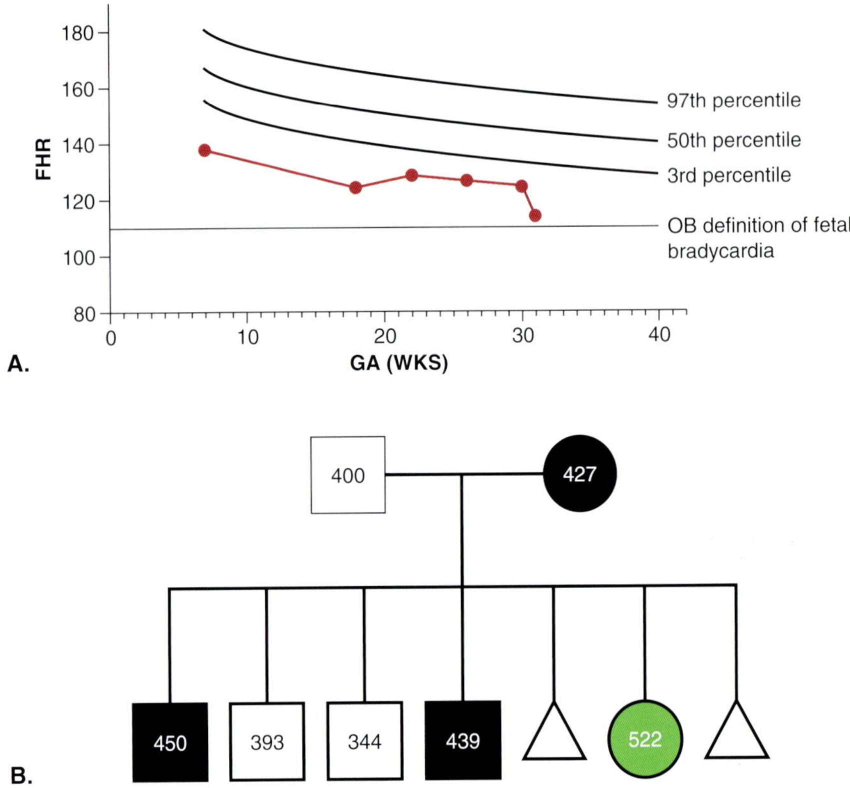

FIGURE 1.2.1 A fetus with sinus bradycardia. **A:** Graph depicting fetal heart rates (FHR, beats per minute [bpm]) versus gestational age (GA, weeks) from 3rd to 97th percentile. A fetus (red dots) with persistent FHR < 3rd percentile for GA but greater than standard definition of fetal bradycardia (FHR < 110 bpm) is shown. There was no family history of long QT syndrome; the mother and father's QTc intervals were normal on 12-lead ECG. The mother had a history of two stillbirths at 21 and 23 weeks GA. **B:** The family pedigree following genetic testing. The fetal proband (green circle) had the longest QTc, but two of her siblings and her mother (black circles and squares) carried with *KCNQ1* inherited variant. The two stillbirths are shown as triangles. The corrected QT intervals of each family member are shown in the circles and squares.

HISTORY OF CURRENT PREGNANCY

The mother should be questioned for a detailed dietary history as well as prescribed and over-the-counter medications, including herbal remedies. Certain maternal medications can cause fetal arrhythmias. For example, beta-adrenergic blocking agents may cause fetal bradycardia, and excessive caffeine or other stimulants can cause tachyarrhythmia or ectopy.

It is helpful to know details about the FHR and rhythm that lead to a suspicion of fetal arrhythmia. If an irregular rhythm was heard prior to a sustained tachyarrhythmia, most likely a premature atrial contraction has initiated a run of supraventricular tachyarrhythmia (SVT). However, if the rhythm was irregular and the rate is now slow, the fetus could have progressed from 2° AV block to complete AV block, or from atrial ectopy to blocked atrial bigeminy.

Fetal arrhythmias can accompany any cardiac defect but can be anticipated with certain ones. AV block is associated with congenitally corrected transposition of the great vessels or left atrial isomerism **(FIG. 1.2.2)**.[5-7] The common association of accessory connections and Ebstein anomaly increases the likelihood of SVT or atrial flutter in a fetus with this defect **(FIG. 1.2.3)**.[8] Sinus bradycardia with normal FHR variability can occur in right and left atrial isomerism, due to abnormalities in the number and location of the sinoatrial node as well as with decreased FHR variability, frequently seen in the fetus with LQTS **(FIG. 1.2.4)**.

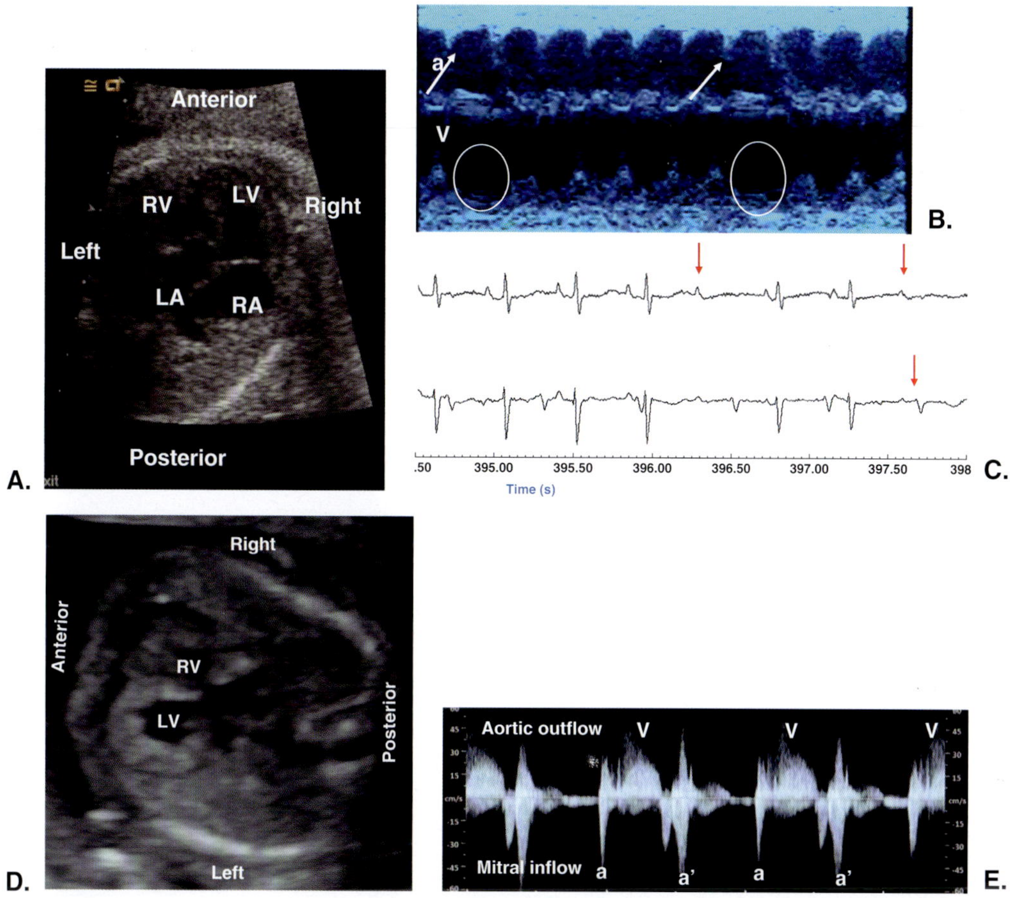

FIGURE 1.2.2 Intermittent and sustained atrioventricular (AV) block with structural cardiac defects. **A:** Congenitally corrected transposition of the great vessels. The right atrium (RA) gives rise to the left ventricle (LV), which is to the right and anterior of the right ventricle (RV). LA, left atrium. (Great vessels not shown.) **B:** Simultaneous atrial (a) and ventricular (V) M-mode of intermittent AV block in the fetus with congenitally corrected transposition of the great vessels. Arrows point to atrial contraction that is not conducted to the ventricle; the circle shows the absence of a ventricular contraction. Note the atrial rate is regular. a, atrium; V, ventricle. **C:** Fetal MCG rhythm tracing showing the intermittent AV block (arrows show p-waves not conducted to QRS). **D:** Left atrial isomerism with sustained AV block at 15 weeks of gestation. Note the thickened spongy-form myocardium especially the left ventricle (LV). RV, right ventricle. **E:** Simultaneous mitral inflow and aortic outflow spectral Doppler demonstrating the fetus in (D) has type 2, 2° AV block: the a-a′ intervals are regular, and every other atrial beat is conducted with an AV interval that is the same as the previous AV interval.

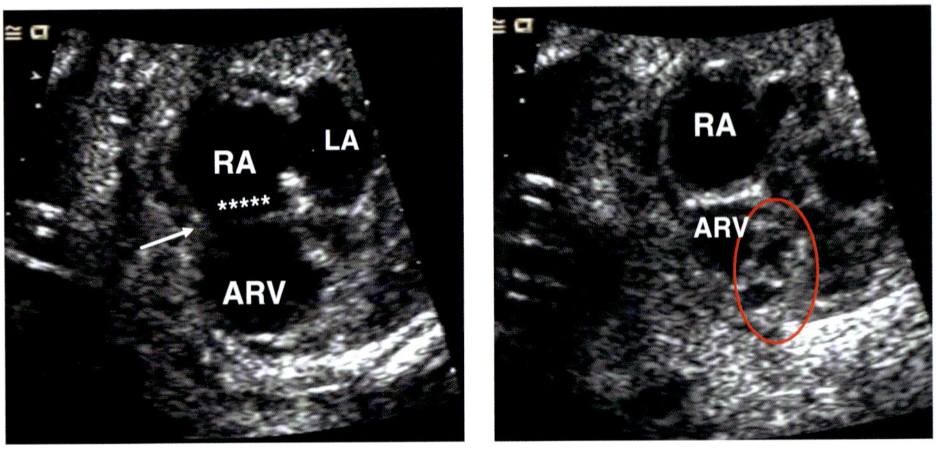

A. B.

FIGURE 1.2.3 A fetus with Ebstein anomaly. **A:** The septal leaflet of the tricuspid valve is so inferiorly displaced the valve cannot be easily seen on the four-chamber view; instead the right atrium (RA), the atrioventricular groove (arrow) and the tricuspid valve orifice (***) are visualized. RA, right atrium. **B:** With slight anterior angulation, the tricuspid valve can be seen (red circle), displaced almost to the RV outflow tract.

The fetal bradycardia associated with maternal anti-Ro/SSA autoantibodies is not always AV block. Rather, affected fetuses can present with sinus bradycardia or a junctional bradycardia, with atrial and ventricular rates being the same, or a junctional bradycardia with AV block (FIG. 1.2.5).[9,10]

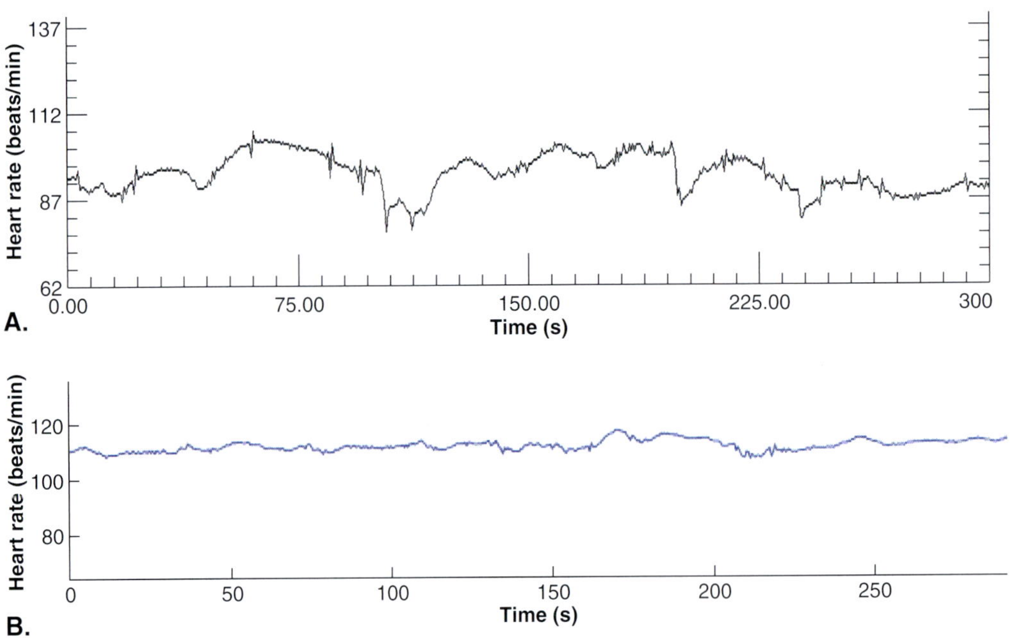

FIGURE 1.2.4 Normal and reduced fetal heart rate (FHR) variability in two bradycardic fetuses at 34 weeks of gestation. **A:** In a fetus with right atrial isomerism, heart rates (HRs) are <100 bpm, but FHR variability is normal. **B:** In contrast, this fetus with the family variant of inherited long QT syndrome had poor HR variability and a FHR < 3rd percentile for gestational age (~115 bpm). However, the biophysical profile score was 8/10, and the mother had a successful vaginal delivery at term.

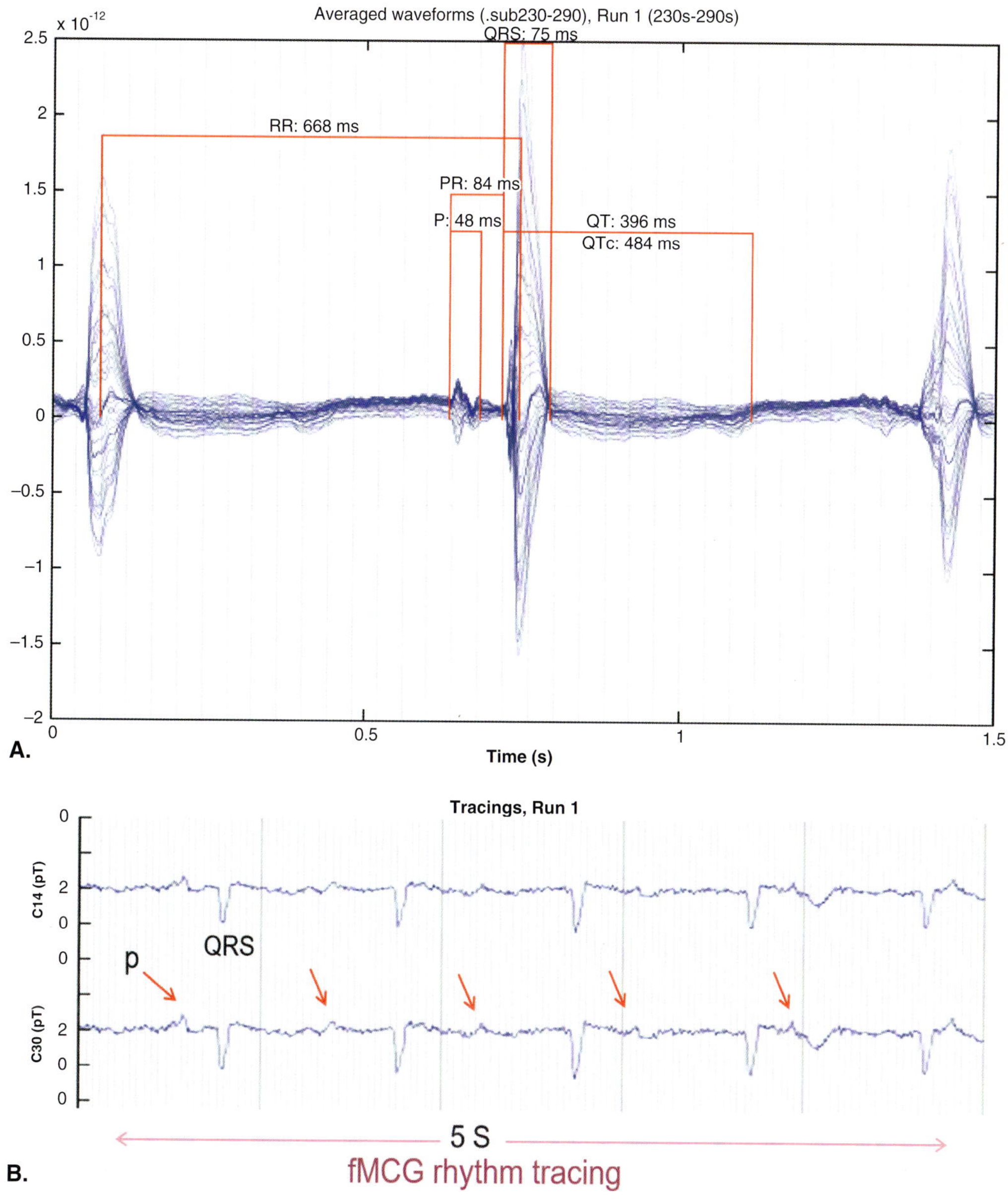

FIGURE 1.2.5 Fetal magnetocardiograms (fMCGs) from two fetuses with bradycardia whose mothers were anti-Ro/SSA antibody positive. **A:** Signal averaged fMCG of sinus bradycardia: one p-wave per QRS complex and a normal PR interval. The cycle length is 668 ms (fetal heart rate 90 bpm). **B:** Rhythm tracing of junctional bradycardia, atrioventricular (AV) dissociation, and AV block.

Viral myocarditis can also present with arrhythmias.[11] If there is a suspicion based on recent maternal illness and echocardiographic features of myocarditis, amniocentesis for culture and PCR of the common viruses, for example, enterovirus, parvovirus, cytomegalovirus, Ebstein-Barr virus, human immunodeficiency virus, coxsackie, and human herpesvirus 6, can be performed.

OBSTETRICAL HISTORY

The outcomes of the mother's past pregnancies are important pieces of information because some arrhythmias, such as junctional ectopic tachycardia and the channelopathies, are heritable[12,13] and others, including anti-Ro/SSA antibody–mediated AV block, have a high (~18%) recurrence rate.[4]

Questions to the mother should include a history of fetal losses or premature deliveries because of congenital heart disease or FHR or rhythm abnormalities. As decreased FHR variability can be part of the LQTS phenotype, a previous urgent delivery for non-reassuring FHR monitoring may be a clue to inherited LQTS (FIG. 1.2.4B).[14] In fact, in a series of *KCNQ1* mothers, fetuses delivered urgently by cesarean delivery for non-reassuring FHR monitoring all carried the maternal LQTS variant.[14] Acquired LQTS may also be heritable, so medication history should be reviewed.[15]

The mother should also be questioned about a previous pregnancy with nonimmune hydrops due to the association of hydrops with cardiac abnormalities, including arrhythmias in 15% to 25%. Nonimmune hydrops due to congestive heart failure secondary to SVT is particularly common. Ten percent of fetuses identified in utero with SVT are found to have pre-excitation, aka Wolff-Parkinson-White syndrome, due to an accessory AV connection. Pre-excitation has been shown by fetal magnetocardiogram (fMCG) in fetuses with structurally normal hearts and as the basis for SVT in fetuses with rhabdomyoma.[16,17] A short PR interval suggestive of pre-excitation has not been diagnosed by echocardiography.

For any fetal loss, gestational age, autopsy report, genetic testing results, and the FHR and rhythms before the loss are important data. For live-born infants, any cardiac issues such as a murmur, syncope, or arrhythmias should be noted.

PAST MEDICAL HISTORY

A detailed maternal past medical history should include any cardiac symptoms such as palpitations, syncope, murmurs, and tachycardia with fevers and any visits to a cardiologist or treatment for a "heart condition." A maternal history of autoimmune thyroid disease also has implications for the development of sinus tachycardia in the fetus.[18]

FAMILY HISTORY

The mother can be questioned for a family history of both cardiac symptoms and cardiac syndromes. Cardiac symptoms include a first-degree relative with slow or fast heart rate, pacemaker, internal cardiac defibrillator or heart surgery, sudden unexplained death at <30 years of age or during intense exercise, drowning, or death in an auto accident. Cardiac conditions include Wolff-Parkinson-White syndrome,[19] short QT syndrome,[20] LQTS,[21] Brugada syndrome,[22] catecholaminergic paroxysmal ventricular tachycardia,[23] cardiomyopathy,[24] or atrial fibrillation.[25] It can be helpful to inquire if anyone else in the family has the same rhythm as the fetus in question. For example, if males in the family have slow heart rates and the fetus is also a male with sinus bradycardia, a mutation in the HCN4 ion channel gene is possible.[26] Finally, it would be appropriate to ask if any family member has undergone genetic testing as part of an arrhythmia evaluation and, if so, what were the results.

OTHER CONSIDERATIONS

It is also important to inquire about serum calcium, magnesium, and vitamin D (25, OH) levels as these can be low in pregnant women. In the pregnancy with or at risk for maternal or fetal arrhythmia, these levels should be corrected to normal. Lastly, it may be appropriate to inquire about current exposure to QT-prolonging medications[27] and if indicated, limit exposures in the future.

SUMMARY

In conclusion, a complete review of maternal, obstetric, and family history is important before performing the echocardiogram on the fetus with a suspected arrhythmia. Diagnosis, prognosis, and treatment may be influenced by a more precise understanding of the underlying cause of an abnormal rate or rhythm.

References

1. Priest JR, Gawad C, Kahlig KM, et al. Early somatic mosaicism is a rare cause of long-QT syndrome. *Proc Natl Acad Sci USA*. 2016;113(41):11555-11560.
2. Miller TE, Estrella E, Myerburg RJ, et al. Recurrent third-trimester fetal loss and maternal mosaicism for long-QT syndrome. *Circulation*. 2004;109:3029-3034.
3. Bhuyan ZA, Momenah TS, Gong Q, et al. Recurrent intrauterine fetal loss due to near absence of HERG: clinical and functional characterization of a homozygous nonsense HERG Q1070X mutation. *Heart Rhythm*. 2008;5(4):553-561.
4. Buyon JP, Hiebert R, Copel J, et al. J Autoimmune-associated congenital heart block: demographics, mortality, morbidity and recurrence rates obtained from a national neonatal lupus registry. *J Am Coll Cardiol*. 1998;31(7):1658-1666.
5. Berg C, Geipel A, Kamil D, et al. The syndrome of left isomerism: sonographic findings and outcome in prenatally diagnosed cases. *J Ultrasound Med*. 2005;24:921-931.
6. Jaeggi ET, Hornberger LK, Smallhorn JF, Fouron JC. Prenatal diagnosis of complete atrioventricular block associated with structural heart disease: combined experience of two tertiary care centers and review of the literature. *Ultrasound Obstet Gynecol*. 2005;26(1):16-21.
7. Cheung Y, Cheng VY, Yung T, Chau AK. Cardiac rhythm and symptomatic arrhythmia in right atrial isomerism. *Am Heart J*. 2002;144:159-164.
8. Delhaas T, Sarvaas GJ, Rijlaarsdam ME, et al. A multicenter, long-term study on arrhythmias in children with Ebstein anomaly. *Pediatr Cardiol*. 2010;31:229-233.
9. Cuneo BF, Strasburger JF, Niksch A, Ovadia M, Wakai RT. An expanded phenotype of maternal SSA/SSB antibody-associated fetal cardiac disease. *J Matern Fetal Neonatal Med*. 2009;22(3):233-238.
10. Jaeggi ET, Chitayat D, Taylor G. Atrial standstill associated with loss of atrial myocytes: a rare cause of fetal bradyarrhythmia. *Heart Rhythm*. 2009;6(9):1370-1372.
11. Thakur V, Fouron JC, Mertens L, Jaeggi ET. Diagnosis and management of fetal heart failure. *Can J Cardiol*. 2013;29(7):759-767.
12. Collins KK, Van Hare GF, Kertesz NJ, et al. Pediatric non post-operative junctional ectopic tachycardia medical management and interventional therapies. *J Am Coll Cardiol*. 2009;53:690-697.
13. Schwartz PJ, Ackerman MJ. The long QT syndrome: a transatlantic approach to diagnosis and therapy. *Eur Heart J*. 2013;34(40):3109-3116.

14. Heradien MJ, Goosen A, Crotti L, et al. Does pregnancy increase cardiac risk for LQT1 patients with the KCNQ1-A341V mutation? *J Am Coll Cardiol.* 2006;48:1410.
15. Itoh H, Crotti L, Aiba T, et al. The genetics underlying acquired long QT syndrome: impact for genetic screening. *Eur Heart J.* 2016;37(18):1456-1464.
16. Naheed ZJ, Strasburger JF, Deal BJ, Benson DW Jr, Gidding SS. Fetal tachycardia: mechanisms and predictors of hydrops fetalis. *J Am Coll Cardiol.* 1996;27(7):1736-1740.
17. Wacker-Gussmann A, Strasburger JF, Cuneo B, Wiggins D, Gotteiner N, Wakai RT. Fetal arrhythmias associated with cardiac rhabdomyomas. *Heart Rhythm.* 2014;11(4):677-683.
18. Galofre JC, Davies TF. Autoimmune thyroid disease in pregnancy: a review. *J Womens Health (Larchmt).* 2009;18(11):1847-1856.
19. Benson DW, Cohen MI. Wolff-Parkinson-White syndrome: lessons learnt and lessons remaining. *Cardiol Young.* 2017;27(S1):S62-S67.
20. Mazzanti A, Underwood K, Nevelev D, Kofman S, Priori SG. The new kids on the block of arrhythmogenic disorders: short QT syndrome and early repolarization. *J Cardiovasc Electrophysiol.* 2017;28(10):1226-1236.
21. Wilde AAM, Amin A. Channelopathies, genetic testing and risk stratification. *Int J Cardiol.* 2017;237:53-55.
22. Gourraud JB, Barc J, Thollet A, Le Marec H, Probst V. Brugada syndrome: diagnosis, risk stratification and management. *Arch Cardiovasc Dis.* 2017;110(3):188-195.
23. Sumitomo N. Current topics in catecholaminergic polymorphic ventricular tachycardia. *J Arrhythm.* 2016;32(5):344-351.
24. Lee TM, Hsu DT, Kantor P, et al. Pediatric cardiomyopathies. *Circ Res.* 2017;121(7):855-873.
25. Baruteau AE, Probst V, Abriel H. Inherited progressive cardiac conduction disorders. *Curr Opin Cardiol.* 2015;30(1):33-39.
26. DiFrancesco D. Funny channel gene mutations associated with arrhythmias. *J Physiol.* 2013;591(17):4117-4124.
27. Woosley RL. *Drugs That Prolong the QT Interval and/or Induce Torsades de Pointes.* Sudden Arrhythmic Deaths Foundation website. Available at sads.org/living-with-sads/Drugs-to-Avoid. Accessed May 15, 2019.

Genetics of Fetal Arrhythmias

Susan Etheridge • Lindsay Meyers

INTRODUCTION

The fetus of a normal pregnancy was delivered emergently by cesarean delivery at 31 weeks' gestation for bradycardia which was thought to be caused by fetal distress. At birth, the infant's Apgar scores were 9 and 9, cord blood pH was 7.27, and the base excess was −5. The 12-lead electrocardiogram (ECG) demonstrated 2:1 atrioventricular (AV) block due to severe QT prolongation (FIG. 1.3.1A), and syndactyly of the fingers on both hands was noted (FIG. 1.3.1B), which are all features of long QT syndrome (LQTS) 8, a channelopathy also known as Timothy syndrome. The infant was intubated due to lung disease of prematurity and numerous episodes of torsades de pointes (TdP) (FIG. 1.3.1C). He ultimately succumbed to complications of prematurity.

The cardiac channelopathies are but one of the inherited arrhythmia disorders. They are caused by disturbed function of cardiac ion channel subunits or the proteins that regulate them and include LQTS, short QT syndrome, Brugada syndrome (BrS), catecholaminergic polymorphic ventricular tachycardia (CPVT), early repolarization syndrome, and some forms of inherited sinus bradycardia. The inherited arrhythmia disorders may be suspected from a detailed family or obstetrical history, supported by features of the current pregnancy including heart rhythm analysis of the fetus and confirmed by genetic testing. While genetic testing for aneuploidy and other chromosome anomalies has become routine in obstetrical practice, and despite availability of gene mutation panels for inherited arrhythmias at commercial laboratories, genetic testing for inherited arrhythmias is vastly underutilized. Given the prevalence of inherited channelopathies, this is an important oversight. By way of comparison, trisomy 21 occurs in 1/700 live births[1] and the prevalence of the most common inherited channelopathy, LQTS, is 1/2000 individuals.[2]

The purpose of this chapter is to outline the fetal presentation of the inherited arrhythmias. We will review current findings of disease inheritance and genetic disease modifiers. Since the most is known about LQTS, we will describe not only the three most common types but also the specific and unique clinical aspects of more uncommon but unique and highly lethal forms including Timothy syndrome and Jervell and Lange-Nielsen syndrome. This is followed by other inherited arrhythmias relevant to the fetus including CPVT, the calmodulinopathies, BrS, and channelopathies of the sinoatrial node resulting in sinus bradycardia. Management of the pregnant mother with channelopathy is discussed in Part 5, Chapter 1, and treatment of the symptomatic fetus with channelopathy is discussed in Part 3, Chapter 6.

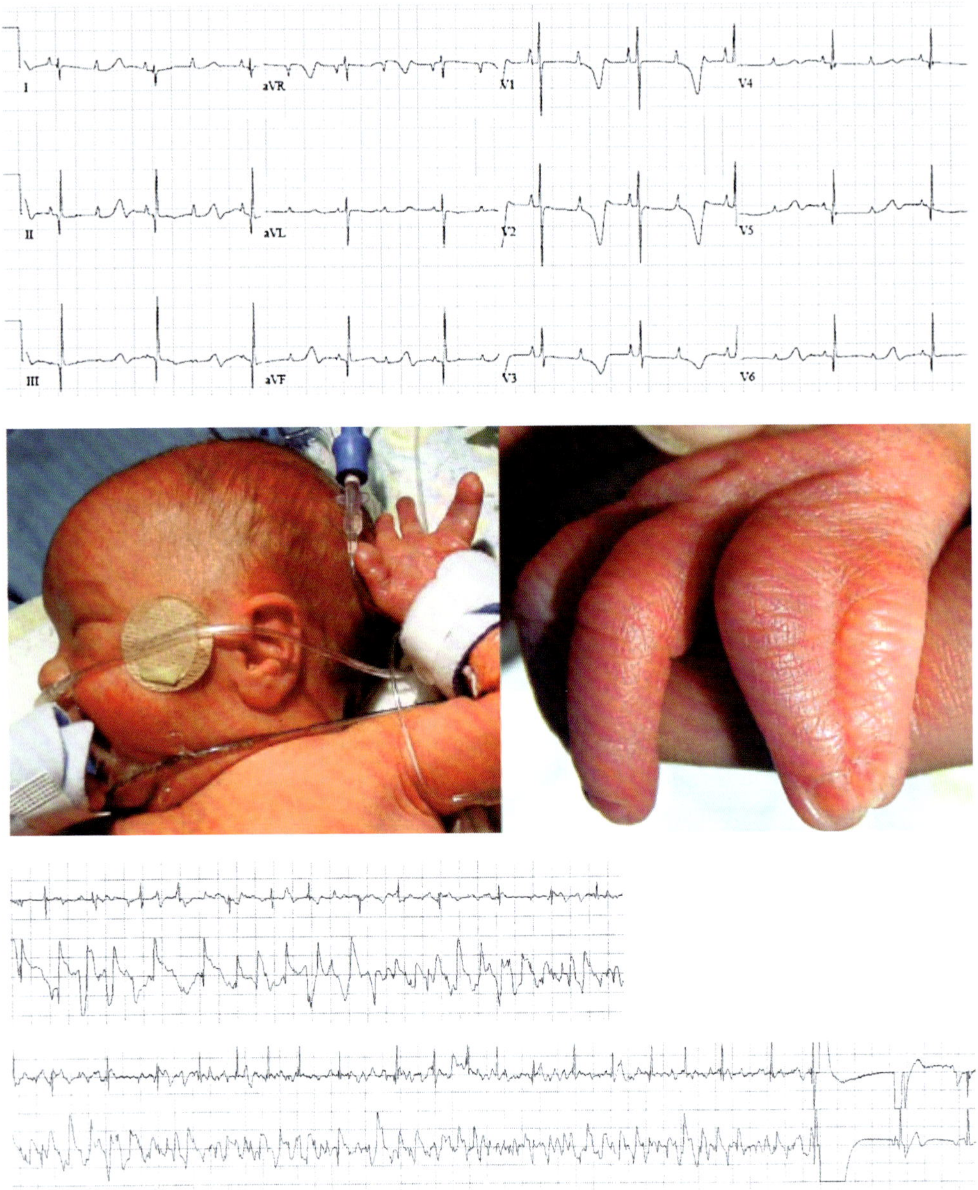

FIGURE 1.3.1 Features of Timothy syndrome. **A:** 12-Lead ECG in a newborn with functional 2:1 atrioventricular block. Note the severe QT prolongation with a sinus P-wave that occurs before each T-wave, that is, before repolarization is complete. **B:** Syndactyly of the fourth and fifth digits in a newborn. Syndactyly can be seen on prenatal ultrasound and should be sought in any fetus with sinus bradycardia or complex arrhythmia. **C:** 2-Lead telemetry demonstrating torsades de pointes degenerating into ventricular fibrillation prior to direct electro-cardioversion. (B, Reprinted from Etheridge SP, Bowles NE, Arrington CB, et al. Somatic mosaicism contributes to phenotypic variation in Timothy syndrome. *Am J Med Genet A.* 2011;155A(10):2578-2583.)

LONG QT SYNDROME (LQTS)

LQTS is an inherited disease of cardiac repolarization characterized by a prolonged QTc interval on the ECG (FIG. 1.3.2). LQTS is usually the result of single pathogenic variant in one of the genes that encode for a cardiac ion channel or an accessory ion channel subunit. These single variants can cause life-threatening arrhythmias, seizures, syncope, and sudden death in heterozygous mutation carriers.[3] The clinical events are a consequence of the signature ventricular arrhythmia, TdP, that can terminate spontaneously or degenerate into ventricular fibrillation (FIG. 1.3.1C). Once recognized, primary prevention with beta-adrenergic blocking agents is highly successful; therefore, early recognition can save lives.

Fetal Presentation

Ideally, LQTS would be diagnosed before birth and primary prevention initiated during infancy, but unless LQTS is suspected because of fetal arrhythmia or a family history, prenatal diagnosis is difficult. One should have a high index of suspicion in the fetus with ventricular tachycardia and/or 2:1 AV block, as the combination of the two arrhythmias is highly suggestive of LQTS. However, these LQTS rhythms occur in <25% of fetal LQTS cases, and the most common presentation is a fetal heart rate <3rd percentile for gestational age. This mild bradycardia can be easily overlooked and felt to be normal.[4,5] In a fetus with mild sinus bradycardia or a signature LQTS rhythm, close attention should be paid to a history of a family member, including the mother, who had syncope without a prodrome, seizures, a history of stillbirth, or multiple fetal losses, and those with an internal cardiac defibrillator or pacemaker. Not only should history be collected for any sudden, unexplained deaths at a young age, but also accidents in the family that include single motor vehicle accidents or drowning/near drowning of an otherwise good swimmer, as these may be a sign of a syncopal event or cardiac arrest. Lastly, if one of the parents has a known LQTS variant, each offspring has a 50% chance of also carrying the variant (see later). If the family history is negative, a de novo LQT variant is possible and should be investigated further, as the arrhythmia profile tends to be more serious and the QTc interval longer than in familial LQTS.[6]

Fetal Diagnosis of LQTS

Fetal LQTS can be diagnosed by fetal magnetocardiography (fMCG).[7,8] Confirmation of the signature rhythms, measurement of the QTc interval, and identification of repolarization abnormalities can all be shown on fMCG performed between 18 to 40 weeks of gestation (FIG. 1.3.3). While the type of LQTS can only be determined by genetic testing (see later), confirming (or refuting) suspected fetal LQTS is invaluable for pregnancy management (discussed in Part 5, Chapter 1). In brief, if LQTS is confirmed by fMCG, fetal surveillance is increased, LQT-prolonging medications are avoided, and delivery is recommended in a cardiac center.[9]

(text continued on page 38)

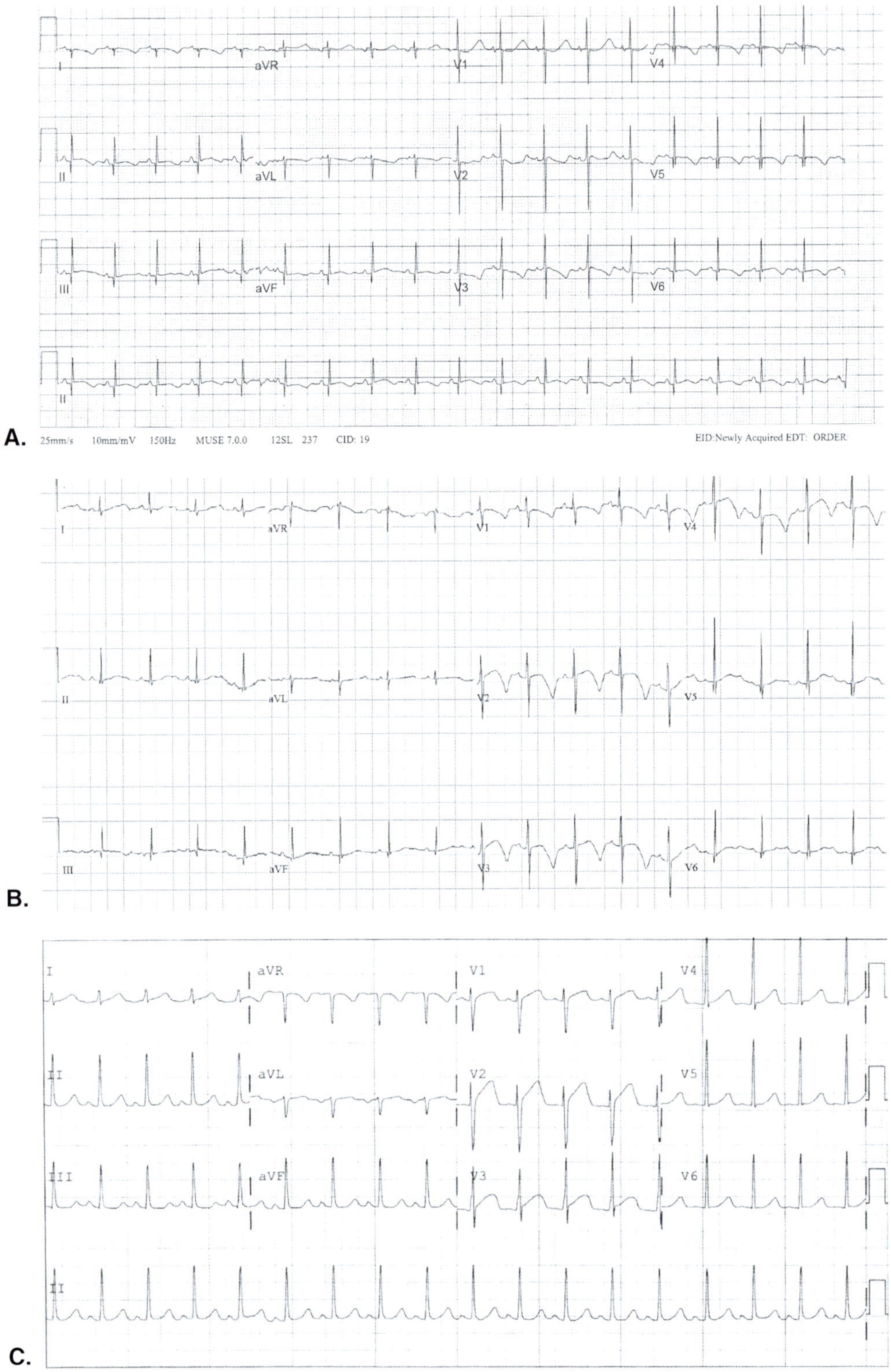

FIGURE 1.3.2 12-Lead ECGs in the three most common types of LQTS. **A:** Newborn with LQT1. The infant is relatively bradycardic (heart rate 110 bpm), and there are prominent U-waves and a prolonged QTc (506 ms). **B:** Infant with LQT2. Note the QT prolongation, the biphasic and somewhat bizarre T-waves in the midprecordial leads V2-V4 and the notched T-waves in many other leads. **C:** Child with LQT3.

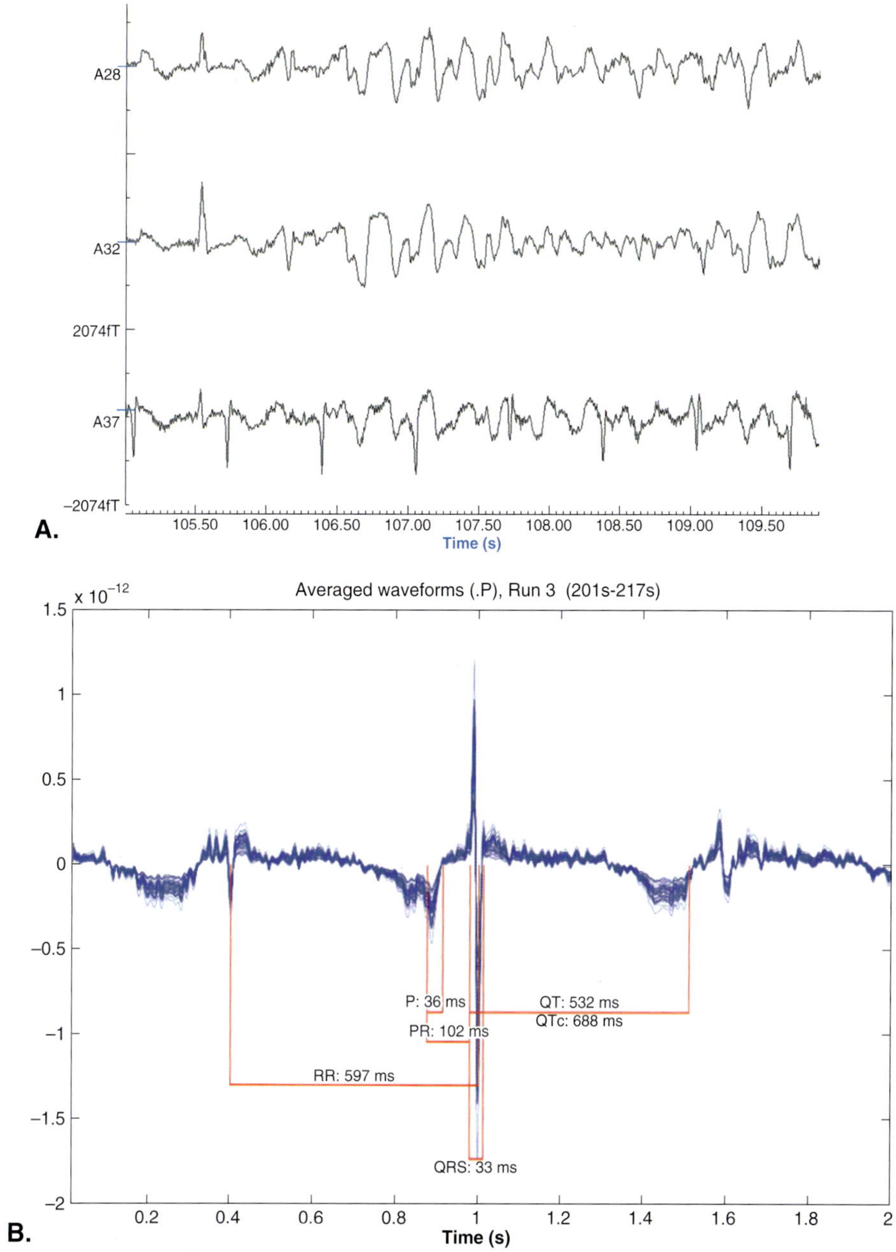

FIGURE 1.3.3 Magnetocardiograms of LQTS. **A:** Rhythm tracing showing torsades de pointes in a 32-week fetus with an SCN5A R1623Q variant and hydrops. **B:** Signal-averaged tracing of a 28-week fetus with CALM-2 mutation, bradycardia (heart rate ~ 100 bpm), and extreme QT prolongation (QTc = 688 ms). **C:** T-wave alternans, a repolarization abnormality common in subjects with LQTS. Note the alternating polarity of the T-waves (red arrows). Top two are the fetal rhythm tracings and the bottom is the maternal and fetal tracing.

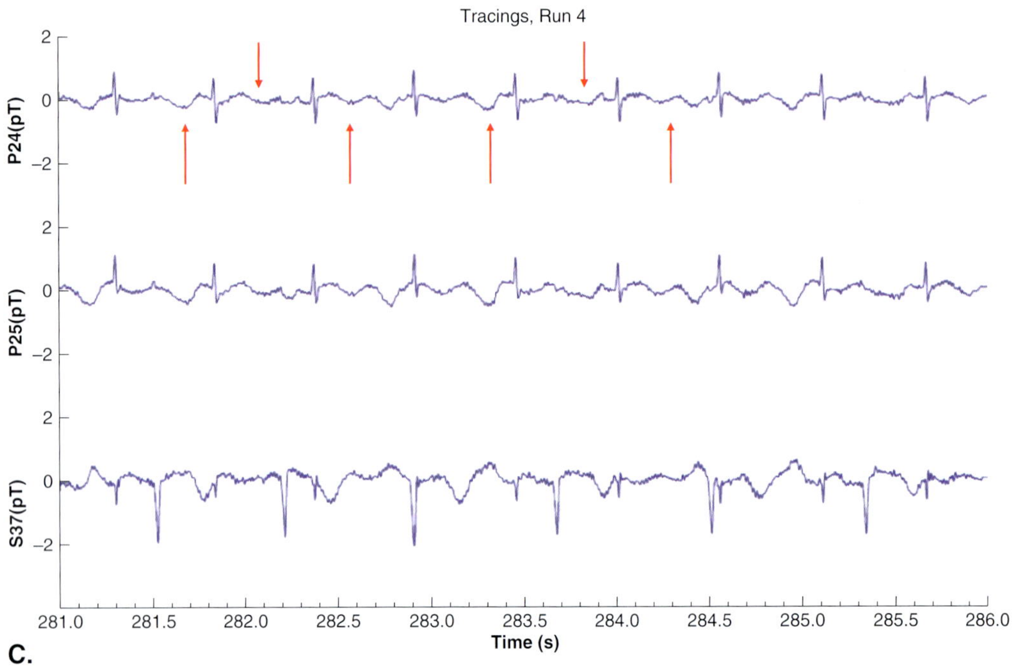

FIGURE 1.3.3 Cont'd

Inheritance

Most commonly, LQTS is inherited in an autosomal dominant fashion. Thus, there is a 50% risk for an individual to inherit a disease-causing variant from an affected parent or to transmit this variant to their offspring. The exceptions are Jervell and Lange-Nielsen syndrome and the newly recognized *TRDN*-related LQTS, both with autosomal recessive inheritance.[10,11] Jervell and Lange-Nielsen syndrome is caused by the presence of two pathogenic variants in *KCNQ1* and/or *KCNE1* **(FIG. 1.3.4)**, and even though it is a recessive disease, parents and siblings may have LQTS having inherited one of the two variants. In these cases, those with a single mutation usually have mild disease.[12]

Occasionally, the fetus can be the proband (the first individual identified with the pathogenic variant). Identifying the underlying genetic variant can aid in treating and counseling the parents of the proband and allows for cascade screening, a process in which at-risk relatives are tested for a known genetic variation in a stepwise fashion until all at-risk individuals are identified. Additionally, guidelines support genetic testing for those with a clinical diagnosis of LQTS.[13,14]

Genetic Testing

To date, at least 17 genes have been reported to be associated with LQTS. However, the majority of known disease-causing variants are identified in genes *KCNQ1* (30%-35%), *KCNQ2* (25%-30%) encoding for potassium channels, and *SCN5A* (5%-10%) encoding for a sodium channel causing LQTS types 1, 2, and 3, respectively.[15] The majority of

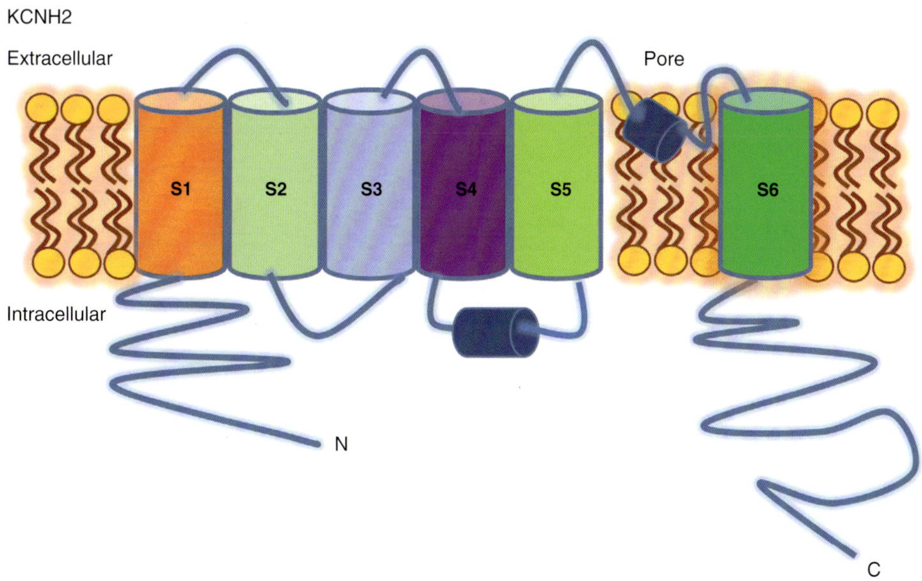

FIGURE 1.3.4 Predicted topology of the iKS (potassium) channel formed by KCNQ1 and KCNE1. Each KCNQ1 subunit contains an NH2 terminus, six membrane-spanning segments S1-S6, a pore loop, two cytoplasmic loops (c loops), and a COOH terminus domain. The KCNE1 subunit contains a single alpha-helical transmembrane domain with an extracellular NH2 terminus and a cytoplasmic COOH terminus domain.

variants identified are single nucleotide variants. Presently, 25% of people with phenotype positive LQTS remain genetically elusive, as commercial gene testing fails to uncover a known pathogenic variant.

Interestingly, the presence of a pathogenic variant alone does not predict clinical outcome because LQTS is characterized by both reduced penetrance and variable expressivity. Reduced penetrance means not every individual who has a pathogenic variant will express the LQTS phenotype. It is estimated that approximately 25% of individuals with a pathogenic variant will have a normal QTc interval on resting ECG.[16] Even though these patients with "concealed" LQTS have a lower risk of sudden cardiac arrest, they do still have an increased risk over the general population.[16] Additionally, almost half of individuals with pathogenic variants will not experience a syncopal episode nor report a family history of either LQTS or sudden death.[17] This highlights the utility of cascade genetic testing in apparently unaffected at-risk relatives, as even though they may be phenotypically negative, they may still be genotype positive and at increased risk for cardiac arrest under certain circumstances. Furthermore, they can pass the variant to future children who may be more severely affected.

Variable expressivity refers to a difference in the clinical phenotypic or the severity of the phenotype, not only between families but also within families (**FIG. 1.3.5**). As an example, one individual may have a normal resting QTc and never develop a symptom over their lifetime and their sibling may experience a sudden cardiac arrest at the age of 16 years. Additionally, the same variant in *SCN5A* may present clinically as LQTS in one individual and as BrS in another. Variable expressivity is likely secondary to other gene-environment interactions that modify a given individual's disease expression.

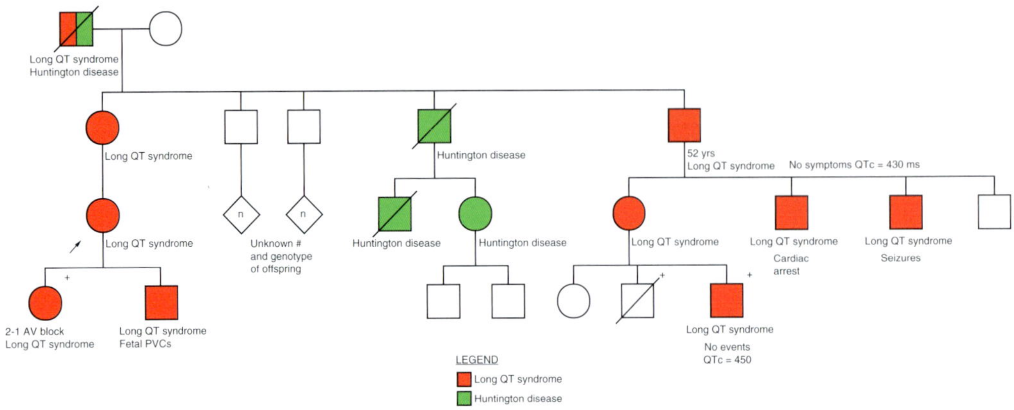

FIGURE 1.3.5 Genetic pedigrees showing reduced penetrance and variable expressivity in a family with long QT syndrome and Huntington disease. Note the difference in symptoms in the family and that some individuals who were gene-positive had normal QTc intervals on 12-lead ECG.

These modifiers include gender, age, and the presence of common variants in the general population that in and of themselves are not disease causing but either act as protective or increase disease susceptibility when in combination with a rare pathogenic variant.[18,19]

Genetic testing for the fetus and newborn suspected of having LQTS is offered by many CLIA-certified labs and available commercially. Prenatal testing can be performed by percutaneous umbilical artery sampling, amniocentesis, or chorionic villus sampling, but prenatal commercial testing is currently limited to the fetus's family variant. Postnatally, testing can be performed using cord or peripheral blood sampling or buccal mucosa swab. The chance of identifying a pathogenic variant on the clinically available multigene panels is approximately 75%, with 90% of patients having a variant in one of the three LQTS-related genes.[20,21]

As with most single-gene disorders, there are three different types of results that can be reported: a clear positive (pathogenic variant), a clear negative, or a variant of uncertain significance. Identification of a pathogenic variant confirms the clinical diagnosis and allows tailored patient management based on the type of LQTS and the specific variant. Since the detection rate of any LQTS multigene panel is not 100%, a negative result does not rule out an underlying genetic etiology. If the fetus/infant has a negative test result, they should be managed based on clinical phenotype and all first-degree relatives should have a clinical evaluation and an ECG.

Genotype-Phenotype Correlations

Aside from the gene-specific genotype-phenotype correlations, there are also genotypic correlates with disease severity, and certain pathogenic variants are associated with a more severe phenotype. These variants are found in the pore region of the *KCNH2* gene[22] and in the transmembrane region or cytoplasmic loop of the *KCNQ1* gene that have a dominant negative effect on the channel and are all associated with increased risk for a cardiac event.[23,24] In addition, individuals who have two pathogenic variants either as a compound heterozygote (two different variants) or homozygote (two of the same variants) in the same gene, or two in two different LQTS-associated genes (digenic) have a higher risk of cardiac events.[25,26]

De novo variants often present with the most severe disease. In one study, fetal presence of TdP with or without 2:1 AV block was highly associated with de novo pathogenic variants (eg, sporadic and not inherited from a parent), most identified in *SCN5A* R1623Q.[6] However, there are also reported cases of variants resulting in severe fetal presentation or recurrent fetal loss that are present in parents in a somatic mosaic state, which include the parental gametes.[27,28] Mosaicism is defined by different cell populations in the body having differing genetic information. This is caused by a genetic variant occurring postzygotically. Depending on the timing of the variant occurrence in embryonic development, the level of mutant genotype may be low enough for an individual to either not show the clinical phenotype or to have a milder phenotype. Mosaicism in relation to LQTS has been found to be present in at least 0.05% of cases, with an estimated prevalence of 0.17% in probands with negative multigene panel testing.[28] While this number is low, it highlights the importance of testing parents of those found to have a severe fetal presentation, even in the absence of parental clinical symptoms. This will impact recurrence risk for the family as well as future pregnancy management. To date, no cases of isolated gonadal mosaicism have been reported in the literature. However, since gonadal mosaicism can never be ruled out, even in apparent de novo inheritance, the recurrence risk is never zero, but typically quoted as <1%.

Disease Modifiers of LQTS

Patient age and sex modify the QT interval and disease expression, and therefore, presentation in utero does not predict childhood or adult phenotype. Those identified in utero and as neonates not surprisingly often have the most concerning disease expression.[6] The severe arrhythmia phenotypes noted in the fetus can be explained in part by pathogenic genetic variants with severe biophysical phenotypes. For example, studies of the *SCN5A* variant R1623Q, noted in sporadic LQTS cases with severe perinatal arrhythmia, identified a novel LQTS mechanism characterized by early channel reopenings and increased probability of long openings.[29] Regardless of the time of diagnosis, individuals with LQTS with TdP in the first year of life are at high risk for poor outcome. Although past data suggest high mortality rates were also high for neonates with LQTS and functional 2:1 AV block, recent publications have shown a more optimistic outcome with use of beta blockers, mexiletine, and pacing.[30] Important in this retrospective review was the observation that 75% of patients have improvement in their conduction (2:1 becomes 1:1) over the first year of life.

Although symptoms can improve, infants with cardiac events in the first year are at very high risk for further events during the first decade of life.[31] LQTS infants with QTc prolongation >500 ms, heart rate <100 beats per minute, and female sex are at increased risk for fatal or near-fatal cardiac arrest during the first year of life. Furthermore, such an event before age 1 year was associated with a hazard ratio of 23.4 ($P < .01$) for an additional fatal or near-fatal cardiac event in the next 10 years.[31]

Rare Forms of LQTS

Timothy Syndrome

This severe and very rare type of LQTS is illustrated in the case at the beginning of this chapter (FIG. 1.3.1). Timothy syndrome, or LQT8, is a disorder of the L-type calcium channels Cav1.2 encoded by *CACNA1C* and is somewhat unique among LQTS types as it is characterized by multisystem involvement. This can be explained by the ubiquitous presence of Cav1.2 throughout the body. Patients have severe QTc prolongation (often with neonatal and fetal 2:1 AV block), congenital heart defects, syndactyly, abnormal facies, hypoglycemia, and neurological disease.[32] Sudden death occurs due to ventricular arrhythmias, but also occurs in the setting of hypoglycemia and during the use of inhalational anesthetics.[33] In the largest study to date of Timothy syndrome, patients were younger at diagnosis (birth to 76 months of age) compared to the overall LQTS population.[33] Timothy syndrome has also been inherited by somatic mosaicism.[34]

Jervell and Lange-Nielsen Syndrome

This is one of the most severe forms of LQTS, characterized by congenital deafness and profound QTc prolongation that often presents in fetal and neonatal life.[35] This autosomal recessive form of LQTS is due to homozygous or compound heterozygous mutations on either *KCNQ1* or a subunit of KCNQ1 called *KCNE1*.[36] Almost 90% of patients become symptomatic, and the sudden death event rate exceeds 25% despite medical therapy.[10] Because of these findings, it is very important to diagnose affected individuals during fetal life so that appropriate treatment can be instituted immediately after birth. Genetic testing may identify both parents carry a pathogenic variant in either *KCNQ1* or *KCNE1*, although individuals with single pathogenic are often only mildly affected or unaffected.

CATECHOLAMINERGIC POLYMORPHIC VENTRICULAR TACHYCARDIA (CPVT)

CPVT is a rare inherited abnormality of calcium-handling proteins most commonly due to pathogenic variants in the ryanodine receptor *RYR2* (~60%), which are inherited in an autosomal dominant fashion. Less common, in about 3% to 5% of cases, is the autosomal recessive form due to compound heterozygous or homozygous pathogenic variants in the *CASQ2* gene. More recently, patients with a clinical diagnosis of CPVT have also been found to have pathogenic variants in the *CALM* genes, as outlined below, as well as rare cases with variants in *TRDN*. There are a few other cases with reported variants in other genes; however, more research is still needed to determine if these genes indeed lead to CPVT phenotype.[37] Approximately 40% of CPVT presents with de novo variants.

While CPVT has not been reported in the fetus, sudden infant death syndrome has been attributed to RYR2 mutation.[38] In addition, the onset of CPVT is at a young age and it is possible that CPVT has unrecognized or undiagnosed symptomatology, including stillbirth, in the fetus. Furthermore, as more survivors are reaching childbearing age,

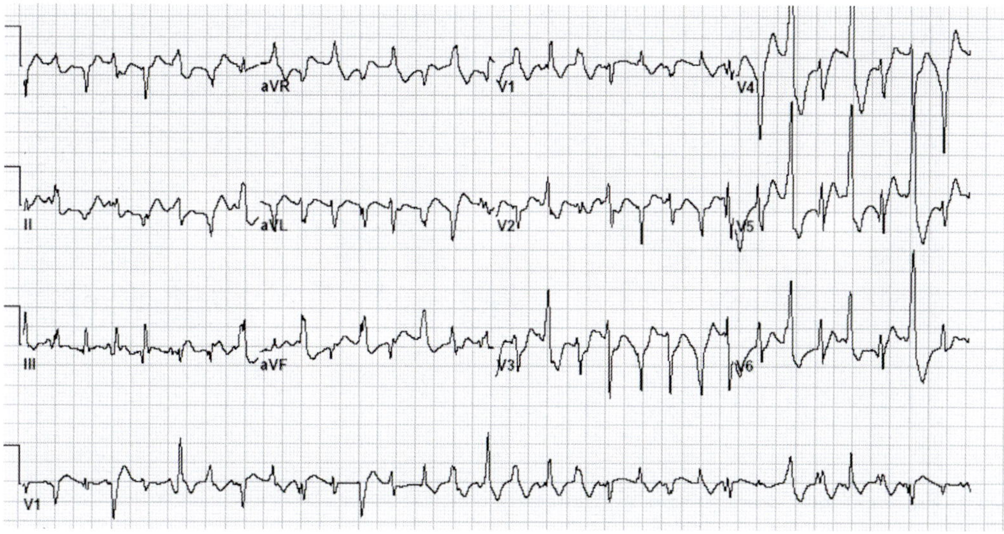

FIGURE 1.3.6 12-Lead ECG and V1 rhythm strip in a child with catecholaminergic polymorphic ventricular tachycardia (CPVT). This is the classic bidirectional ventricular tachycardia in a 6-year-old presenting with syncope due to CPVT. In the V1 rhythm strip, note the upright and negative QRS complexes characterizing bidirectional ventricular tachycardia.

evaluation by fMCG may uncover previously unrecognized or undiagnosed findings in the fetus, including bidirectional ventricular tachycardia, the signature rhythm of CPVT **(FIG. 1.3.6)**.

CALMODULINOPATHIES

There are three calmodulin genes *CALM1* (chr14q31), *CALM2* (Chr2p21), and *CALM3* (chr19q13) that all encode for an identical calmodulin protein, CaM.[39-43] CaM has direct interaction with Cav1.2 L-type calcium channels, deactivating Cav1.2 when CaM binds to free calcium.[3] Pathogenic variants in the *CALM* genes are referred to as calmodulinopathies, since individuals with pathogenic variants in one of the three *CALM* genes can present with a range of phenotypes including LQTS, CPVT, idiopathic ventricular fibrillation, and sudden death. Calmodulinopathies appear to have two general phenotypes: CALM-LQTS and CALM-CPVT.[43] Individuals with CALM-LQTS phenotype have an earlier onset of symptoms, with over half in the perinatal period, a younger onset of major arrhythmic events (1.5 years), and nearly 80% experienced a life-threatening arrhythmia. Individuals with CALM-LQTS are also more likely to have a congenital heart defect, mainly septal defects. In contrast, the age of first major cardiac event of CALM-CPVT individuals was 6 years and few of them experience a life-threatening event. Most (78% CPVT and 93% LQTS) calmodulinopathies are de novo variants. There is report of parental mosaicism, again highlighting the important of parental testing even in the absence of an overt phenotype. Data on fetal presentation of CALM variants are limited but have been described[42] **(FIG. 1.3.7)**.

(text continued on page 46)

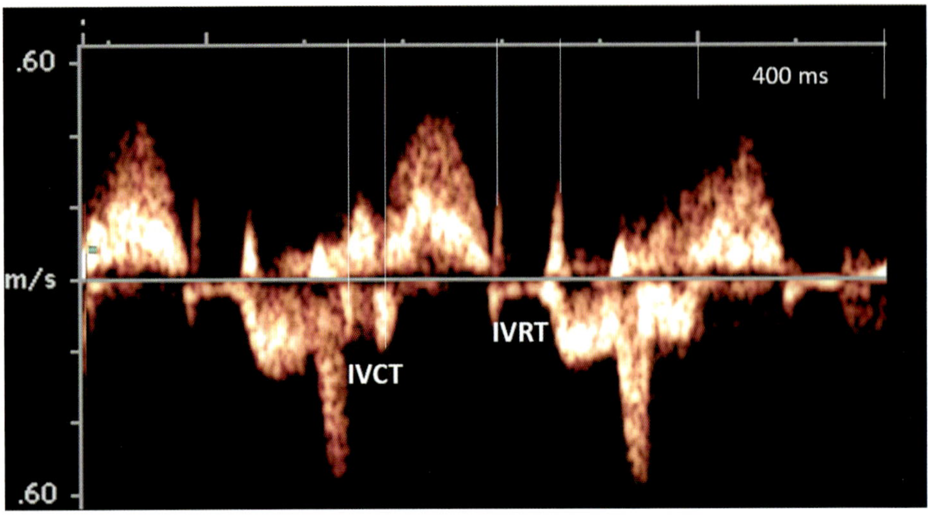
.60
m/s
.60
400 ms
IVCT
IVRT

A.

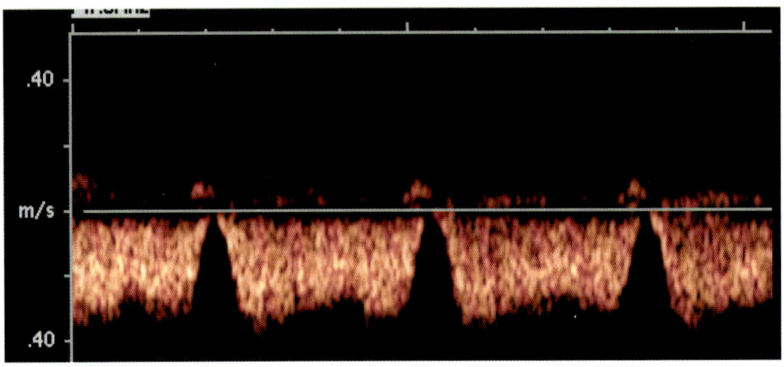
.40
m/s
.40

B.

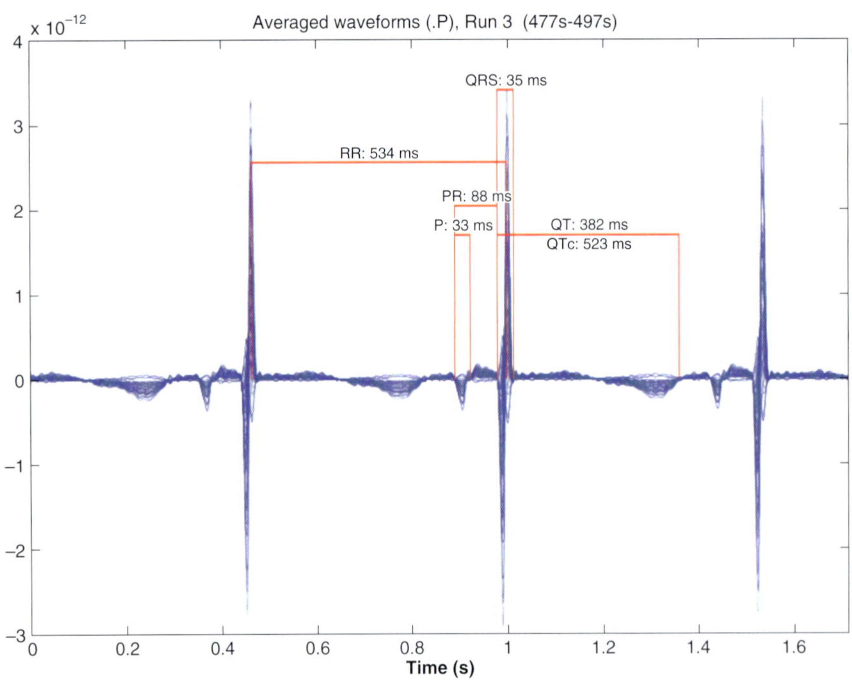
Averaged waveforms (.P), Run 3 (477s-497s)
x 10^-12
QRS: 35 ms
RR: 534 ms
PR: 88 ms
P: 33 ms
QT: 382 ms
QTc: 523 ms
4
3
2
1
0
−1
−2
−3
0
0.2
0.4
0.6
0.8
1
1.2
1.4
1.6
Time (s)

C.

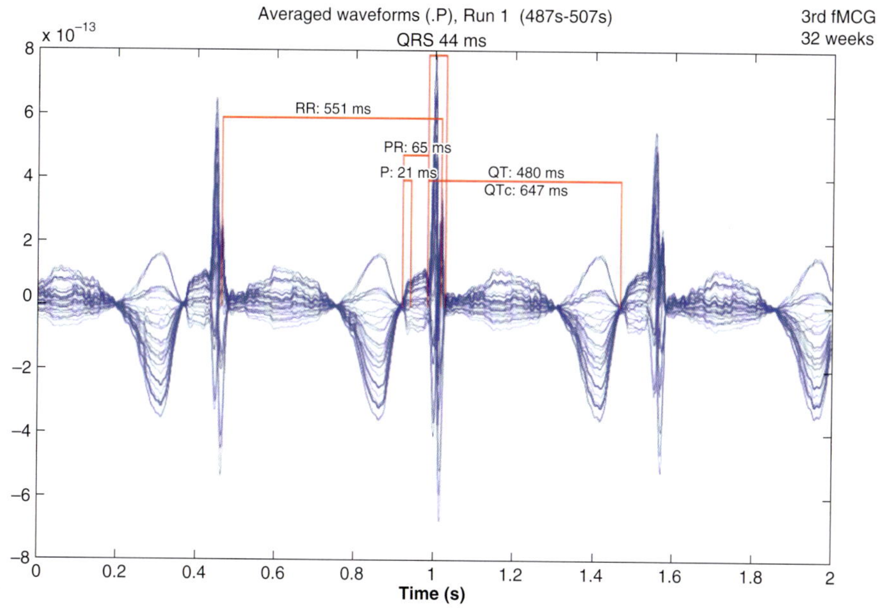

D.

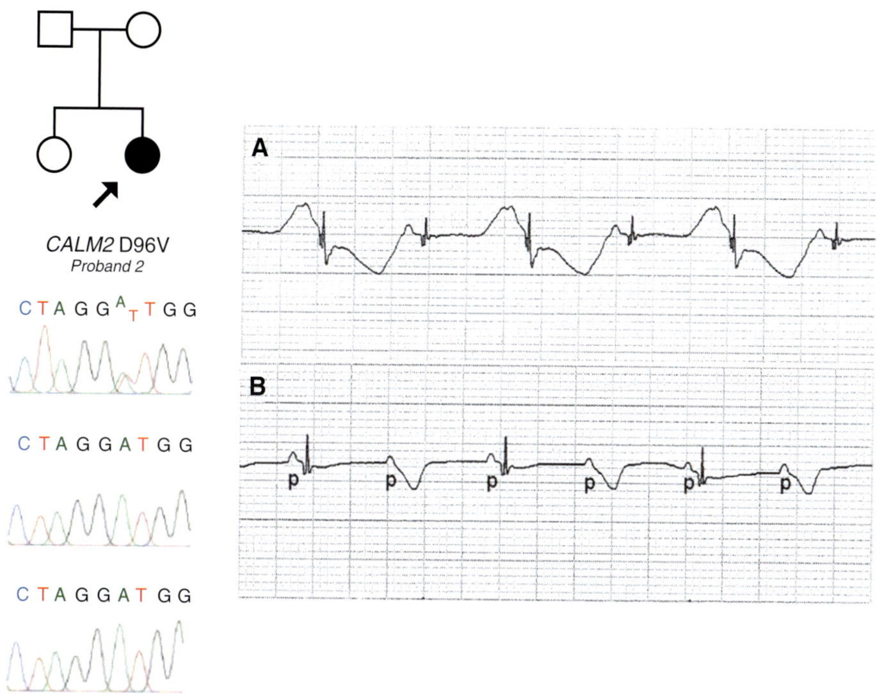

E.

FIGURE 1.3.7 Fetal and neonatal findings in a subject diagnosed after birth with a *CALM2* variant. **A:** Spectral Doppler showing mitral inflow (above baseline) and aortic outflow (below baseline) spectral Doppler of a 28-week fetus that presented at 25 weeks with sinus bradycardia (heart rate 100 bpm). Note the exceedingly prolonged isovolumic relaxation time (IVRT) (~120 ms, normal < 50 ms) and long isovolumic contraction time (IVCT), suggestive of both electrical and mechanical abnormalities of repolarization. **B:** Spectral Doppler of flow in the ductus venosus at 32 weeks. Despite subjectively normal systolic flow, A-wave reversal (above baseline) implies decreased right ventricular compliance. **C and D:** Signal-averaged fMCG at 25 and 32 weeks. Note the extremely prolonged QTc interval in both tracings, and the variability in the T-wave, present only in the tracing at 32 weeks **(D)** and it indicates T-wave alternans. **E:** Genetic pedigree, *CALM2* variant and ECG findings at birth. Note the marked T-wave alternans and prolonged QT interval during sinus rhythm **(A)**. The infant soon developed functional 2° atrioventricular block due to extreme QT interval prolongation **(B)**. (E, Reprinted from Crotti L, Johnson CN, Graf E, et al. Calmodulin mutations associated with recurrent cardiac arrest in infants. *Circulation*. 2013;127:1009-1012.)

BRUGADA SYNDROME (BRS)

While BrS is an autosomal dominant channelopathy most often due to loss-of-function variants of the sodium channel gene *SCN5A*, BrS has not yet been described in the fetus. As with CPVT, this may be because fetuses at risk due to maternal or paternal BrS have not been evaluated by fMCG or there are no fetal electrophysiological manifestations of BrS in the baseline state. Generally, in children the "Brugada pattern" seen on ECG (incomplete right bundle branch block and ST changes in the anterior precordial leads V1-V3) occurs with provocation, such as fever **(FIG. 1.3.8)**. Unlike LQTS, the calmodulinopathies, and CPVT, the first manifestations of BrS occur in late childhood and early adulthood.

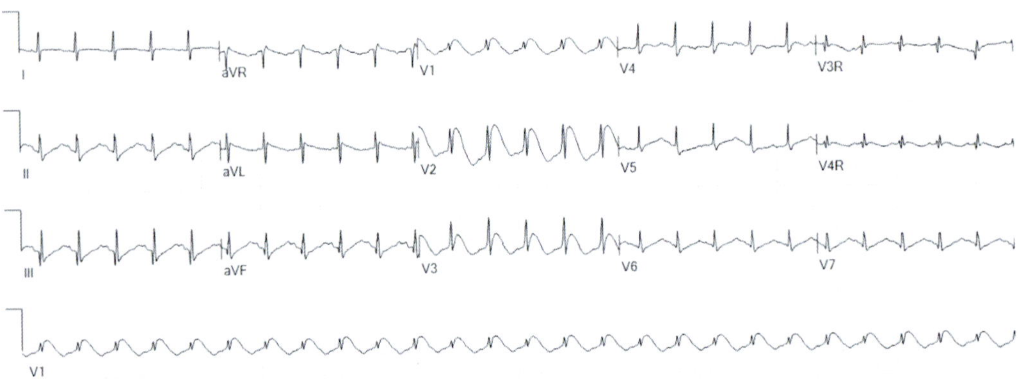

FIGURE 1.3.8 12-Lead ECG in Brugada syndrome. ST- and T-wave changes that occurred during fever in an infant with presumed Brugada syndrome. The ECG normalized once the patient was afebrile.

PATHOGENIC VARIANTS IN HCN4 AND SCN5A

While not typically thought of as a channelopathy, variants in the gene encoding the HCN4 ion channel are associated with inherited sinus bradycardia. *HCN4* pathogenic variants have not been well described, but bradycardia was detected in a male fetus in a multigenerational family with an HCN4 mutation (B. Cuneo, personal communication). *HCN4* encodes the protein that contributes to formation of channels important for spontaneous diastolic membrane depolarization of sinoatrial node cells. Familial sinus bradycardia associated with a pathogenic variant mutation in the cardiac pacemaker channel was first described in 2006.[44] Another heritable cause of sinus bradycardia is compound heterozygous mutation in the sodium channel gene *SCN5A*.[45] In general, isolated sinus node dysfunction is rare in the fetus and unusual in children and should alert the clinician to the possibility of either an *HCN4* or a sodium channel mutation.[46]

SUMMARY

Inherited abnormalities of cardiac ion channel subunits or the proteins that regulate them can result in arrhythmias—AV block, ventricular tachycardia, ventricular ectopy, and sinus bradycardia—during fetal life. The fetal manifestations of the channelopathies, except for LQTS, are not well described, and more research into pregnancies with unexplained and atypical arrhythmias, unexplained stillbirths, as well as those with a family history of CPVT and BrS is necessary to describe the phenotypes. Increased awareness and recognition of the inherited arrhythmia syndromes and the noninvasive diagnosis by fMCG have already had profound impact on fetal and neonatal management of affected individuals. For example, ventricular tachycardia will not be misdiagnosed as supraventricular tachycardia and treated with QT-prolonging anti-arrhythmic agents. Recognition that sinus bradycardia is the most common fetal manifestation of LQTS may alert the medical team to the possibility of this diagnosis and not fetal distress.

However, fetal diagnosis of even LQTS has not kept pace with genetic advances. We speculate in the next 10 years with increased awareness, advances in fetal ECG and MCG, and noninvasive genetic testing, many more fetuses with inherited arrhythmias will be identified and treated in utero.

References

1. Parker SE, Mai CT, Canfield MA, et al. Updated national birth prevalence estimates for selected birth defects in the United States, 2004-2006. *Birth Defects Res A Clin Mol Teratol*. 2010;88:1008-1016.
2. Schwartz PJ, Stramba-Badiale M, Crotti L, et al. Prevalence of the congenital long-QT syndrome. *Circulation*. 2009;120:1761-1767.
3. Moss AJ, Schwartz PJ, Crampton RS, Locati E, Carleen E. The long QT syndrome: a prospective international study. *Circulation*. 1985;71(1):17-21.
4. Mitchell JL, Cuneo BF, Etheridge SP, Horigome H, Weng HY, Benson DW. Fetal heart rate predictors of long QT syndrome. *Circulation*. 2012;126:2688-2695.
5. Winbo A, Fosdal I, Lindh M, et al. Third trimester fetal heart rate predicts phenotype and mutation burden in the type 1 long QT syndrome. *Circ Arrhythm Electrophysiol*. 2015;8(4):806-814.

6. Cuneo BF, Etheridge SP, Horigome H, et al. Arrhythmia phenotype during fetal life suggests long-qt syndrome genotype: risk stratification of perinatal long-QT syndrome. *Circ Arrhythm Electrophysiol.* 2013;6(5):946-951.
7. Cuneo BF, Strasburger JF, Yu S, et al. In utero diagnosis of long QT syndrome by magnetocardiography. *Circulation.* 2013;128:2183-2191.
8. Hamada H, Horigome H, Asaka M, et al. Prenatal diagnosis of long QT syndrome using fetal magnetocardiography. *Prenat Diagn.* 1999;19:677-680.
9. Donofrio MT, Moon-Grady AJ, Hornberger LK, et al. Diagnosis and treatment of fetal cardiac disease: a scientific statement from the American Heart Association. *Circulation.* 2014;129(21):2183-2242.
10. Schwartz PJ, Spazzolini C, Crotti L, et al. The Jervell and Lange-Nielsen syndrome: natural history, molecular basis, and clinical outcome. *Circulation.* 2006;113(6):783-790.
11. Altmann HM, Tester DJ, Will ML, et al. Homozygous/compound heterozygous triadin mutations associated with autosomal recessive long QT syndrome and Pediatric sudden cardiac arrest: elucidation of triadin knockout syndrome. *Circulation.* 2015;131(23):2051-2060.
12. Tranebjaerg L, Bathen J, Tyson J, Bitner-Glindzicz M. Jervell and Lange-Nielsen syndrome: a Norwegian perspective. *Am J Med Genet.* 1999;89(3):137-146.
13. Ackerman MJ, Priori SG, Willems S, et al. HRS/EHRA expert consensus statement on the state of genetic testing for the channelopathies and cardiomyopathies: this document was developed as a partnership between the Heart Rhythm Society (HRS) and the European Heart Rhythm Association (EHRA). *Europace.* 2011;13(8):1077-1109.
14. Al-Khatib SM, Stevenson WG, Ackerman MJ, et al. 2017 AHA/ACC/HRS guideline for management of patients with ventricular arrhythmias and the prevention of sudden cardiac death: a report of the American College of Cardiology/American Heart Association Task Force on Clinical Practice Guidelines and the Heart Rhythm Society. *J Am Coll Cardiol.* 2018;72(14):e91-e220.
15. Crotti L, Celano G, Dagradi F, Schwartz PJ. Congenital long QT syndrome. *Orphanet J Rare Dis.* 2008;3:18.
16. Goldenberg I, Horr S, Moss AJ, et al. Risk for life-threatening cardiac events in patients with genotype-confirmed long-QT syndrome and normal-range corrected QT intervals. *J Am Coll Cardiol.* 2011;57(1):51-59.
17. Riuró H, Campuzano O, Berne P, et al. Genetic analysis, in silico prediction, and family segregation in long QT syndrome. *Eur J Hum Genet.* 2015:23(1):79-85.
18. Napolitano C, Novelli V, Francis MD, Priori SG. Genetic modulators of the phenotype in the long QT syndrome: state of the art and clinical impact. *Curr Opin Genet Dev.* 2015;33:17-24.
19. Coll M, Pérez-Serra A, Mates J, et al. Incomplete penetrance and variable expressivity: hallmarks in channelopathies associated with sudden cardiac death. *Biology (Basel).* 2018;7(1):3. doi:10.3390/biology7010003.
20. Tester DJ, Will ML, Haglund CM, Ackerman MJ. Compendium of cardiac channel mutations in 541 consecutive unrelated patients referred for long QT syndrome genetic testing. *Heart Rhythm.* 2005;2(5):507-517.
21. Kapplinger JD, Tester DJ, Salisbury BA, et al. Spectrum and prevalence of mutations from the first 2,500 consecutive unrelated patients referred for the FAMILION long QT syndrome genetic test. *Heart Rhythm.* 2009;6(9):1297-1303.
22. Moss AJ, Zareba W, Kaufman ES, et al. Increased risk of arrhythmic events in long-QT syndrome with mutations in the pore region of the human ether-a-go-go–related gene potassium channel. *Circulation.* 2002;105(7):794-799.
23. Moss AJ, Shimizu W, Wilde AA, et al. Clinical aspects of type-1 long-QT syndrome by location, coding type, and biophysical function of mutations involving the KCNQ1 gene. *Circulation.* 2007;115(19):2481-2489.
24. Barsheshet A, Goldenberg I, O-Uchi J, et al. Mutations in cytoplasmic loops of the KCNQ1 channel and the risk of life-threatening events: implications for mutation-specific response to β-blocker therapy in type 1 long-QT syndrome. *Circulation.* 2012;125(16):1988-1996.
25. Itoh H, Shimizu W, Hayashi K, et al. Long QT syndrome with compound mutations is associated with a more severe phenotype: a Japanese multicenter study. *Heart Rhythm.* 2010;7(10):1411-1418.
26. Mullally J, Goldenberg I, Moss AJ, et al. Risk of life-threatening cardiac events among patients with long QT syndrome and multiple mutations. *Heart Rhythm.* 2013;10(3):378-382.
27. Miller TE, Estrella E, Myerburg RJ, et al. Recurrent third-trimester fetal loss and maternal mosaicism for long-QT syndrome. *Circulation.* 2004;109(24):3029-3034.
28. Priest JR, Gawad C, Kahlig KM, et al. Early somatic mosaicism is a rare cause of long-QT syndrome. *Proc Natl Acad Sci USA.* 2016;113(4):11555-11560.

29. Kambouris NG, Nuss HB, Johns DC, et al. A revised view of cardiac sodium channel "blockade" in the long-QT syndrome. *J Clin Invest.* 2000;105(8):1133-1140.
30. Aziz PF, Tanel RE, Zelster IJ, et al. Congenital long QT syndrome and 2:1 atrioventricular block: an optimistic outcome in the current era. *Heart Rhythm.* 2010;7(6):781-785.
31. Spazzolini C, Mullally J, Moss AJ, et al. Clinical implications for patients with long QT syndrome who experience a cardiac event during infancy. *J Am Coll Cardiol.* 2009;54(9):832-837.
32. Splawski I, Timothy KW, Sharpe LM, et al. Ca(V)1.2 calcium channel dysfunction causes a multisystem disorder including arrhythmia and autism. *Cell.* 2004;119(1):19-31.
33. Dufendach KA, Timothy K, Ackerman MJ, et al. Clinical outcomes and modes of death in Timothy syndrome: a multicenter international study of a rare disorder. *JACC Clin Electrophysiol.* 2018;4(4):459-466.
34. Etheridge SP, Bowles NE, Arrington CB, et al. Somatic mosaicism contributes to phenotypic variation in Timothy syndrome. *Am J Med Genet A.* 2011;155A(10):2578-2583.
35. Jervell A, Lange-Nielsen F. Congenital deaf-mutism, functional heart disease with prolongation of the Q-T interval and sudden death. *Am Heart J.* 1957;54(1):59-68.
36. Schulze-Bahr E, Wang Q, Wedekind H, et al. KCNE1 mutations cause Jervell and Lange-Nielsen syndrome. *Nat Genet.* 1997;17(3):267-268.
37. Lieve KV, van der Werf C, Wilde AA. Catecholaminergic polymorphic ventricular tachycardia. *Circ J.* 2016;80(6):1285-1291.
38. Tester DJ, Dura M, Carturan E, et al. A mechanism for sudden infant death syndrome (SIDS): stress-induced leak via ryanodine receptors. *Heart Rhythm.* 2007;4(6):733-739.
39. Nyegaard M, Overgaard MT, Søndergaard MT, et al. Mutations in calmodulin cause ventricular tachycardia and sudden cardiac death. *Am J Hum Genet.* 2012;91(4):703-712.
40. Makita N, Yagihara N, Crotti L, et al. Novel calmodulin mutations associated with congenital arrhythmia susceptibility. *Circ Cardiovasc Genet.* 2014;7(4):466-474.
41. Reed GJ, Boczek NJ, Etheridge SP, Ackerman MJ. CALM3 mutation associated with long QT syndrome. *Heart Rhythm.* 2015;12(2):419-422.
42. Crotti L, Johnson CN, Graf E, et al. Calmodulin mutations associated with recurrent cardiac arrest in infants. *Circulation.* 2013;127(9):1009-1017.
43. Crotti L, Spazzolini C, Tester DJ, et al. Calmodulin mutations and life-threatening cardiac arrhythmias: insights from the International Calmodulinopathy Registry. *Eur Heart J.* 2019;40(35):2964-2975.
44. Milanesi R, Baruscotti M, Gnecchi-Ruscone T, DiFrancesco D. Familial sinus bradycardia associated with a mutation in the cardiac pacemaker channel. *N Engl J Med.* 2006;354(2):151-157.
45. Benson DW, Wang DW, Dyment M, et al Congenital sick sinus syndrome caused by recessive mutations in the cardiac sodium channel gene (SCN5A). *J Clin Invest.* 2003;112(7):1019-1028.
46. Ishikawa T, Ohno S, Murakami T, et al. Sick sinus syndrome with HCN4 mutations shows early onset and frequent association with atrial fibrillation and left ventricular noncompaction. *Heart Rhythm.* 2017;14(5):717-724.

PART

2

Techniques to Analyze Fetal Rhythm

Electronic Monitoring

Rachel L. Rodel • Henry L. Galan

INTRODUCTION

The two most common obstetrical means to assess fetal well-being are electronic fetal heart rate (FHR) monitoring and the biophysical profile (BPP). Electronic FHR monitoring is the cornerstone of fetal well-being assessment before birth and during labor but is unreliable and uninterpretable in the presence of many arrhythmias. On the other hand, the BPP, an ultrasound evaluation of amniotic fluid, fetal breathing, movement, and tone, most accurately assesses well-being of the fetus with arrhythmia, especially in the late preterm fetus when survival is generally high and morbidity is relatively low.

While FHR monitoring is of limited use to assess well-being in the fetus with arrhythmia, FHR monitoring can characterize the frequency and duration of the arrhythmia and some of its characteristics, which, in turn, guide management. Is the arrhythmia intermittent or incessant? Does it start and stop suddenly or gradually? With treatment, are there periods of normal FHR and how long do they last? Does treatment restore FHR variability or just change the rate?

This chapter will first review the current recommended terminology and the standard practices for assessing fetal well-being by electronic FHR monitoring and the BPP score. Second, it will review how these practices can be applied in the face of fetal arrhythmias and review FHR patterns in various arrhythmias.

STANDARD PRACTICES

Electronic FHR Monitoring

FHR testing, including the nonstress test (NST), is routinely used in the antepartum and intrapartum periods.[1-4] The normal baseline FHR tracing is 110 to 160 beats per minute (bpm) with a beat to beat variability of 6 to 25 bpm. FHR tracings are classified as either "reactive" or "nonreactive." Reactive tracings demonstrate moderate FHR variability with a normal baseline FHR and at least two FHR accelerations ≥15 bpm above the baseline lasting ≥15 seconds within a 20-minute period. The two accelerations in the 20-minute period must occur within a 40-minute window of time. If the fetus is < 32 weeks, acceptable accelerations are ≥10 bpm above the baseline for ≥10

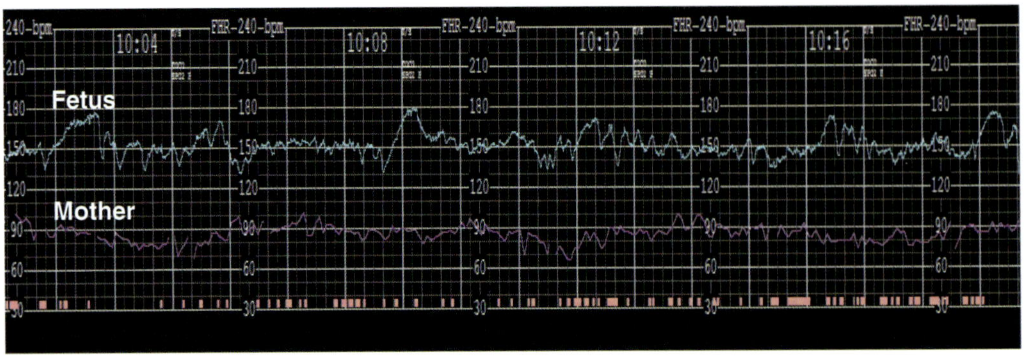

FIGURE 2.1.1 A reactive nonstress test (NST) is demonstrated with a normal baseline fetal heart rate (FHR), moderate variability, accelerations, and no decelerations. The maternal and FHR tracings are shown in pink and aqua, respectively.

seconds. A NST not meeting the criteria for reactivity is defined as nonreactive and typically requires additional evaluation of the fetus: either additional time for the NST to become reactive or performing a BPP. **FIG. 2.1.1** demonstrates a reactive and normal fetal NST, and reflects a normal acid-base balance in the fetus.

Certain fetal arrhythmias may undermine the overall utility of electronic fetal monitoring. These arrhythmias include very short lived tachycardias and bradycardias, arrhythmias with beat to beat irregularities such as premature atrial and ventricular contractions **(FIG. 2.1.2)**, and tachycardias that exceed the upper and lower rate limits of the monitoring. For example, if the monitor records a consistent FHR of 60 to 120 bpm

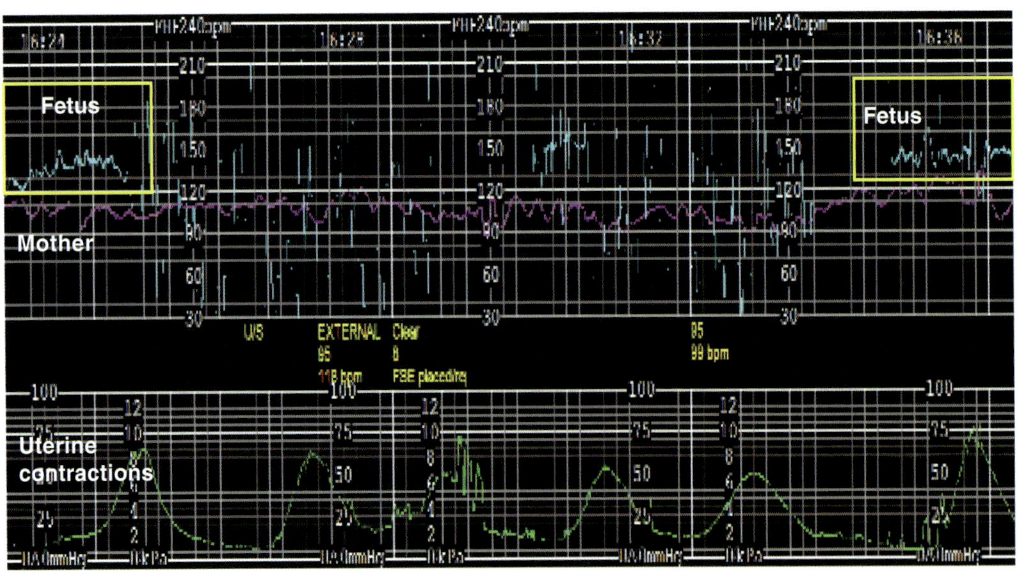

FIGURE 2.1.2 This tracing demonstrates premature atrial contractions in a term laboring patient. The maternal and FHR tracings are shown in pink and aqua, respectively. Uterine monitoring is shown as a green line in the bottom panel. The FHR tracing begins at a normal baseline (in yellow box) but then becomes uninterpretable. A return to a normal baseline with moderate variability was captured in the second yellow box, and afterward, the ectopy resolved and the fetus was able to be monitored adequately for a safe vaginal delivery.

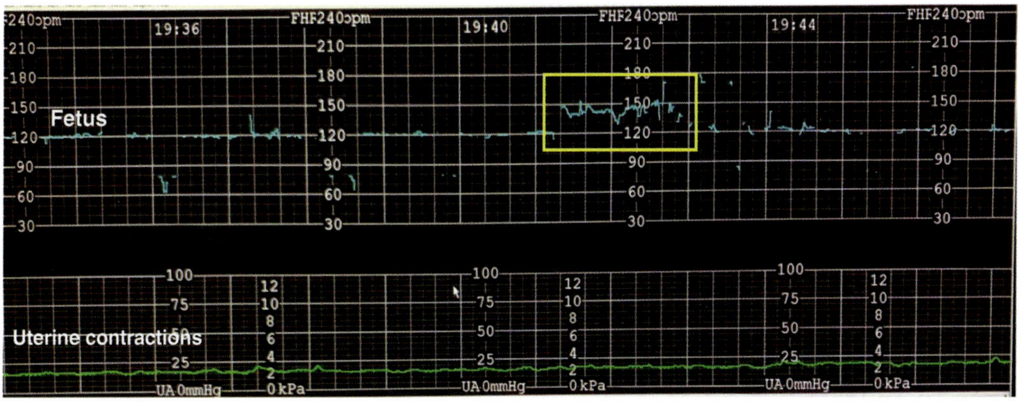

FIGURE 2.1.3 This is a classic tracing of a fetus with supraventricular tachycardia. The FHR tracing is shown in aqua. Uterine monitoring is shown as a green line in the bottom panel. On the right is a nonreactive FHR tracing at a rate of 120 bpm (in reality the monitor has cut the rate in half and FHR is 240 bpm). In the yellow box, the fetus has converted abruptly to sinus rhythm, as seen by the normal FHR variability. The abrupt transition suggests a reentrant mechanism of tachycardia.

with absent variability, the rhythm is probably a supraventricular tachycardia (SVT) at a rate of 240 bpm (FIG. 2.1.3). The true FHR, as well as the atrioventricular (AV) relationship, can be determined by ultrasound examination.

Biophysical Profile

The premature and late preterm (34-36 6/7 weeks) fetus with arrhythmia benefits from delayed delivery as long as fetal well-being can be assured. In the presence of an arrhythmia, frequent BPPs—modified to exclude FHR parameters because they will not reflect fetal state—are the most reliable method to indicate fetal distress necessitating delivery. In the presence of an arrhythmia, the BPP has a maximum score of 8, with 0 to 2 points for each of four components[5] (TABLE 2.1.1). Both the 10-point (including FHR) and the 8-point BPP perform similarly in predicting fetal well-being.[5] A BPP score of 0 to 4 typically indicates fetal distress and delivery is recommended. For example, in a case series of fetuses with anti-Ro/SSA–mediated AV block, two fetuses with 2° AV block and ventricular rates in the 70s were delivered in the late preterm period because of an abnormal BPP and did well.[6]

TABLE 2.1.1 COMPONENTS OF THE 8-POINT BIOPHYSICAL PROFILE SCORE

Component	Points	Requirements
Fetal tone	2/2	At least one episode of extension and flexion of an extremity or spine.
Fetal movement	2/2	At least three discrete body or limb movements.
Fetal breathing	2/2	At least one episode of rhythmic breathing ≥30 s.
Amniotic fluid volume	2/2	Deepest vertical pocket ≥2 cm with horizontal dimension of ≥1 cm.
Total biophysical profile score	8/8	

In addition to helping with the timing of delivery, BPP of the tachycardic fetus can help direct therapy. For example, transplacental antiarrhythmic therapy alone would be appropriate for a hydropic preterm fetus with tachycardia and a BPP score of 8/8, but for the same fetus with a score of 4/8, escalation to include direct intramuscular or intracordal therapy may be indicated for a more rapid conversion to sinus rhythm.[7,8]

IRREGULAR CARDIAC RHYTHMS

Premature Atrial Contractions and Premature Ventricular Contractions

The most common fetal arrhythmias are premature atrial or ventricular contractions (PACs or PVCs; also known as ectopic beats or extra-systoles) (FIG. 2.1.2).[9] These rhythms do not benefit from FHR monitoring as the results are uninterpretable since ectopy presents as "dropped" or "skipped" beats (TABLE 2.1.2), unless the ectopy is very intermittent. Blocked (or nonconducted) atrial bigeminy (BAB) presents as an intermittent or sustained bradycardia of 60 to 80 bpm. If sustained, it is impossible to differentiate BAB from AV block by monitoring alone. Structural congenital heart disease is seen uncommonly (0.3%-2.0%) in fetuses with atrial or ventricular ectopy. In general, limiting maternal stimulants such as excessive caffeine or sugar and listening to the FHR each week Doppler until the ectopy is resolved is recommended. Antepartum testing with NST or BPP is not required. A detailed discussion of ectopy is found in Part 3, Chapter 1.

TABLE 2.1.2 MONITORING CHARACTERISTICS OF ARRHYTHMIAS

Arrhythmia	Baseline HR (bpm)	Variability	Tracing Notes
Atrial or ventricular ectopy	Unchanged	Indeterminable	Discontinuous
Sinus tachycardia	160-200	Normal	Normal
SVT, atrial flutter, JET, PJRT, some VT	120-140	Decreased or none	Halving of FHR. Abrupt initiation and termination of tachycardia
JET, some VT	190-220	Decreased or none	Warm up and cool down of tachycardia
Sinus bradycardia	<110	Normal	Normal
BAB	70-90	None	Continuous if sustained BAB, irregular if PACs
AV block	30-70	Decreased or none	Continuous

AV, atrioventricular; AET, atrial ectopic tachycardia; BAB, blocked atrial bigeminy; FHR, fetal heart rate; HR, heart rate; JET, junctional ectopic tachycardia; PAC, premature atrial contraction; PJRT, permanent junctional reciprocating tachycardia; SVT, supraventricular tachycardia; VT, ventricular tachycardia.

Fetal Tachycardias

Sinus Tachycardia

Sinus tachycardia is defined as a baseline FHR greater than 160 bpm minute sustained for at least 10 minutes.[2] Fetal tachycardia can be caused by many factors, including fetal infection, medications, obstetric hemorrhage, or maternal medical disorders including hyperthyroidism.[10] If the mother is symptomatic or has a history of thyroid disease, even if she has had a thyroidectomy, maternal thyroid-stimulating antibody (TSAb) levels should be checked as they cross the placenta and can cause fetal tachycardia.[11] Sinus tachycardia usually shows some baseline variability, but this variability becomes more difficult to assess with higher heart rates and does diminish with fetal acidemia (FIG. 2.1.4). More information on sinus tachycardia can be found in Part 3, Chapter 3.

Supraventricular Tachycardias

The supraventricular arrhythmias include "SVT" with a 1:1 AV relationship (see Part 1, Chapter 1) and atrial flutter. Typical monitoring of supraventricular arrhythmias includes sustained tachycardia, absent FHR variability, and a fixed baseline.[12] One caveat for electronic FHR monitoring is that monitoring may split or halve the true baseline FHR as demonstrated in FIG. 2.1.5. The FHR in SVT is typically 240 to 260 bpm but can range from 200 to 300 bpm. Continuous electronic FHR monitoring is a useful adjunct to fetal tachycardia management as it can:

1. Measure duration of tachycardia (intermittent or sustained) during a 12- to 24-hour period to see if treatment is required;
2. Provide clues to the mechanism of tachycardia; and
3. Determine the effects of treatment.

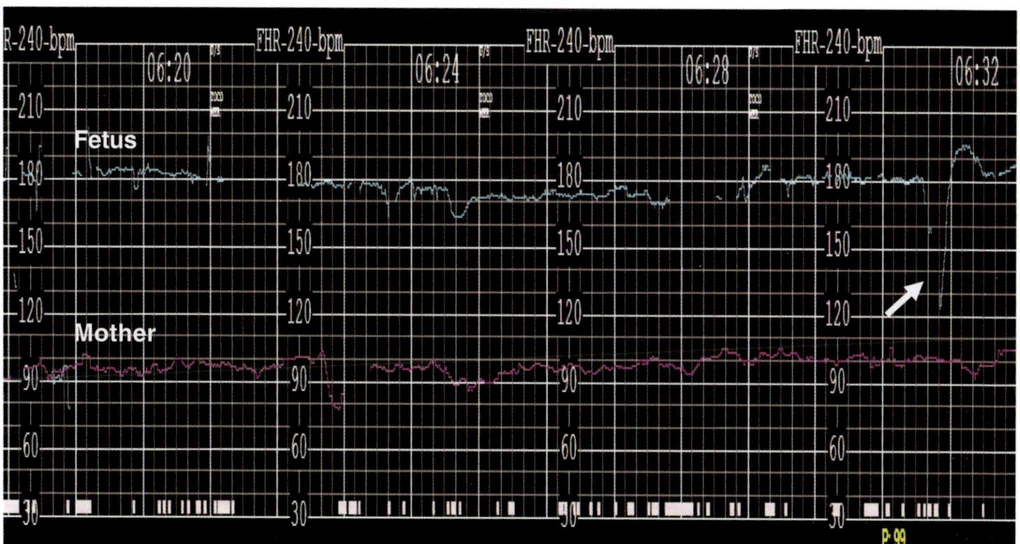

FIGURE 2.1.4 This tracing is from a fetus with sinus tachycardia due to chorioamnionitis at 24 weeks' gestation. The maternal and FHR tracings are shown in pink and aqua, respectively. Minimal variability with a variable deceleration (white arrow) demonstrates the concern for abnormal oxygenation in this fetus with intra-amniotic infection and maternal fever.

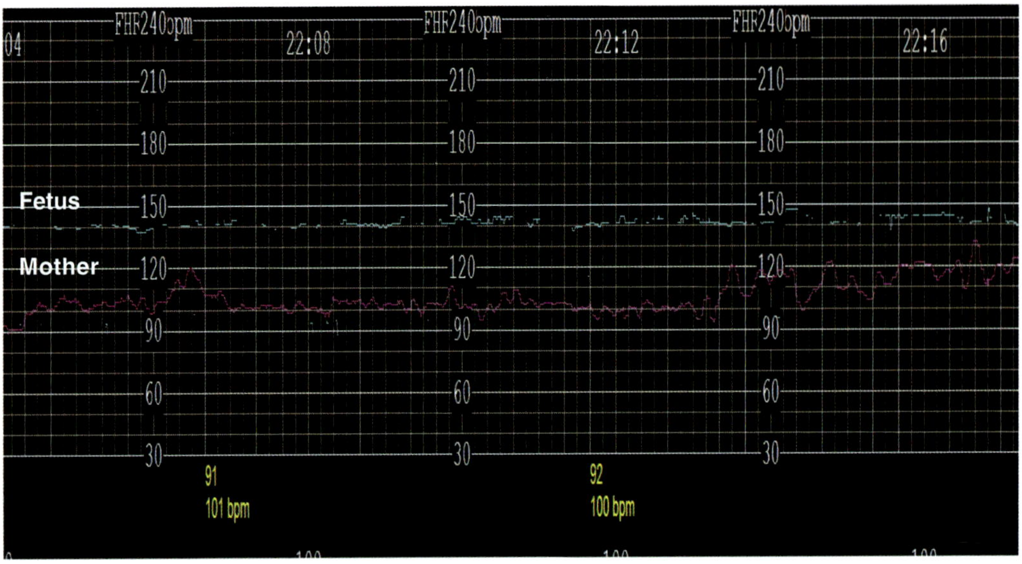

FIGURE 2.1.5 A fetus with supraventricular tachycardia and a rate of 280 bpm. The maternal and FHR tracings are shown in pink and aqua, respectively. The true ventricular rate has been halved by the monitor. The lack of FHR variability at 140 bpm is the clue that the monitor is not capturing the true baseline.

If the tachycardia duration is more than half of the monitoring period, treatment is generally indicated as effusions or even hydrops can occur after a few days in sustained tachycardia. On the other hand, intermittent tachycardia only occasionally becomes sustained[13] and can often be managed by vigilant FHR monitoring by the mother at home or by the provider in the office. The mechanism of tachycardia is either reentrant, manifest by abrupt onset and cessation of tachycardia, or automatic, with a gradual increase and decrease in FHR.[14] A positive response of SVT to antiarrhythmic therapy is evidenced either as slowing of the tachycardia rate or longer periods of normal FHR with variability (FIG. 2.1.6).

Atrial flutter, the other type of SVT, cannot be distinguished from 1:1 "SVT" by electronic FHR monitoring because ventricular rate is similar. There can be some variability of the ventricular rate in atrial flutter because the AV relationship can vary from 2:1 to 4:1 (FIG. 2.1.7). It is important to recognize that only the ventricular, not the atrial, beats are detected by electronic FHR monitoring, and that in atrial flutter, the atrial rate can range from 360 to >500 bpm.

Rare Tachycardias

There are several rare nonsinus tachycardias characterized by slower ventricular rates (190-230 bpm) than "SVT" and atrial flutter. These include junctional ectopic tachycardia (FIG. 2.1.6), atrial ectopic tachycardia, accelerated ventricular rhythm, and permanent junctional reciprocating tachycardia. Ventricular tachycardia is also an unusual tachycardia with baseline FHR from 200 to 400 bpm. The SVTs will be discussed in more detail in Part 3, Chapter 2.

A.

B.

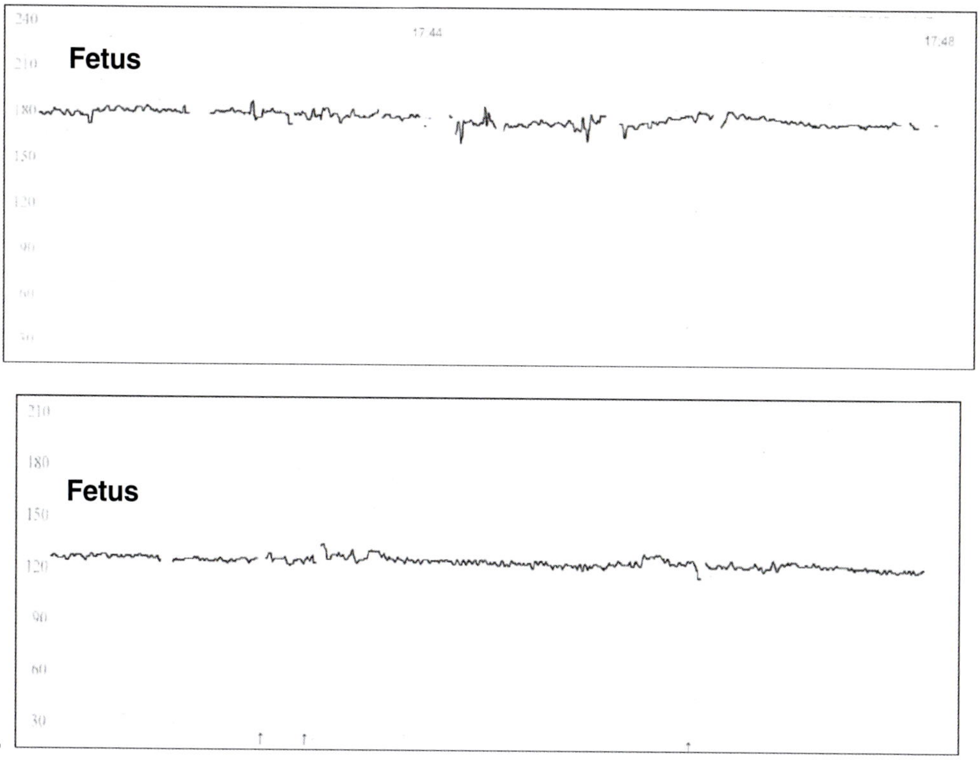

FIGURE 2.1.6 This is a tracing of a fetus with junctional ectopic tachycardia (JET). The initial baseline FHR was 180 bpm and after treatment, decreased to 150 bpm (not shown), then 130 bpm. However, the fetus is still in JET as shown by minimal variability and absence of accelerations and decelerations in this tracing.

Fetal Bradycardias

Sinus Bradycardia

Bradycardia is defined as a baseline FHR of less than 110 bpm sustained for at least 10 minutes.[2] This differs from a deceleration, which resolves in less than 10 minutes.[12] Although fetal bradycardia can be caused by many acute events in labor, it may also be seen in the antepartum period related to congenital heart disease associated with heterotaxy, myocardial conduction disease caused by maternal anti-Ro/SSA antibodies (FIG. 2.1.8),[15-17] and long QT syndrome (LQTS).[18,19] With the exception of fetal LQTS, fetal sinus bradycardia typically shows normal variability and reactivity. The rhythms of fetal LQTS will be further described in Part 3, Chapter 6.

Atrioventricular Block

AV block due to maternal anti-Ro typically presents between 18- and 26-weeks' gestation[20,21] while AV block associated with structural cardiac defects presents much earlier, often at <15 weeks of gestation.[22,23] Typical structural defects presenting with AV block are congenitally corrected transposition of the great vessels and left atrial isomerism. Regardless of the etiology, complete (3°) AV block results in the lowest

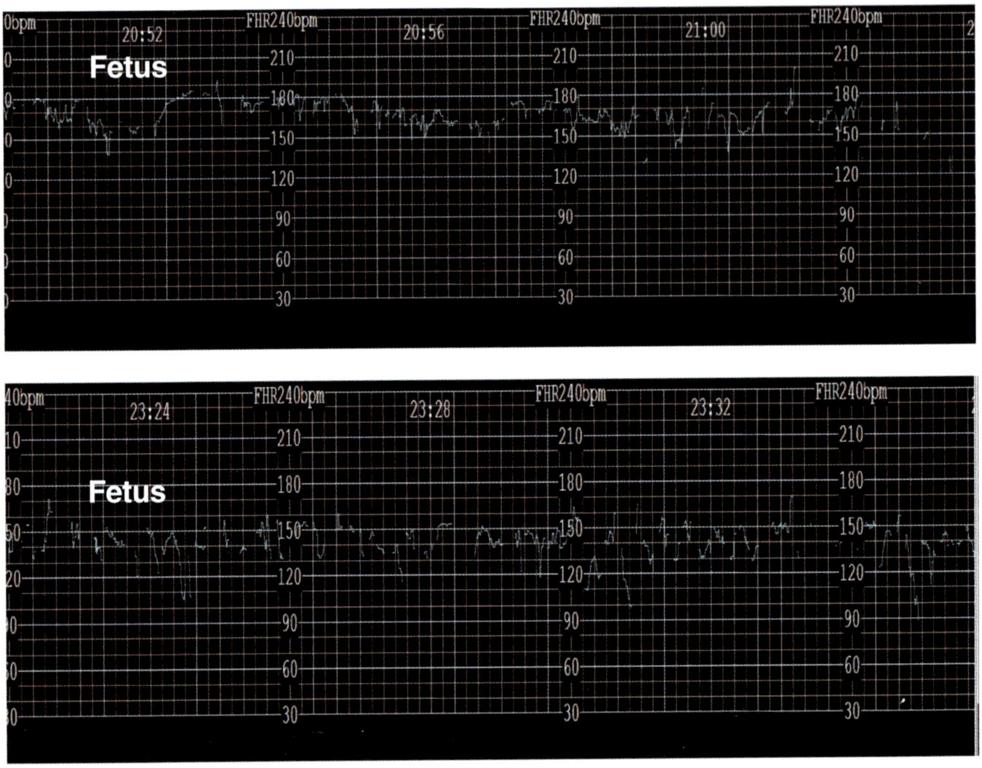

A.

B.

FIGURE 2.1.7 This tracing demonstrates atrial flutter with a varying atrioventricular relationship. The fetal echocardiogram showed frequent short runs of atrial flutter with a variable atrial rate 300 to 400 bpm (not shown on monitoring) and a ventricular rate of 180 to 220 bpm.

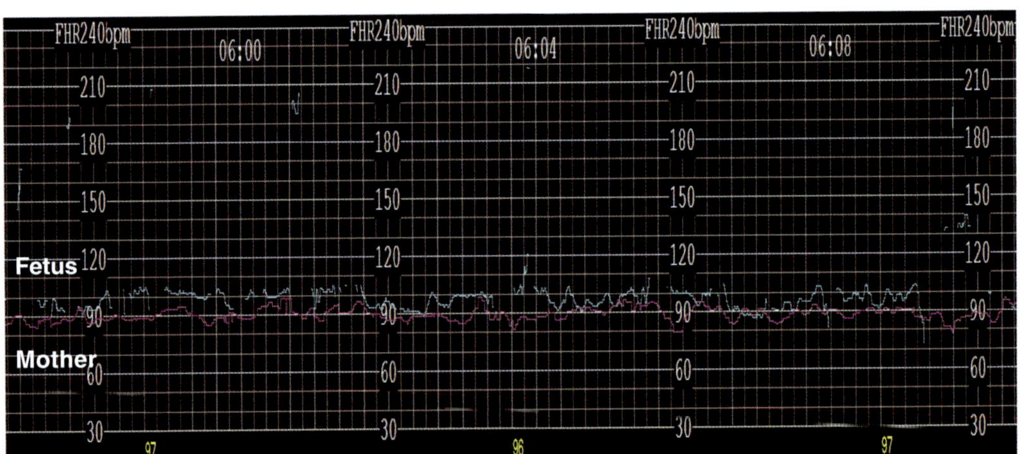

FIGURE 2.1.8 This tracing demonstrates fetal bradycardia with a baseline FHR ~95 to 100 bpm and moderate variability. The maternal and FHR tracings are shown in pink and aqua, respectively. The mother had anti-Ro/SSA antibodies, which had affected the sinoatrial node.

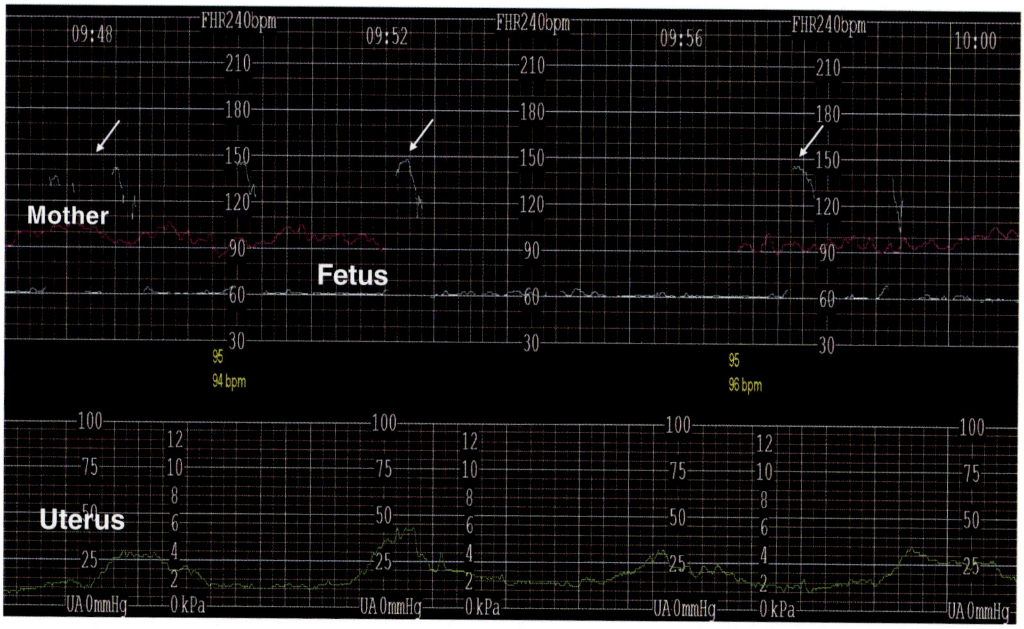

FIGURE 2.1.9 This tracing demonstrates atrioventricular block in a 33-week fetus affected by maternal anti-Ro/SSA antibodies. The maternal and FHR tracings are shown in pink and aqua, respectively. Uterine monitoring is shown as a green line in the bottom panel. Although there are brief periods of a "normal" FHR (white arrows), by echocardiography, the rhythm during the "normal" FHR was a junctional ectopic tachycardia, not sinus rhythm.

baseline FHR, usually between 30 and 70 bpm, and absent FHR variability.[19] In some cases of AV block, the ventricular rate appears to normalize for short periods of time **(FIG. 2.1.9)**. However, fetal echocardiography reveals the rhythm not to be sinus, but rather a junctional tachycardia. The FHR in 3° AV block can be even lower than the maternal heart rate **(FIG. 2.1.10)**. More information on AV block can be found in Part 3, Chapters 4 and 5.

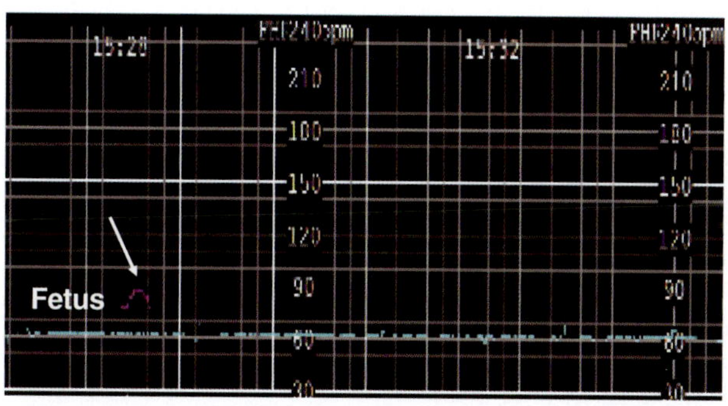

FIGURE 2.1.10 A baseline FHR of 60 bpm with absent variability is identified in a fetus with complex congenital heart disease and left atrial isomerism. The maternal and FHR tracings are shown in pink and aqua, respectively. The rhythm was found to be complete (3°) atrioventricular block by echo. The mother's heart rate (white arrow) briefly seen in this tracing is higher than the FHR.

SUMMARY

Although electronic FHR monitoring can present a challenge in fetuses with arrhythmias, valuable information can be gained from detailed analysis of the tracings. While not always able to provide evidence of fetal well-being, FHR monitoring can guide the necessity for and assess the success of antiarrhythmic drug therapy. If an abnormal FHR tracing is the first sign of a fetal arrhythmia, the patient should undergo a detailed obstetrical ultrasound including hydrops assessment and be referred for fetal echocardiography to have further interrogation of the rhythm and to rule out associated structural cardiac malformations. During labor, continuous electronic fetal monitoring is recommended for pregnancies complicated by fetal arrhythmia. Initial data from a small study show promise for improved assessment of well-being in fetuses with arrhythmias during labor using fetal electrocardiographic heart rate,[20] but until then, if the well-being of the fetus cannot be established using electronic FHR monitoring or the tracing is uninterpretable, cesarean delivery may be indicated.

References

1. American College of Obstetricians and Gynecologists. Practice bulletin No. 145: antepartum fetal surveillance. *Obstet Gynecol.* 2014;124(1):182-192.
2. American College of Obstetricans and Gynecologists. Practice Bulletin No. 106: intrapartum fetal heart rate monitoring: nomenclature, interpretation, and general management principles. *Obstet Gynecol.* 2009;114(1):192-202.
3. Macones GA, Hankins GD, Spong CY, Hauth J, Moore T. The 2008 National Institute of Child Health and Human Development workshop report on electronic fetal monitoring: update on definitions, interpretation, and research guidelines. *Obstet Gynecol.* 2008;112(3):661-666.
4. Macones GA, Hankins GD, Spong CY, Hauth J, Moore T. The 2008 National Institute of Child Health and Human Development workshop report on electronic fetal monitoring: update on definitions, interpretation, and research guidelines. *J Obstet Gynecol Neonatal Nurs.* 2008;37(5):510-515.
5. Graham N, Harman CR. Antepartum testing. In: Bergella V, ed. *Maternal-Fetal Evidence Based Guidelines.* 3rd ed. Boca Raton, FL: CRC Press; 2017:499-501.
6. Cuneo BF, Lee M, Roberson D, et al. A management strategy for fetal immune-mediated atrioventricular block. *J Matern Fetal Neonatal Med.* 2010;23(12):1400-1405.
7. Strasburger JF, Cuneo BF, Michon MM, et al. Amiodarone therapy for drug-refractory fetal tachycardia. *Circulation.* 2004;109(3):375-379.
8. Parilla BV, Strasburger JF, Socol ML. Fetal supraventricular tachycardia complicated by hydrops fetalis: a role of direct fetal intramuscular therapy. *Am J Perinatol.* 1996;13(8):463-486.
9. Fouron JC. Fetal arrhythmias: the Saint-Justine hospital experience. *Prenat Diagn.* 2004;24:1068-1080.
10. Larmay HJ, Strasburger JF. Differential diagnosis and management of the fetus and newborn with an irregular or abnormal heart rate. *Pediatr Clin North Am.* 2004;51(4):1033-1050.
11. Peleg D, Cada S, Peleg A Ben-Ami M. The relationship between maternal serum thyroid-stimulating immunoglobulin and fetal and neonatal thyrotoxicosis. *Obstet Gynecol* 2002;99:1040-1043.
12. American College of Obstetricians and Gynecologists. Practice Bulletin No. 116: management of intrapartum fetal heart rate tracings. *Obstet Gynecol.* 2010;116(5):1232-1240.
13. Cuneo BF, Strasburger JF. Management strategy for fetal tachycardia. *Obstet Gynecol.* 2000;96(4):575-581.
14. Simpson JL. Fetal supraventricular tachycardias: diagnosis and management. *Semin Perinatol.* 2000;24(5):360-372.
15. Brucato A, Cimaz R, Catelli L, Meroni P. Anti-Ro-associated sinus bradycardia in newborns. *Circulation.* 2000;102(11):E88-E89.
16. Cuneo BF, Strasburger JF, Niksch A, Ovadia M, Wakai RT. An expanded phenotype of maternal SSA/SSB antibody-associated fetal cardiac disease. *J Matern Fetal Neonatal Med.* 2009;22(3):233-238.
17. Chockalingam P, Jaeggi ET, Rammeloo LA, et al. Persistent fetal sinus bradycardia associated with maternal anti-SSA/Ro and anti-SSB/La antibodies. *J Rheumatol.* 2011;38(12):2682-2685.

18. Mitchell J, Cuneo BF, Etheridge SP, Horigome H, Weng HY, Benson DW. Fetal heart rate predictors of long QT syndrome. *Circulation.* 2012;126(23):2688-2695.
19. Beinder E, Grancay T, Menendez T, Singer H, Hofbeck M. Fetal sinus bradycardia and the long QT syndrome. *Am J Obstet Gynecol.* 2001;185(3):743-747.
20. Wacker-Gussmann A, Strasburger JF, Cuneo BF, Wakai RT. Diagnosis and treatment of fetal arrhythmia. *Am J Perinatol.* 2014;31(7):617-628.
21. Jaeggi ET, Fouron JC, Silverman ED, Ryan G, Smallhorn J, Hornberger LK. Transplacental fetal treatment improves the outcome of prenatally diagnosed complete atrioventricular block without structural heart disease. *Circulation.* 2004;110(12):1542-1548.
22. Pepes S, Zidere V, Allan LD. Prenatal diagnosis of left atrial isomerism. *Heart.* 2009;95(24):1974-1977.
23. Jaeggi ET, Hornberger LK, Smallhorn JF, Fouron JC. Prenatal diagnosis of complete atrioventricular block associated with structural heart disease: combined experience of two tertiary care centers and review of the literature. *Ultrasound Obstet Gynecol.* 2005;26(1):16-21.

Echocardiography

Lisa Willis Howley

INTRODUCTION

Fetal arrhythmias, accounting for ~10% to 20% of referrals to fetal cardiologists, can be accurately diagnosed in the prenatal period.[1-4] Clinical detection and diagnosis of fetal rhythm abnormalities is important as some may cause fetal hemodynamic compromise and increase the risk of in utero or postnatal demise of the affected fetus, while others are benign. Because direct examination of fetal cardiac electrical activity remains a challenge, M-mode and Doppler echocardiography are the most widely used tools to evaluate fetal rhythm and define the arrhythmia mechanism. These techniques, which are described in detail later, are the mechanical surrogates of fetal electrophysiological cardiac events.

M-MODE

M-mode imaging was one of the first echocardiographic modalities used to assess fetal arrhythmias. Because of its high temporal resolution and ability to visualize atrial and ventricular events simultaneously, M-mode is excellent for assessing the atrial and ventricular beat rates and the AV relationship. M-mode is not as helpful in determining ejection, filling, and isovolumic contraction times or duration of the atrioventricular (AV) interval. Electrical events are inferred from the motion of the cardiac chambers.[5-9] The M-mode cursor can be positioned to evaluate only atrial or ventricular activity, or it can be positioned so that both atrial and ventricular activity can be recorded simultaneously (FIG. 2.2.1A-C). M-mode imaging is dependent on favorable fetal position and good image quality and is limited by poor image resolution or a hypocontractile myocardium. Atrial contractions can be difficult to visualize, especially with simultaneous interrogation of atrium and ventricles, thus simultaneous right and left atrial M-mode obtained from the sagittal view of the aortic arch can give very clear imaging of atrial contraction.

Simultaneous atrial and ventricular M-mode can differentiate AV block from blocked atrial bigeminy in the bradycardic fetus (FIG. 2.2.2A and B). The nonconducted ("blocked") atrial beat (a′) is seen closely following the conducted atrial beat (a), in comparison to the regular atrial contractions and AV dissociation seen with AV block. Similarly, two common causes of nonsinus tachycardia can be differentiated by M-mode: the rapid atrial contractions of atrial flutter with 2:1 or 3:1 block and the 1:1 AV

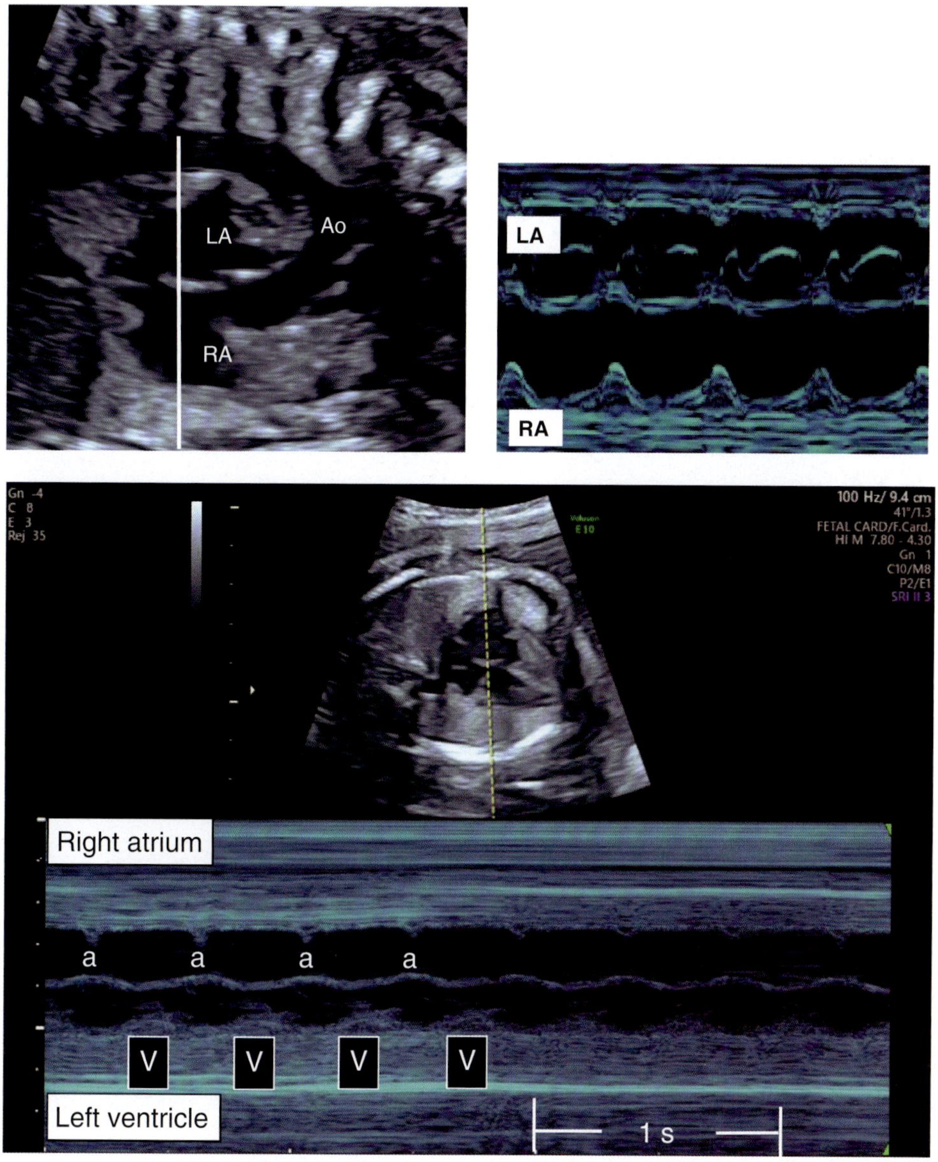

FIGURE 2.2.1 **A:** Sagittal view of the atria and the aortic arch, highlighting an optimal image to evaluate biatrial motion using M-mode (M-mode line extending through the right atrial appendage). **B:** The expected M-mode tracing from **A**. Ao, aorta; LA, left atrium; RA, right atrium. **C:** Cursor position to sample atrium and ventricle for M-mode interrogation. M-mode tracing depicting the atrial activity (a) and ventricular contraction (V) seen in a normal 1:1 pattern.

relationship from reentrant supraventricular tachycardia **(FIG. 2.2.2C** and **D)**. Lastly, isolated atrial M-Mode can give valuable clues to the diagnosis of an irregular (ventricular) fetal rhythm. If the atrial rate is normal and the atrial defections are regular, the fetus most likely has AV block **(FIG. 2.2.2E)**. In contrast, premature beats can be easily visualized as two atrial defections (premature atrial contractions) close together (a and a′) or a gap in the atrial contractions when the ventricle beats prematurely **(FIG. 2.2.2F** and **G)**.

(text continued on page 66)

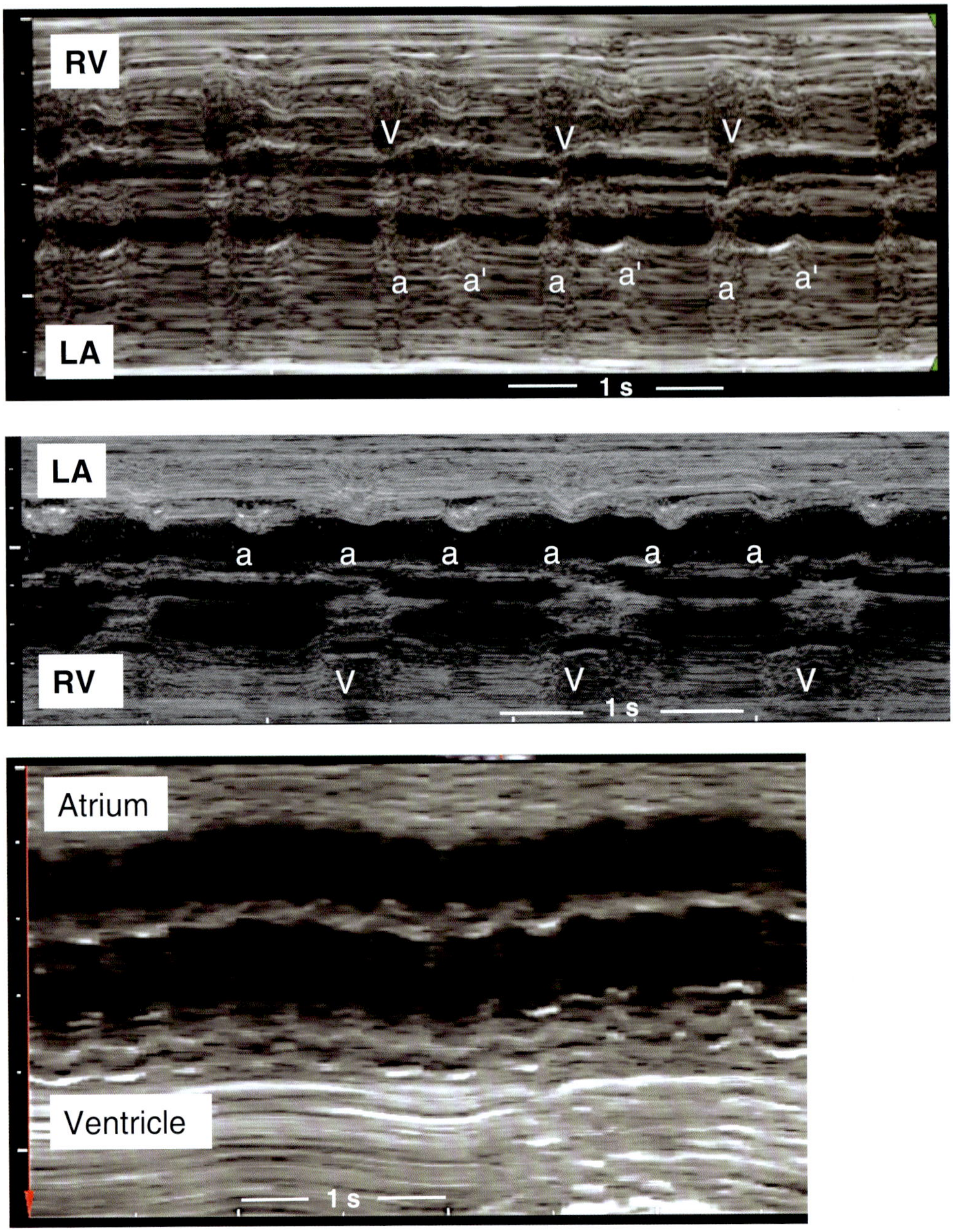

A.
B.
C.

FIGURE 2.2.2 Simultaneous atrial and ventricular M-modes. **A:** A fetus with blocked atrial bigeminy with a typical long-short-long pattern (a-a′ interval = 290 ms, a′-a interval 498 ms). **B:** A fetus with Mobitz type 2, 2°heart block with a regular atrial rate (A-A interval = 407 ms) and a bradycardic ventricular rate (R-R interval = 795 ms). **C:** This fetus is in supraventricular tachycardia with equal atrial and ventricular rates. **D:** This fetus has atrial flutter; note the faster atrial rate compared to ventricular rate. **E:** A fetus with an irregular rhythm. The atrium rate is completely regular, diagnostic of type 1 or intermittent type 2 atrioventricular block. **F:** Another fetus with an irregular rhythm due to premature atrial contractions (red arrows). **G:** A third fetus with irregular rhythm due to premature ventricular contractions (arrows). There is retrograde conduction to the atrium (stars) resulting in a regular atrial rate, but the shape and size of the atrial contractions are different from the normal atrial contractions (compared to the atrial contractions in **E,** which are all the same).

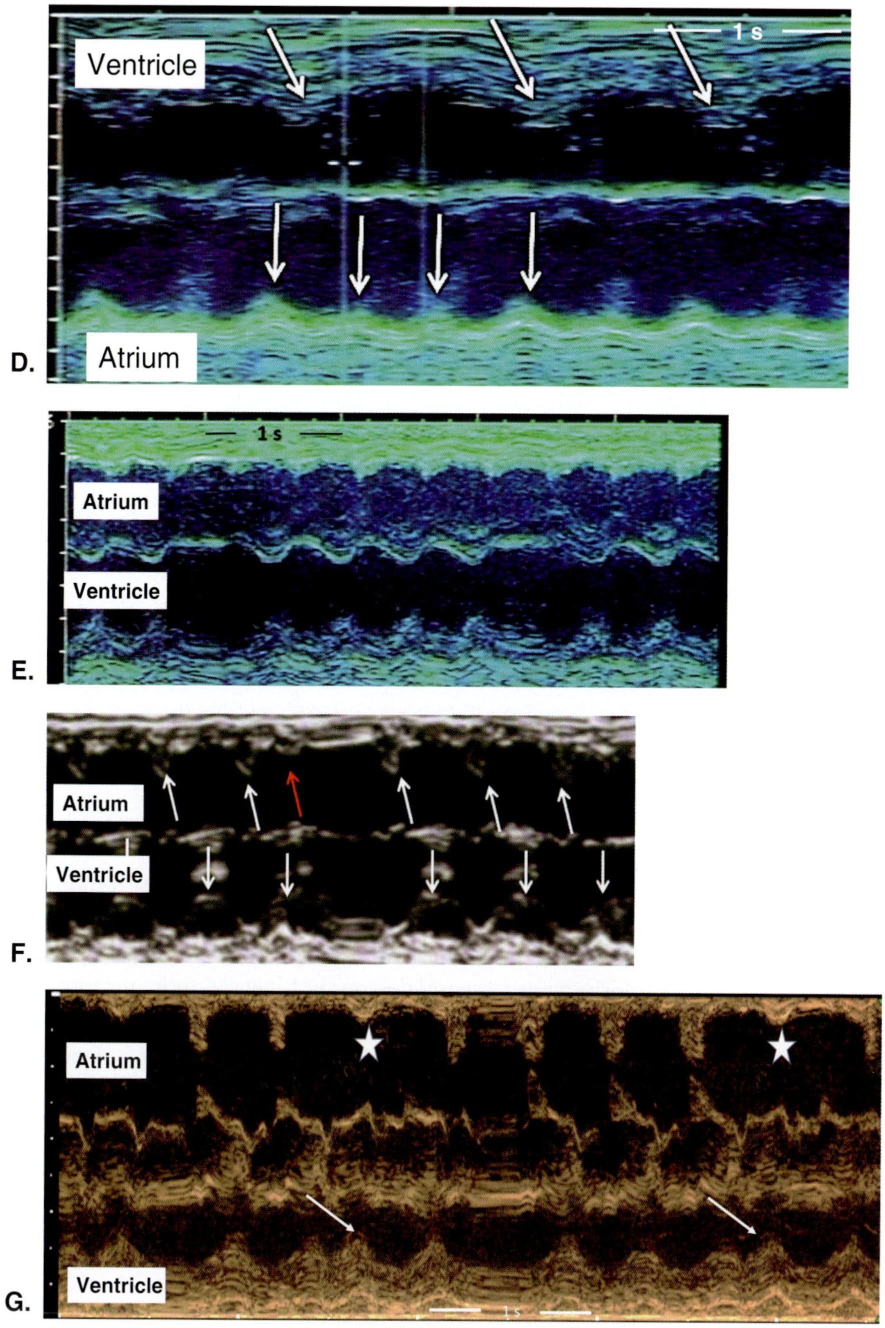

FIGURE 2.2.2 Cont'd

Another helpful technique to better assess simultaneous atrial and ventricular contractions is using the so-called anatomic M-mode feature, which is available on most ultrasound platforms and can improve atrial image quality.

SPECTRAL DOPPLER

The simultaneous display of atrial and ventricular mechanical activities and the timing and duration of these events is best seen using spectral Doppler (SD).[3,10-13] There are several fetal cardiac sites where SD can be performed: the goal is to measure atrial and ventricular contraction in the same cycle. Conventionally, SD has been performed in the apex up or down in the left ventricular five-chamber view with the cursor parallel to the mitral and aortic valves. Displayed in this view is the mitral a-wave (atrial systole) and the aortic outflow (ventricular systole) **(FIG. 2.2.3A-C)**. Notably, SD sampling in the left ventricular chamber is primarily useful in fetal arrhythmias with a 1:1 AV relationship. When the atrial rate exceeds the ventricular rate, such as atrial flutter or AV block, simultaneous SD of a vein and an artery may better define atrial and ventricular contractions. In fetuses where the atrial rate exceeds the ventricular rate, atrial contraction may occur against a closed mitral valve, interrupting flow from the atrium to the ventricle and limiting atrial Doppler information reaching the left ventricle.

Simultaneous SD interrogation of venous and arterial flow in an adjacent vein and artery has been incorporated into the evaluation of fetal arrhythmia. This technique demonstrates the relationship between atrial contraction (blood flow reversal in the vein) and ventricular contraction (forward flow in the artery). The advantage of this method over using SD in the left ventricular chamber is the lack of an AV valve which, when present, may disrupt the atrial Doppler signal. Sampling sites for simultaneous interrogation of venous and arterial flow include superior vena cava and adjacent ascending aorta[11] **(FIG. 2.2.4)**, the pulmonary vein and branch pulmonary artery[12] **(FIG. 2.2.5)**, and rarely the inferior vena cava and descending aorta. A more recently described technique, simultaneously recording pulsed-wave Doppler signals in the innominate vein and transverse aortic arch, has become favored as it allows for a near-zero angle of insonation of the innominate vein, which optimizes visualization of the retrograde atrial systolic flow[13,14] **(FIG. 2.2.6)**.

(text continued on page 76)

A.

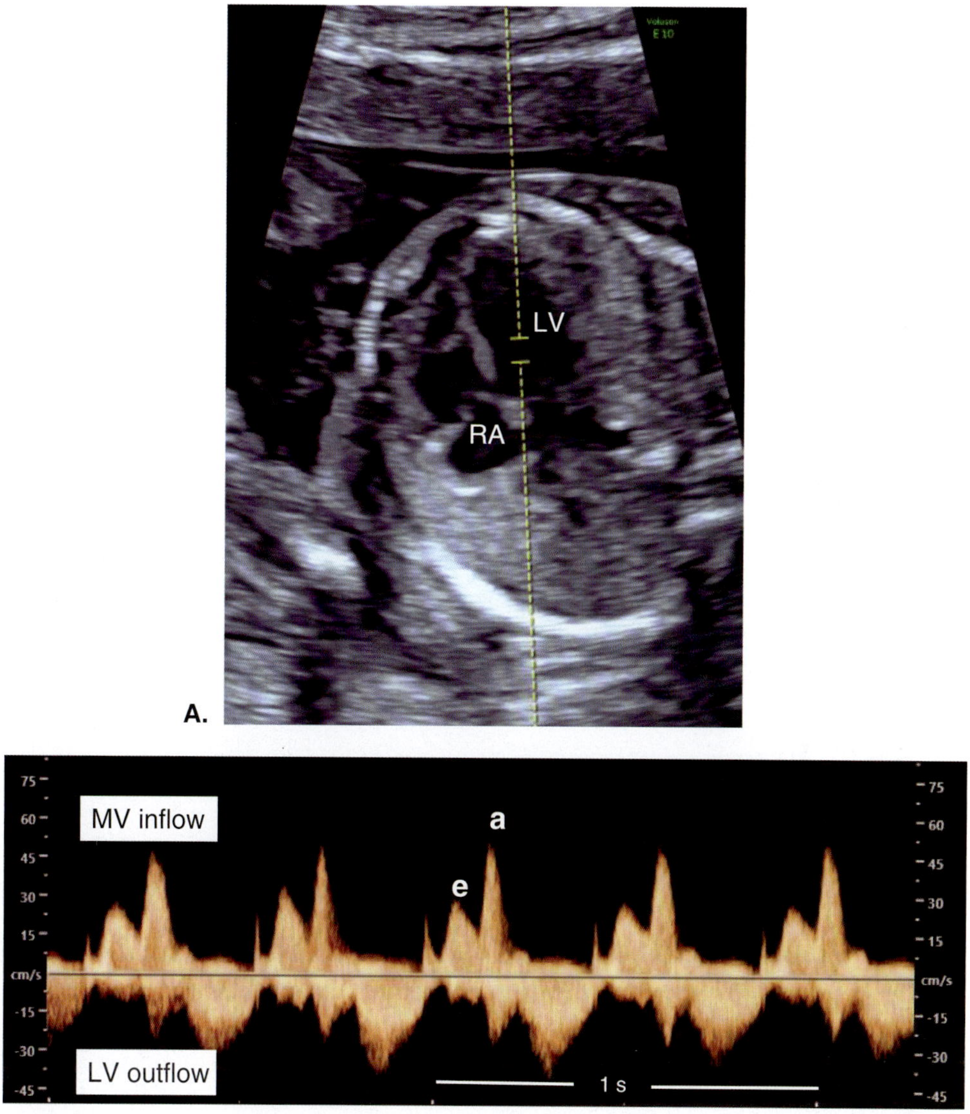

B.

FIGURE 2.2.3 **A:** Apical five-chamber view with the sample gate positioned in the left ventricle (LV) between the mitral valve and ventricular outflow tract to obtain simultaneous left ventricular inflow and outflow pulsed Doppler patterns. **B** and **C:** Normal pulsed Doppler tracing of the mitral valve (MV) inflow and left ventricular (LV) outflow Doppler pattern at two different heart rates. The flow above the baseline is normal biphasic MV inflow with an e-point (e) and a-point (a). The e represents passive diastolic inflow and the a represents atrial contraction. **D:** Pulsed-wave Doppler tracing of the MV inflow and LV outflow in a fetus with anti-Ro/SSA–mediated complete AV block with absence of fetal AV synchrony. The atrial rate is regular (A-A interval = 445 ms) and the R-R interval is 1164 ms.

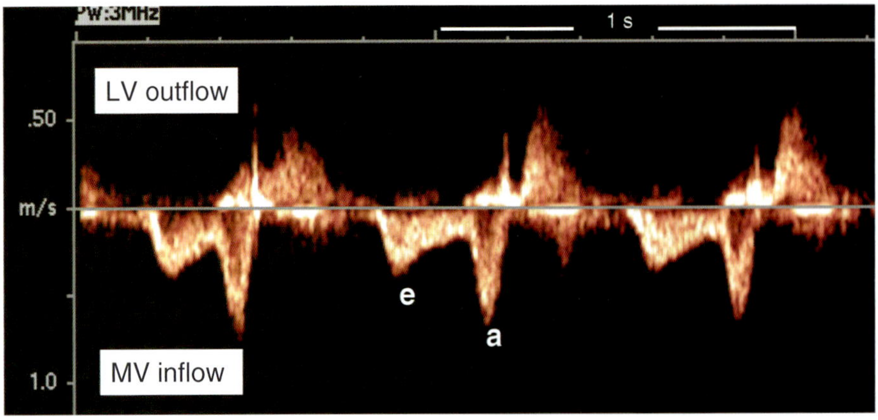

C.

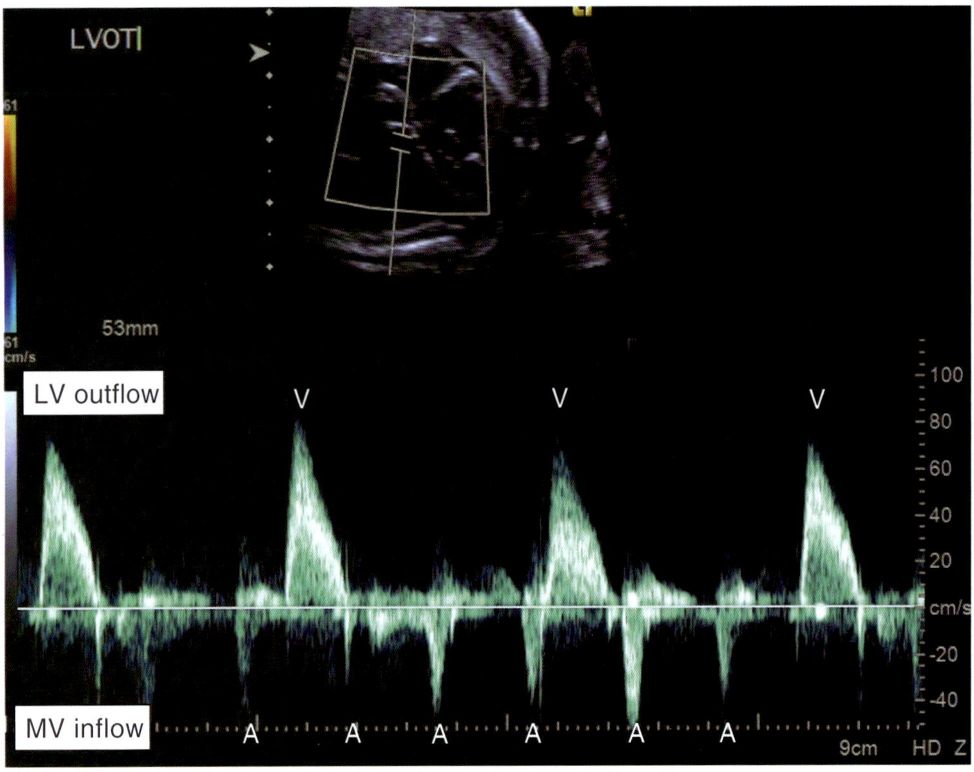

D.

FIGURE 2.2.3 Cont'd

A.

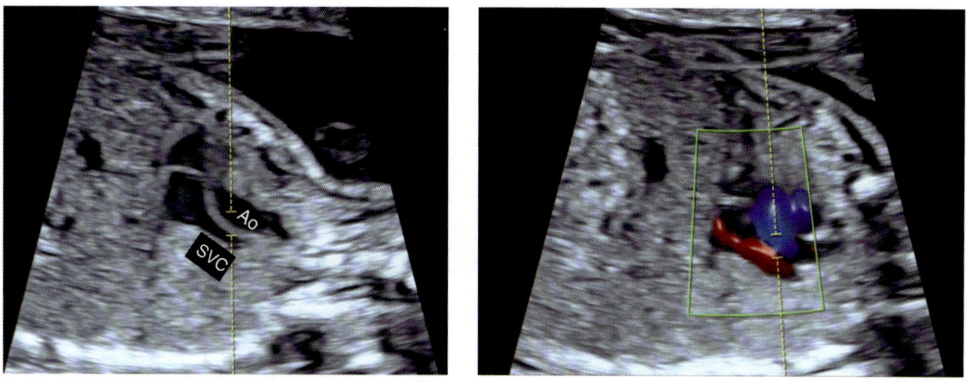

FIGURE 2.2.4 **A:** Sample gate position to obtain a pulsed Doppler tracing using the SVC/Ao method. The sample volume is widened to simultaneously include both the superior vena cava (SVC) and ascending aorta (Ao) pulsed Doppler flow signals. **B:** Normal fetal rhythm using the SVC/Ao technique where the SVC Doppler waves appear above the zero-velocity line and the aortic waves are below this line. In this normal rhythm, each atrial systole (A) is followed by a ventricular contraction (V). **C:** SVC/Ao technique demonstrating 1:1 reciprocating supraventricular tachycardia with a long VA interval (VA = 155 ms and AV = 130 ms). The ventricular rate is regular with an R-R interval of 287 ms. **D:** Atrial flutter with 2:1 AV conduction using the SVC/Ao technique. The atrial rate is regular (A-A interval = 132 ms) and the R-R interval is 256 ms. **E:** Pulsed wave Doppler tracing using the SVC/Ao technique in a fetus with anti-Ro/SSA–mediated complete AV block with the absence of fetal AV synchrony. Note the variation in the A-wave velocity with larger A-waves seen at the time of ventricular systole (mitral valve closed).

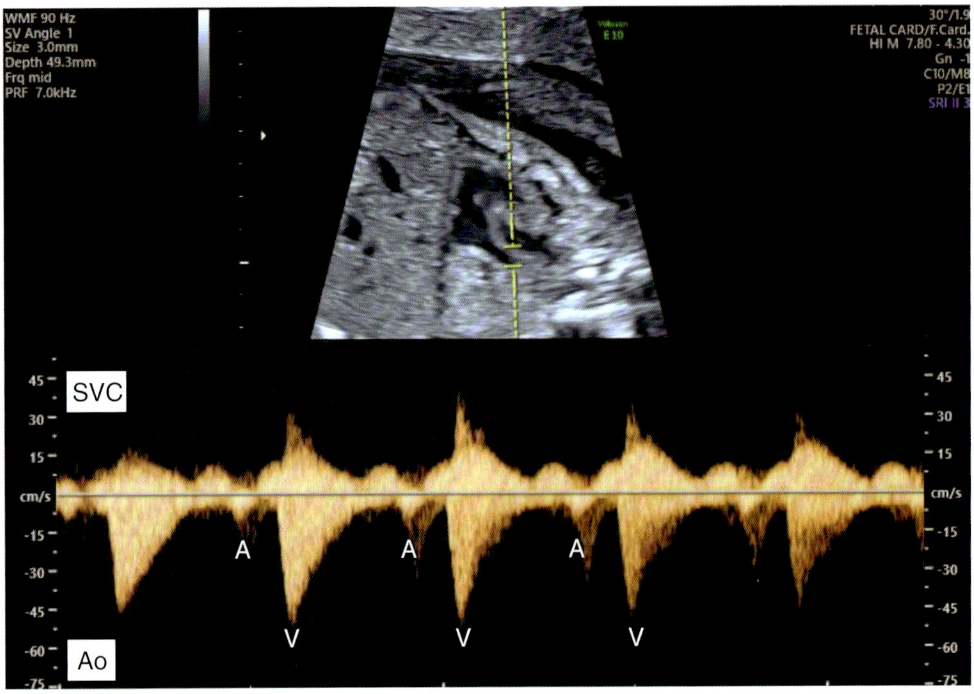

B.

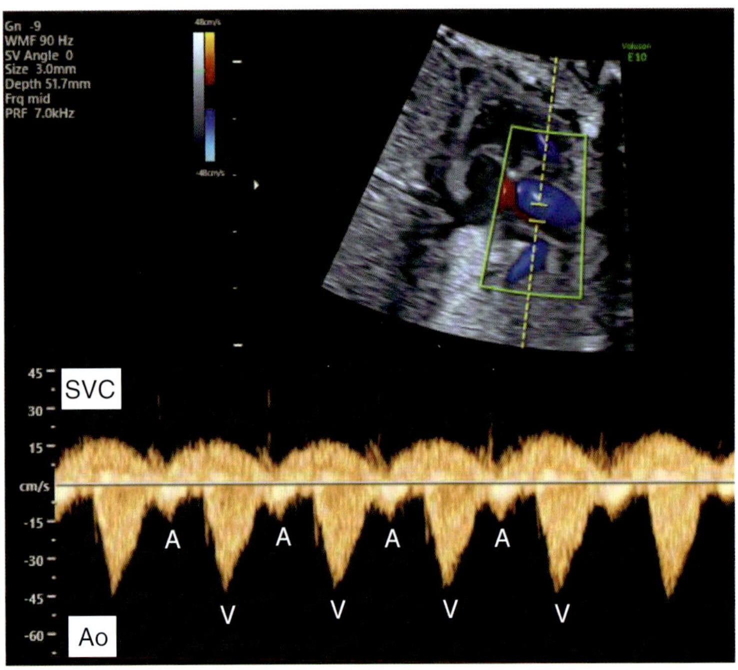

C.

FIGURE 2.2.4 Cont'd

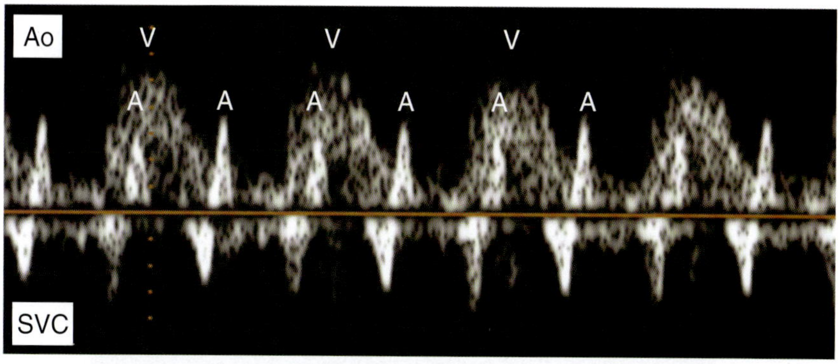

D.

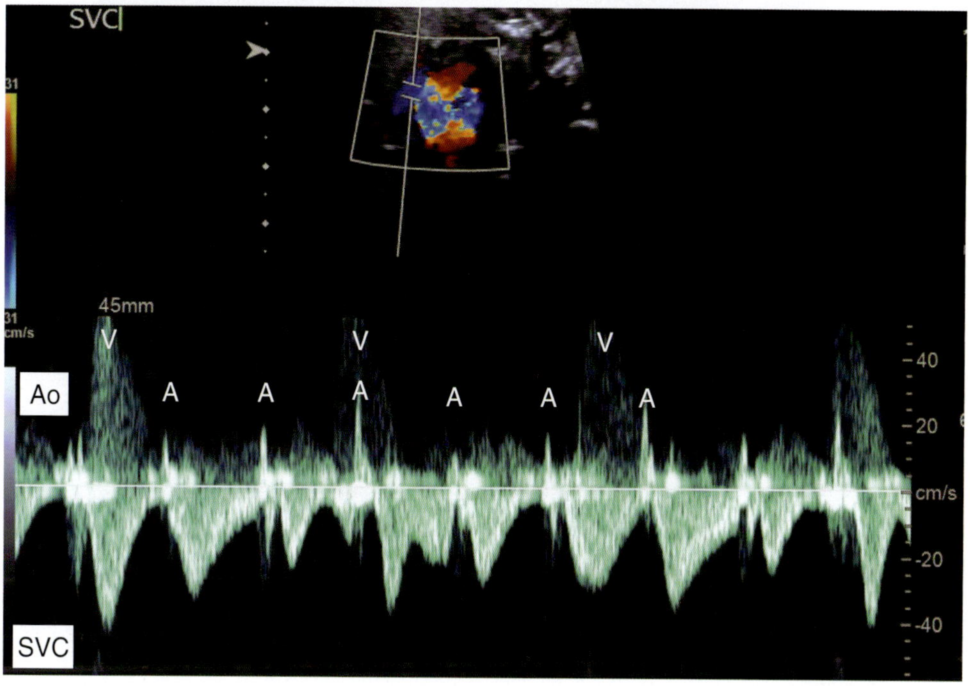

E.

FIGURE 2.2.4 Cont'd

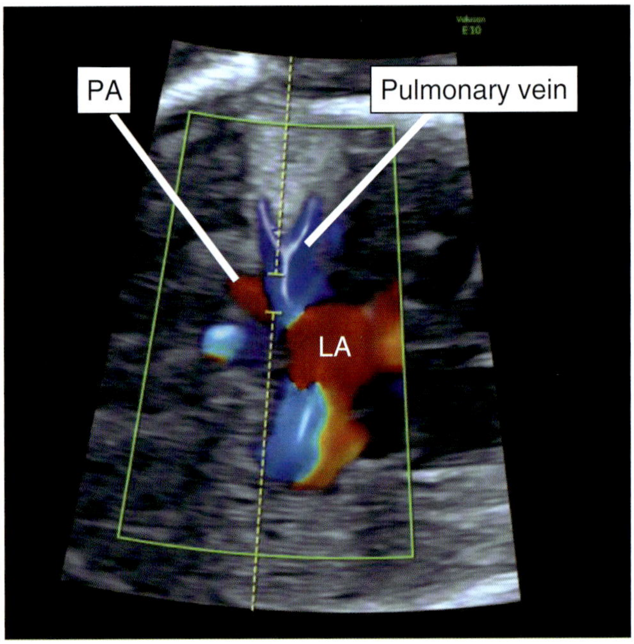

A.

FIGURE 2.2.5 A: Sample gate position to obtain a pulsed-wave Doppler tracing using the pulmonary vein/pulmonary artery (PA) method. The sample volume is widened to simultaneously include both the pulmonary venous pulsed Doppler returning to the atrium and the pulmonary artery pulsed Doppler flow signal leaving the heart. **B:** Simultaneous pulsed Doppler sampling of a pulmonary artery (above the zero-velocity line) and a pulmonary vein (below the zero-velocity line) with each atrial systole (A) followed by a ventricular contraction (V). **C:** Simultaneous pulsed Doppler sampling of a pulmonary artery and pulmonary vein, initially starting in normal rhythm and then transitioning to blocked atrial bigeminy. While in blocked atrial bigeminy, the atrial rate is regularly irregular with a long-short-long pattern (A-A′ interval = 202 ms, A′-A interval 523 ms). The ventricular rate is regular with an R-R interval of 719 ms.

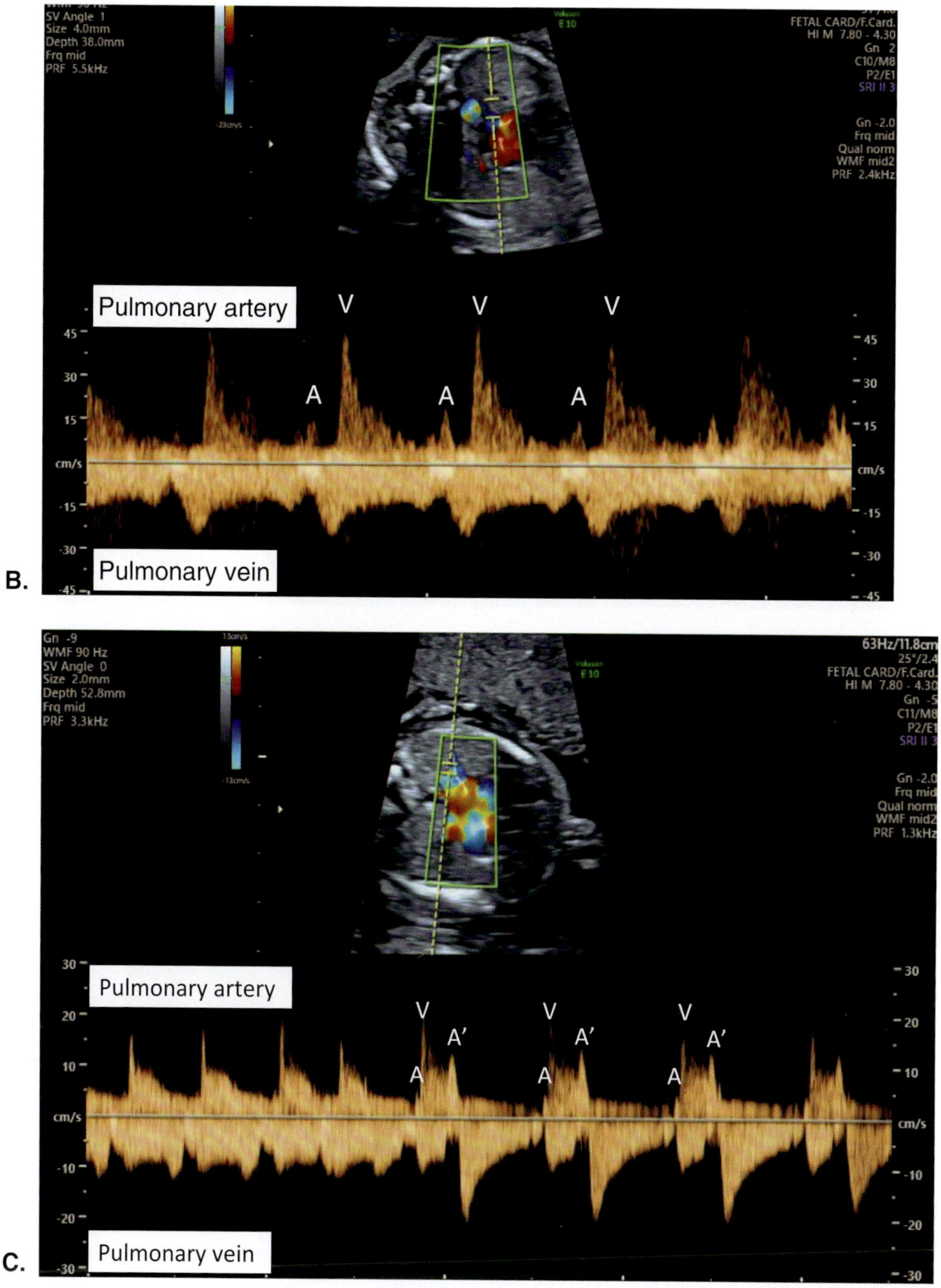

FIGURE 2.2.5 Cont'd

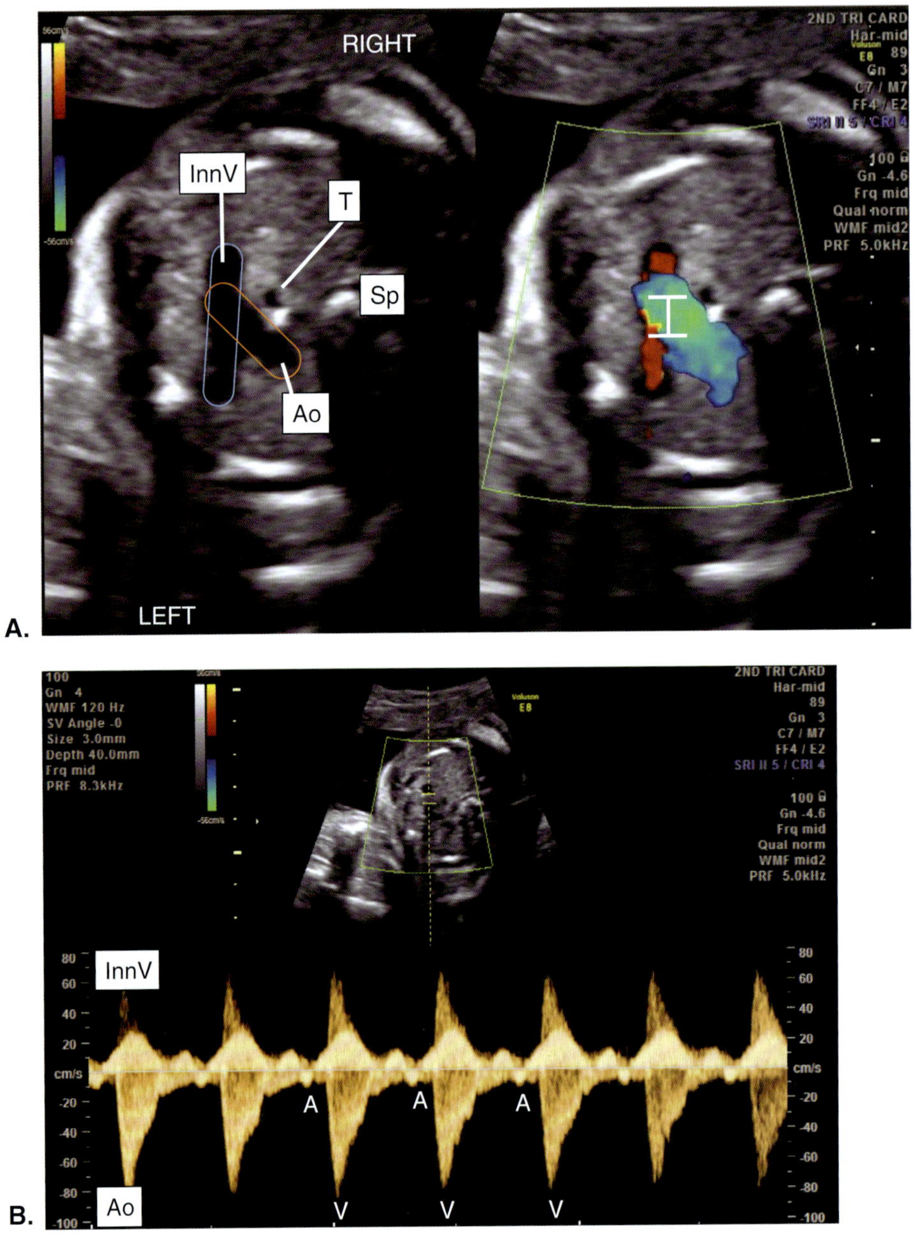

FIGURE 2.2.6 **A:** Axial 2D and color Doppler image of the fetal thorax demonstrating the position and relationship of the innominate vein (InnV), the transverse aortic arch (Ao), the trachea (T), and the spine (Sp). The sample gate is placed simultaneously over the InnV and the Ao to determine the mechanical relationship between the atria and the ventricles, respectively. **B:** Simultaneous pulsed Doppler sampling of the innominate vein and transverse aorta (InnV/Ao) demonstrating a fetus in sinus rhythm with a normal AV interval of 88 ms. **C:** Simultaneous pulsed Doppler sampling of the InnV/Ao demonstrating an isolated conducted premature atrial contraction (*PAC). **D:** Simultaneous pulsed Doppler sampling of the InnV/Ao in a fetus with 1:1 reciprocating supraventricular tachycardia with a short VA interval (VA = 54 ms and AV = 230 ms). The ventricular rate is regular with an R-R interval of 278 ms. **E:** Simultaneous pulsed Doppler sampling of the InnV and Ao in a fetus with type 2, 2° AV block. The atrial rate is regular (A-A interval = 451 ms). Every other atrial beat is conducted to the ventricle; the R-R interval is 902 ms.

C.
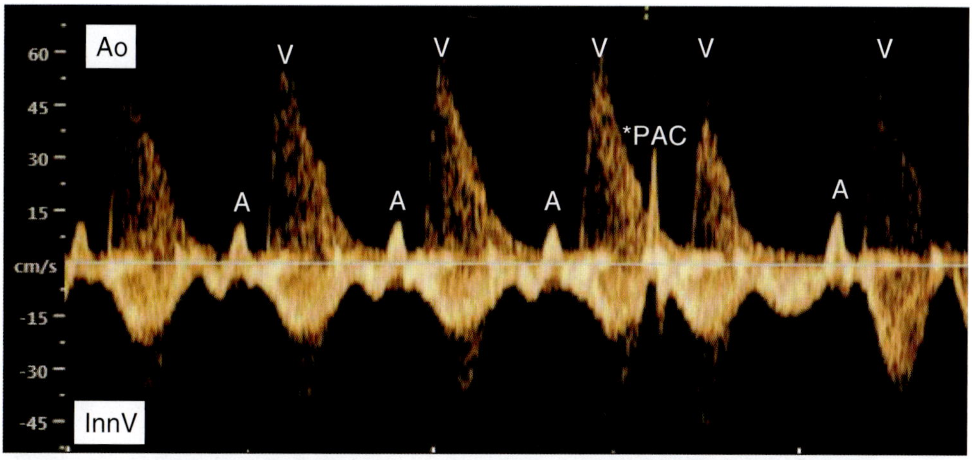

D.
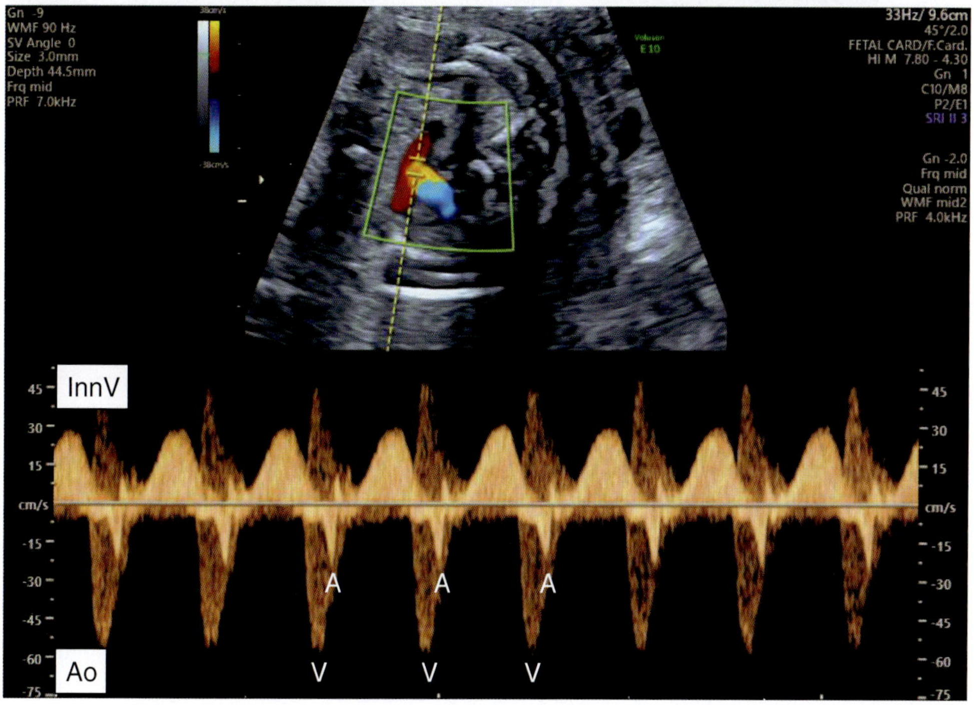

FIGURE 2.2.6 Cont'd

E.
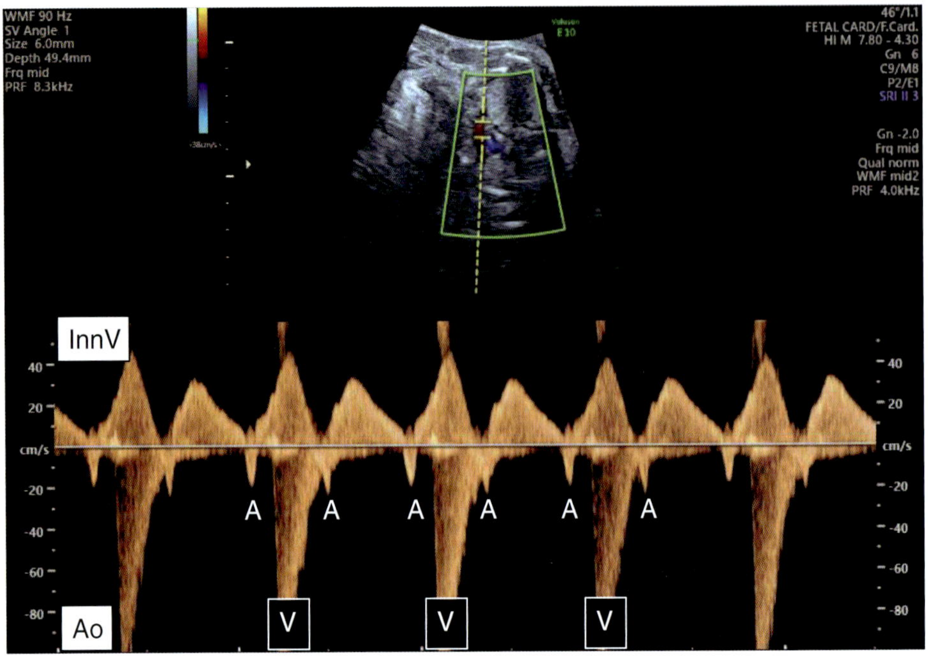

FIGURE 2.2.6 Cont'd

TISSUE DOPPLER IMAGING

Pulsed-wave tissue Doppler imaging (p-TDI), like M-mode, simultaneously records atrial and ventricular tissue motion and can be used in the assessment of fetal heart rhythm.[15] To perform this technique, the fetal heart must be positioned in an apical view within the fetal chest with a near-zero angle of insonation. A single pulsed Doppler sample volume is positioned at the lateral annulus of either AV valve, and motion curves caused by atrial and ventricular contraction can be collected and measured to evaluate fetal arrhythmias **(FIG. 2.2.7)**. In order to optimize the fetal rhythm data collected using p-TDI, the ultrasound system presets must be modified for tissue motion as opposed to blood flow including: selection of a low Doppler receive gain (typical peak velocities for p-TDI are in the range of 10-15 cm/s), reduction of the pulse repetition frequency, and minimizing the wall filter.

Color Doppler tissue imaging (c-DTI), also referred to as tissue velocity imaging, is another echocardiographic modality that can be used in fetal rhythm assessment.[16-19] This technique measures the motion of the fetal myocardium and allows for precise timing of the atrial and ventricular events. To perform c-DTI, a four-chamber view of the fetal heart must be obtained in any orientation with visualization of one atrial wall, one AV valve, and one ventricular wall and cine clips collected. Offline analysis of c-DTI clips must be performed with independent analysis of atrial contraction and ventricular contraction. Once both atrial systole and ventricular systole are independently confirmed, simultaneous assessment of the atrial and ventricular activity can be performed and fetal rhythm determined. Advantages of c-DTI include its excellent temporal resolution and lack of angle-dependence as there is only need to demonstrate wall motion and not peak myocardial velocities. c-DTI can define the mechanical relationship of the atrial and ventricular wall motion[17] and has the capability to analyze the activity of several regions of the heart within the same cardiac cycle. Although c-DTI can be very effective at defining arrhythmias, this echocardiographic modality is currently not universally available, may be time-intensive, and is dependent upon good fetal image quality (FIG. 2.2.8).

Tissue velocity imaging (TVI) is particularly helpful in identifying atrial ectopy. Sampling at the level of the lateral tricuspid or mitral valve annulus, atrial contraction is represented by the a′ wave and can be used to localize the origin of the ectopic atrial activation (the mechanical equivalent of an abnormal p-wave axis on electrocardiogram) and could accurately diagnose PACs, even those occurring during ventricular contraction.[15] Cannon "a" waves on venous Doppler and fused AV valve inflows are also suggestive of a diagnosis of PACs even in the absence of simultaneous assessment of ventricular contraction.

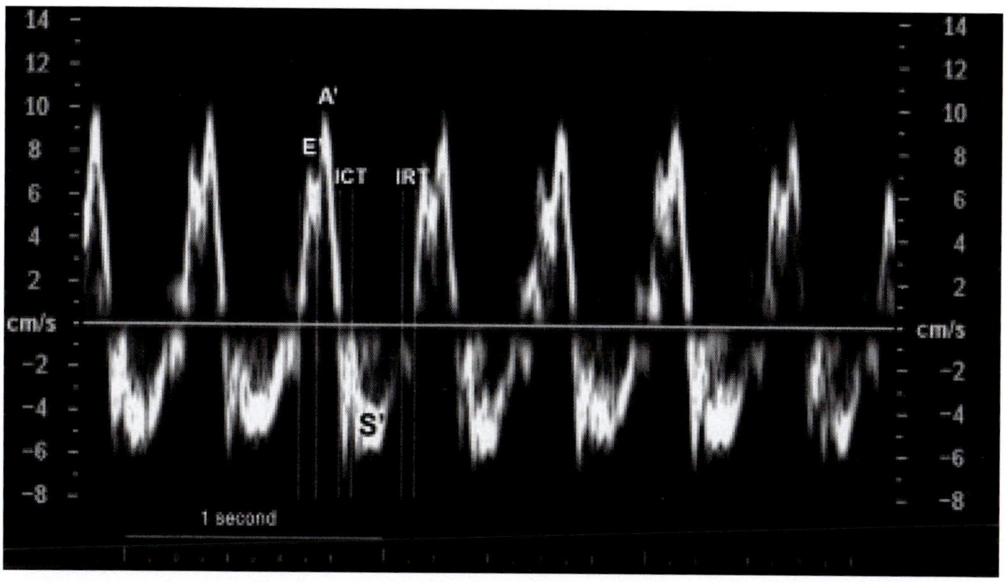

FIGURE 2.2.7 Normal fetal pulsed-wave tissue Doppler echocardiography tracing with insonation of the right atrioventricular valve annulus from the base of the heart, where systolic wall movements appear below the baseline. During each cardiac cycle, there is a systolic movement toward the apex of the heart (S′, below baseline) and two diastolic movements away from the apex (E′, A′, above baseline). The intervals denote (from left to right) the first (E′) and second (A′) diastolic excursions, the isovolumic contraction time (ICT) between the end of A′ and the onset of S′, and the isovolumic relaxation time (IRT) between the end of S′ and the subsequent E′. In this recording, a medium sweep speed was used to record a longer "rhythm strip." For analysis of intervals, the highest sweep speed should be selected. (Reprinted from Tutschek B, Schmidt KG. Pulsed-wave tissue Doppler echocardiography for the analysis of fetal cardiac arrhythmias. *Ultrasound Obstet Gynecol*. 2011;38(4):406-412.)

A.

B.

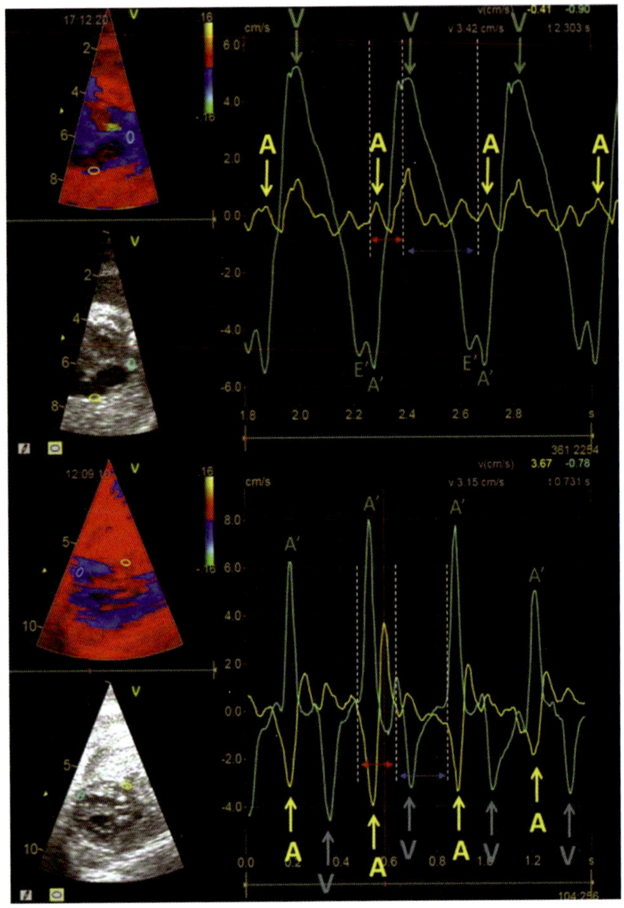

FIGURE 2.2.8 Color Doppler tissue imaging (c-DTI) in sinus rhythm. The yellow curves represent atrial wall motion (A) and the green curves ventricular (V) wall motion. The yellow arrows point to the peak of atrial systole and the green arrows, the peak of ventricular systole. The dotted lines mark the intervals between atrial and ventricular systole. E0 reflects passive ventricular filling and A0 reflects ventricular filling secondary to atrial contraction. **A:** Doppler tissue imaging curves derived from a fetal four-chamber view in apical orientation. A-V interval (red arrow) = 120 ms, V-A interval (blue arrow) = 240 ms. **B:** Doppler tissue imaging curves derived from a fetal four-chamber view perpendicular to the cardiac axis. A-V interval (red arrow) = 130 ms, V-A interval (blue arrow) = 250 ms. Note how depending on the orientation of the heart and how close it is to the atrioventricular valve, the wave format on the cTDI tracing changes, reflecting direction of the wall motion. This illustrates the need to analyze the rhythm frame by frame on the two-dimensional image to confirm the timing of the beginning of the atrial and ventricular contraction when using this method. (Reprinted from Alvarez SGV, Khoo NS, Colen T, et al. The incremental benefit of color tissue Doppler in fetal arrhythmia assessment. *J Am Soc Echocardiogr.* 2019;32(1):145-156.)

Confusing Arrhythmias

As previously mentioned, arrhythmia interpretation by echo assumes that mechanical events are the surrogate for electrical events. However, there are certain situations where "mechanical rhythm" does not reflect electrical rhythm. Electromechanical dysfunction has been reported with several types of arrhythmias, including atrial flutter and atrial contractions in AV block. Intermittent myocardial akinesia or sustained hypokinesia can mimic absence of P or QRS waves when they are truly present. Atrial and ventricular events can occur simultaneously, as in junctional ectopic tachycardia and AV block with junctional escape rhythm. In these situations, the most complete evaluation using spectral Doppler of mitral inflow/aortic outflow, a vein/artery, M-mode, and if possible, fMCG will be a helpful adjunct in rhythm analysis.

SUMMARY

It is very helpful to practice the different ways of assessing fetal arrhythmias during scanning of the normal fetus. Many of these views take practice but can be mastered. The mitral inflow/left ventricular outflow is probably the most straightforward and helpful in measurements of the AV interval. We have found the simultaneous venous/arterial Doppler to be most helpful in distinguishing atrial from ventricular ectopy and defining the mechanism of supraventricular tachycardia. M-mode is very helpful in distinguishing blocked atrial bigeminy from AV block. However, the most helpful techniques may vary and some familiarity with all will improve fetal arrhythmia diagnosis and understanding.

References

1. Hornberger LK, Sahn DJ. Rhythm abnormalities of the fetus. *Heart.* 2007;93(10):1294-1300.
2. Strasburger J, Wakai RT. Fetal cardiac arrhythmia detection and in utero therapy. *Nat Rev Cardiol.* 2010;7(5):277-290.
3. Jaeggi E, Nii M. Fetal brady- and tachyarrhythmias: new and accepted diagnostic and treatment methods. *Semin Fetal Neonatal Med.* 2005;10(6):504-514.
4. Fouron JC. Fetal arrhythmias: the Saint-Justine hospital experience. *Prenat Diagn.* 2004;24(13):1068-1080.
5. Steinfeld L, Rappaport HL, Rossbach HC, Martinez E. Diagnosis of fetal arrhythmias using echocardiographic and Doppler techniques. *J Am Coll Cardiol.* 1986;8(6):1425-1433.
6. Kleinman CS, Donnerstein RL, Jaffe CC, et al. Fetal echocardiography. A tool for evaluation of in utero cardiac arrhythmias and monitoring of in utero therapy: analysis of 71 patients. *Am J Cardiol.* 1983;51(2):237-243.
7. Strasburger JF, Huhta JC, Carpenter RJ Jr, Garson A Jr, McNamara DG. Doppler echocardiography in the diagnosis and management of persistent fetal arrhythmias. *J Am Coll Cardiol.* 1986;7(6):1386-1391.
8. Kleinman CS, Hobbins JC, Jaffe CC, Lynch DC, Talner NS. Echocardiographic studies of the human fetus: prenatal diagnosis of congenital heart disease and cardiac dysrhythmias. *Pediatrics.* 1980;65(6):1059-1067.
9. Allan LD, Anderson RH, Sullivan ID, Campbell S, Holt DW, Tynan M. Evaluation of fetal arrhythmias by echocardiography. *Br Heart J.* 1983;50(3):240-245.
10. Huhta JC, Strasburger JF, Carpenter RJ, Reiter A, Abinader E. Pulsed Doppler fetal echocardiography. *J Clin Ultrasound.* 1985;13(4):247-254.
11. Fouron JC, Fournier A, Proulx F, et al. Management of fetal tachyarrhythmia based on superior vena cava/aorta Doppler flow recordings. *Heart.* 2003;89(10):1211-1216.
12. Carvalho JS, Prefumo F, Ciardelli V, Sairam S, Bhide A, Shinebourne EA. Evaluation of fetal arrhythmias from simultaneous pulsed wave Doppler in pulmonary artery and vein. *Heart.* 2007;93(11):1448-1453.
13. Howley LW, Schuchardt E, Park D, Gilbert L, Gruenwald J, Cuneo BF. Simultaneous recording of pulsed-wave Doppler signals in innominate vein and transverse aortic arch: new technique to evaluate atrioventricular conduction and fetal heart rhythm. *Ultrasound Obstet Gynecol.* 2018;52(4):544-545.
14. Mosimann B, Arampatzis G, Amylidi-Mohr S, et al. Reference ranges for fetal atrioventricular and ventriculoatrial time intervals and their ratios during normal pregnancy. *Fetal Diagn Ther.* 2018;44(3):228-235.

15. Tutschek B, Schmidt KG. Pulsed-wave tissue Doppler echocardiography for the analysis of fetal cardiac arrhythmias. *Ultrasound Obstet Gynecol.* 2011;38(4):406-412.
16. Rein AJ, O'Donnell C, Geva T, et al. Use of tissue velocity imaging in the diagnosis of fetal cardiac arrhythmias. *Circulation.* 2002;106(14):1827-1833.
17. Alvarez SGV, Khoo NS, Colen T, et al. The incremental Benefit of color tissue Doppler in fetal arrhythmia assessment. *J Am Soc Echocardiogr.* 2019;32(1):145-156.
18. Nii M, Hamilton RM, Fenwick L, Kingdom JC, Roman KS, Jaeggi ET. Assessment of fetal atrioventricular time intervals by tissue Doppler and pulse Doppler echocardiography: normal values and correlation with fetal electrocardiography. *Heart.* 2006;92(12):1831-1837.
19. Herling L, Johnson J, Ferm-Widlund K, et al. Automated analysis of fetal cardiac function using color tissue Doppler imaging. *Ultrasound Obstet Gynecol.* 2018;52(5):599-608.

Magnetocardiography

Ronald Wakai

INTRODUCTION

Electrocardiography (ECG) is the gold standard for rhythm assessment; however, fetal ECG (fECG) is not used clinically for assessment of fetal rhythm due to its limited signal quality and success rate. The subject of this chapter is a relatively new technique, fetal magnetocardiography (fMCG), FMCG is the magnetic analogue of fECG; that is, the same cardiac currents that generate the fECG also give rise to magnetic signals that comprise the fMCG. The fMCG and fECG are both directly proportional to the net heart current; thus, they are similar in appearance and information content. The fECG, however, suffers from a low and/or variable signal amplitude, especially during the critical period of pregnancy from about 26 to 35 weeks when the fetal skin is covered by the vernix caseosa. The high electrical resistance of the fetal skin and vernix impedes the transmission of currents to the maternal surface. Magnetic signals, in contrast, do not rely on volume conduction and thus are less affected.

The last decade has seen considerable progress in demonstrating the utility of fMCG for evaluation of fetal arrhythmia. Although fMCG is not widely used, its efficacy has been acknowledged in leading clinical journals and in the first-ever American Heart Association Scientific Statement on Fetal Diagnosis and Treatment.[1] This chapter introduces readers to the basic principles, technical aspects, and clinical application of fMCG. The main objective is to describe the advantages of fMCG and the rationale for its use as an adjunct to fetal echocardiography.

ADVANTAGES OF FMCG

Currently, echocardiography is the only method used clinically to diagnose fetal arrhythmia; however, it is important to bear in mind that the mechanical rhythm assessed by echocardiography is a surrogate for electrical rhythm and has significant limitations.

The main advantage of fMCG is its ability to provide waveform information. This is critical for accurate diagnosis of ventricular rhythms, such as premature ventricular contractions (PVCs) and ventricular tachycardia (VT). Perhaps the most compelling advantage of fMCG is its ability to assess repolarization, which is mechanically silent and therefore cannot be assessed by echocardiography. fMCG can detect QTc prolongation, T-wave alternans, ST depression, and other important phenomena associated with abnormal repolarization.

fMCG is also more precise than echocardiography. It has been shown that in some cases the mechanical rhythm does not always accurately reflect the underlying electrical rhythm,[2,3] which can result in an ambiguous or inaccurate diagnosis. In addition, fMCG offers some practical advantages. It is well suited for extended, Holter-like monitoring. This makes it highly useful for assessment of complex rhythms that change over time. It is also useful for detection of brief, transient rhythms, such as brief runs of VT, which are critical to catch at an early stage.

SIGNAL CHARACTERISTICS OF THE FMCG

The fECG and fMCG show similar temporal behavior; however, their signal topographies differ substantially. Electric signals are due to potential differences along the direction of the current, as described by Ohm's law. Magnetic signals are composed of flux lines that encircle the net current, as described by Ampere's (FIG. 2.3.1). The polarity of the signal depends on whether the flux lines are entering or exiting the body surface; therefore, the polarity of the detected signal is reversed on opposite sides of the current.

Although fMCG is an effective technique, it has significant limitations relative to postnatal ECG. The main limitation is that the signal-to-noise ratio (SNR) is exceedingly low at early gestational ages due to the small size of the developing heart. Typically, studies are performed after about 20 weeks when the success rate is high. In addition to the gestational age dependence, the rapid falloff of the signal with distance is an important consideration. Thus, the lie of the fetus, the placement of the sensors, and the body mass ratio of the mother are factors that can influence the signal quality or the timing of a study.

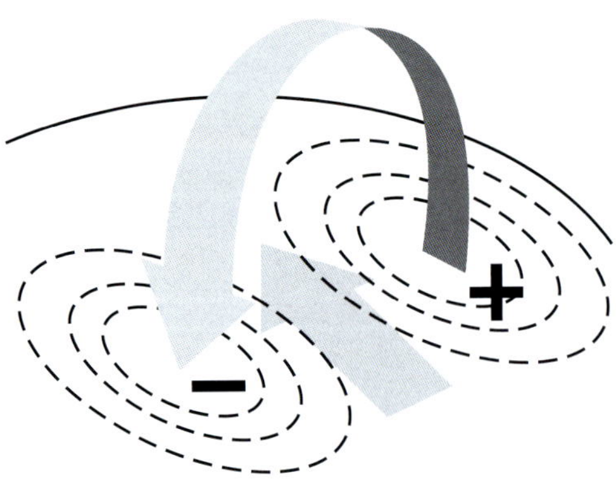

FIGURE 2.3.1 Magnetic flux line (curved arrow) encircling cardiac current, represented by the straight arrow. The dashed elliptical curves are the isofield lines of the magnetic signal, which are analogous to the equipotential lines of electric signals. The polarity of the signal is positive for flux lines emerging from the body surface and negative for flux lines entering the body.

A further limitation is that the configuration of fMCG waveforms is ambiguous because the position and orientation of the sensors with respect to the fetus depends on fetal lie and, therefore, may differ from subject to subject. In practice, recordings are made at several positions to capture a range of waveform configurations.

INSTRUMENTATION

The main drawback of fMCG is the high cost and complexity of the instrumentation. Until recently, the only detectors with sufficient sensitivity to record the fMCG were SQUID (Superconducting QUantum Interference Device) magnetometers (**FIG. 2.3.2A**). The principles of operation of SQUIDs are beyond the scope of this work and can be found elsewhere.[4] They are superconductor devices and require liquid helium, a vanishing resource. In 2016, a SQUID fMCG system (Tristan 621/624 Biomagnetometer, Tristan Technologies, San Diego) received FDA 510(k) clearance. The combined cost of this system and a magnetically shielded room is approximately $1M.

Recently, however, there has been a breakthrough in magnetic sensor technology. The new sensors, known as an optically pumped magnetometers (OPMs; **FIG. 2.3.2B**), are compact and perform similarly to SQUIDs without the need for liquid helium.[5] Their small size enables the use of person-sized shields, which allows the entire system to be portable and much less expensive. Currently, there are no commercial vendors of OPM fMCG systems, but it is likely that OPMs will replace SQUIDs in the foreseeable future and that the eventual cost of an OPM fMCG system will be several times less than that of current SQUID fMCG systems.

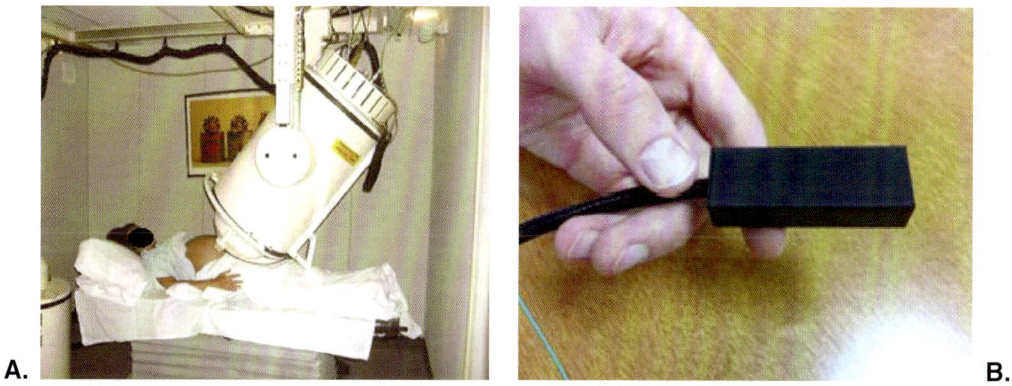

FIGURE 2.3.2 A: Multichannel SQUID magnetometer positioned on maternal abdomen. **B:** Optically pumped magnetometer sensor.

DATA COLLECTION

Recording the fMCG is relatively straightforward. Typically, a brief ultrasound examination is performed to locate the fetal heart, and the detector is placed on the maternal surface in close proximity to the fetal heart. The operator sits at a computer console outside the shielded room, and the mother is instructed to lie quietly on the patient table for the duration of the recording.

The recordings typically last 5 to 10 minutes; however, typically several recordings are taken, moving the sensor position at least once in between. For cases involving complex or intermittent arrhythmias, the recording time can exceed 1 hour. For cases involving obstetrical high-risk conditions, the recording time should be at least 20 minutes so that fetal heart rate reactivity can be assessed.

In principle, only a few channels are required to capture the information contained in the signal. In practice, however, fMCG sensor arrays may comprise a dozen or more channels to facilitate the use of signal processing, which is essential for removing interference.

SIGNAL PROCESSING

The raw fMCG signals are contaminated with large interference. The main interference is the maternal MCG, which is typically larger than the fMCG unless the fetus is near term. Multichannel sensors enable the use of a signal processing technique known as spatial filtering,[6,7] which is the spatial analogue of temporal filtering; that is, the filter output is a linear combination of the spatial samples. The method is able to separate the fetal signal from the maternal MCG and other interferences based on differences in their spatial characteristics. These differences result largely because the fetal heart is much closer to the sensors than the maternal heart and other sources of interference.

DATA ANALYSIS

The signal-processed recordings are used to generate fetal heart rate and fetal activity tracings, averaged fMCG waveforms, and rhythm strips. These data are used for clinical interpretation.

Actocardiograms

The combination of fetal heart rate and fetal activity monitoring is known as fetal actocardiography (FIG. 2.3.3). In obstetrics, fetal actocardiography is synonymous with nonstress testing, the primary method of assessing fetal well-being. Actocardiograms are obtained by detecting the fetal QRS complexes, which can be performed in an automated fashion using a computer program.[8] The QRS times are used to compute fetal heart rate tracings and the QRS amplitudes are used to compute actogram tracings, that is, tracings of fetal activity. The basis of fMCG actography is the variation in signal amplitude that results from changes in the position and orientation of the fetal heart due to fetal trunk movement.[9]

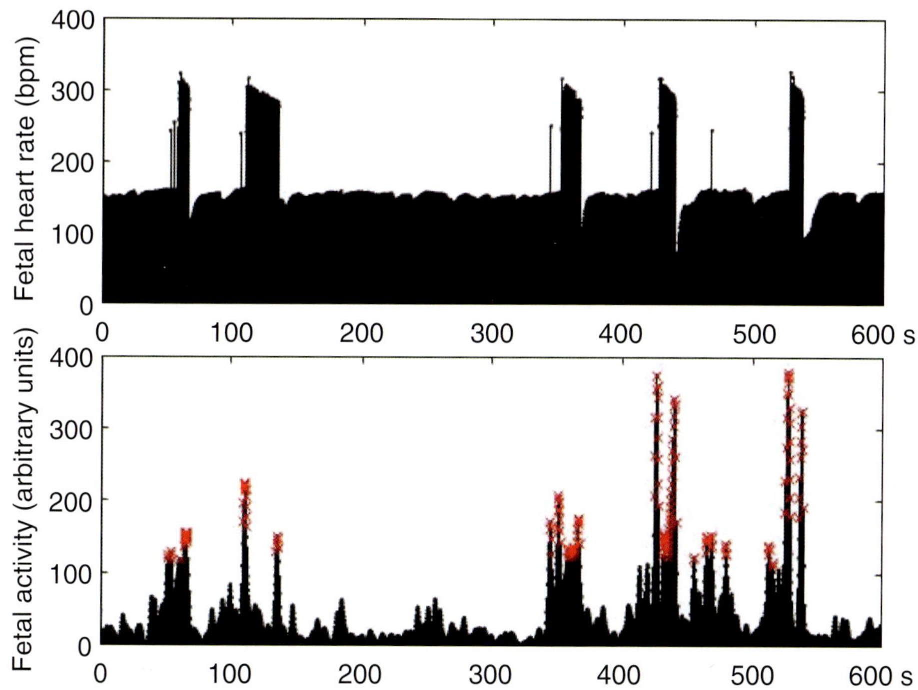

FIGURE 2.3.3 Fetal actocardiogram. The top panel shows the fetal heart rate tracing of a fetus with intermittent supraventricular tachycardia (SVT). The bottom panel shows a tracing of fetal activity (actogram), obtained from changes in the QRS amplitudes of the channels. Notice that the episodes of SVT are associated with fetal activity and that the activity is often strongest around the initiation and termination of SVT.

Although actocardiograms are not commonly used postnatally, they are a useful adjunct for assessment of fetal rhythm. Changes in rhythm are often accompanied by changes in fetal activity, as well as fetal heart rate. For example, the onset and cessation of supraventricular tachycardia (SVT) is commonly associated with fetal movement[10] as shown in FIG. 2.3.3. This implies that changes in autonomic activity are often involved in the initiation and termination of SVT.

An important advantage of fMCG actocardiography is the ability to accurately assess beat-to-beat fetal heart rate variability (FHRV).[11] FHRV is a major diagnostic parameter. Persistently minimal or absent FHRV is among the most ominous indicators of fetal compromise; however, ultrasound lacks the precision to accurately assess beat-to-beat FHRV.

Averaged Waveforms

As noted above, the SNR of the fMCG is typically less than that of postnatal ECG; however, if the rhythm is regular, averaging can be used to increase the SNR (FIG. 2.3.4). This is accomplished by averaging consecutive fetal complexes during a period of 20 seconds or longer when the heart rate is near baseline and the fetus is

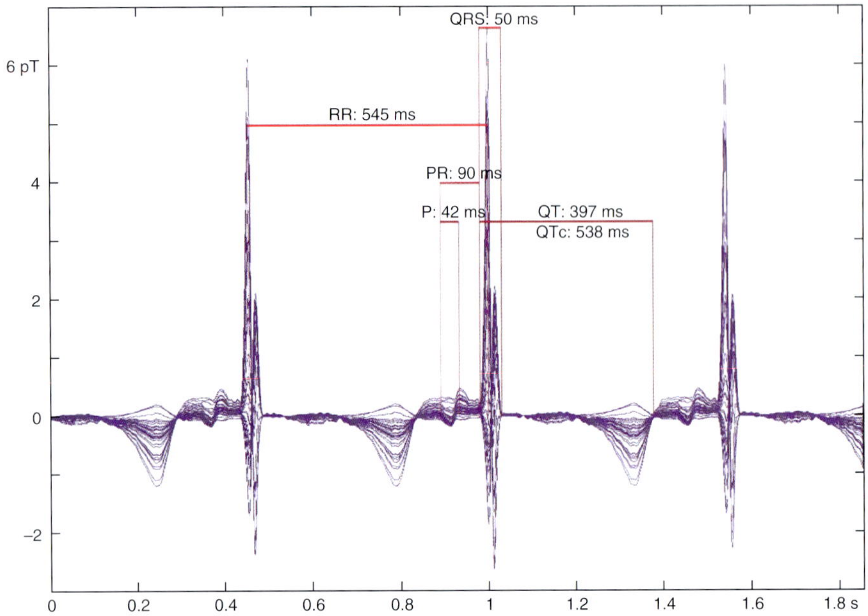

FIGURE 2.3.4 Averaged fetal magnetocardiogram waveform from fetus with long QT syndrome (LQTS). The waveform shows QTc prolongation (QTc > 500 ms) and a late-peaking T-wave morphology, which is characteristic of LQTS. The RR interval is also long-for-gestational-age. The other waveform intervals are normal.

quiescent. Averaging allows precise measurement of waveform intervals, which are the main quantitative data used to diagnose rhythm abnormalities. The PR, QRS, and QT intervals are most important. PR is measured from the beginning of the P-wave to the beginning of the QRS complex. QRS is measured from the beginning to the end of the QRS complex. QT is measurement from the beginning of the QRS complex to the end of the T-wave. Bazett formula, $QTc = QT/(RR)^{1/2}$, is used to compute QTc, the heart rate–corrected QT interval. The PR interval has a mechanical analogue, the AV interval. These intervals are used to diagnose AV block. The QRS and QTc intervals have no mechanical analogue, which makes it difficult or impossible for echocardiography to detect many important arrhythmias associated with abnormal QRS morphology, such as VT and Wolff-Parkinson-White (WPW) syndrome, or abnormal T-wave morphology, such as long QT syndrome (LQTS). The averaged waveform in FIG. 2.3.4 exhibits QTc prolongation and a late-peaking T-wave. These are hallmarks of LQTS and exemplify the efficacy of fMCG for evaluation of fetuses at risk of LQTS.

Rhythm Tracings

fMCG rhythm strips display short segments of the recordings, similar to 12-lead ECGs. FIG. 2.3.5 shows one such example from a fetus with rhabdomyomas. The QRS complexes show an abnormal, slurred QRS morphology indicative of WPW. WPW is mediated by an accessory connection and therefore is strongly associated

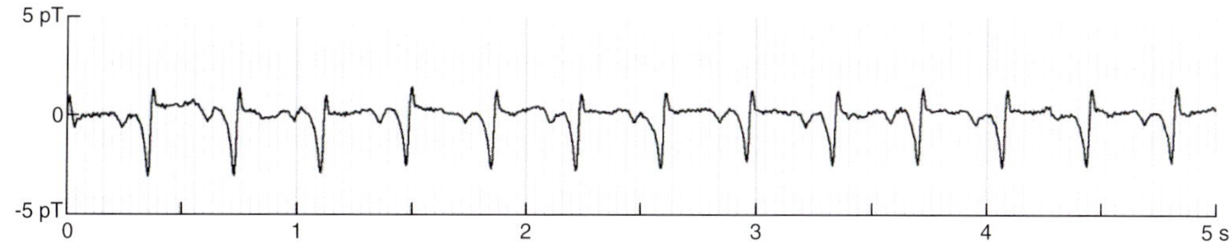

FIGURE 2.3.5 Rhythm strip from fetus with rhabdomyomas. The initial segment of the QRS complex shows slurring (preexcitation) due to Wolff-Parkinson-White syndrome.

with atrioventricular reentrant tachycardia, the most common form of fetal SVT. fMCG studies have shown that the incidence of WPW is even higher (approximately 80%) in fetuses with rhabdomyomas.[12]

It is also useful to display long continuous tracings, similar to Holter tracings, by stacking the tracings from a single channel to display several minutes of data. **FIG. 2.3.6** shows a rather dramatic example from a fetus with LQTS. The tracings are dominated by brief episodes of torsade de pointes (TdP), a lethal, polymorphic VT.

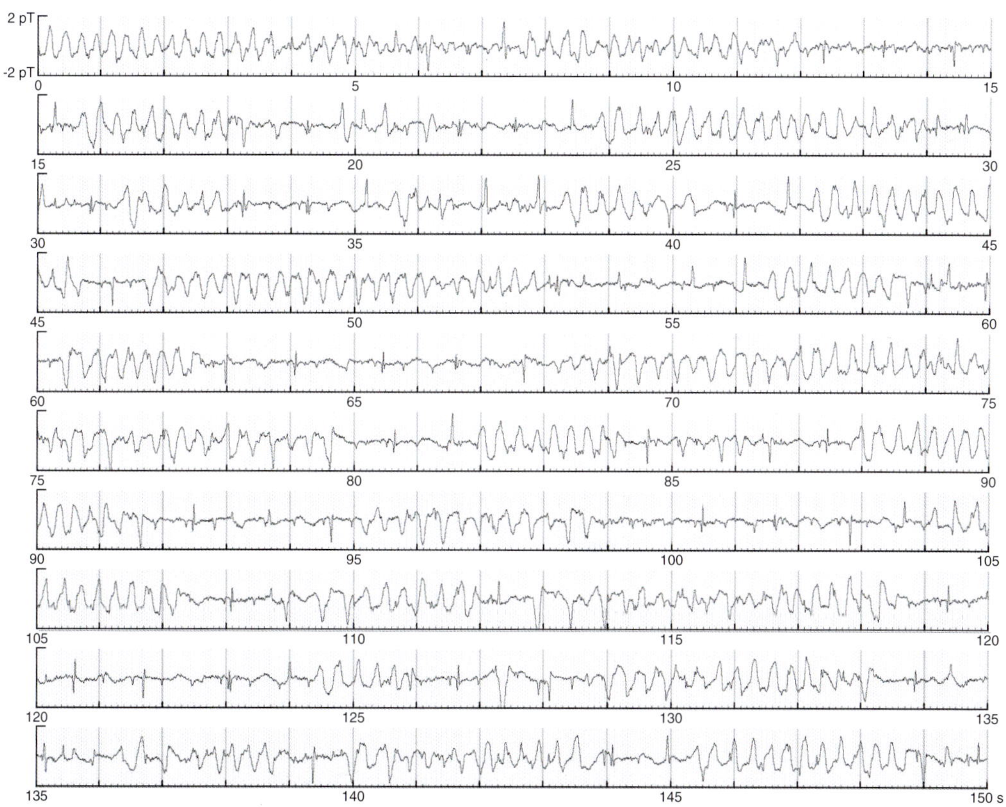

FIGURE 2.3.6 Holter-like fetal magnetocardiography tracing of duration 150 s from a fetus with long QT syndrome showing continual episodes of torsade de pointes.

CLINICAL EXAMPLES

There are many different forms of arrhythmia, most of which are described in detail in other chapters. The main role of fMCG is to provide an accurate differential diagnosis. This is especially important when prescribing therapy.

Tachycardia

The most common type of fetal arrhythmia is SVT (FIG. 2.3.7A). VT (FIG. 2.3.7B) is rarer, but much more malignant. When therapy is contemplated, it is critical to distinguish between the two since the type of tachycardia will significantly influence the choice of drug. Echocardiography can usually distinguish SVT from VT, but in some cases can be ambiguous. fMCG is definitive because it can differentiate narrow and wide QRS morphologies, which are defining characteristics of SVT and VT, respectively.

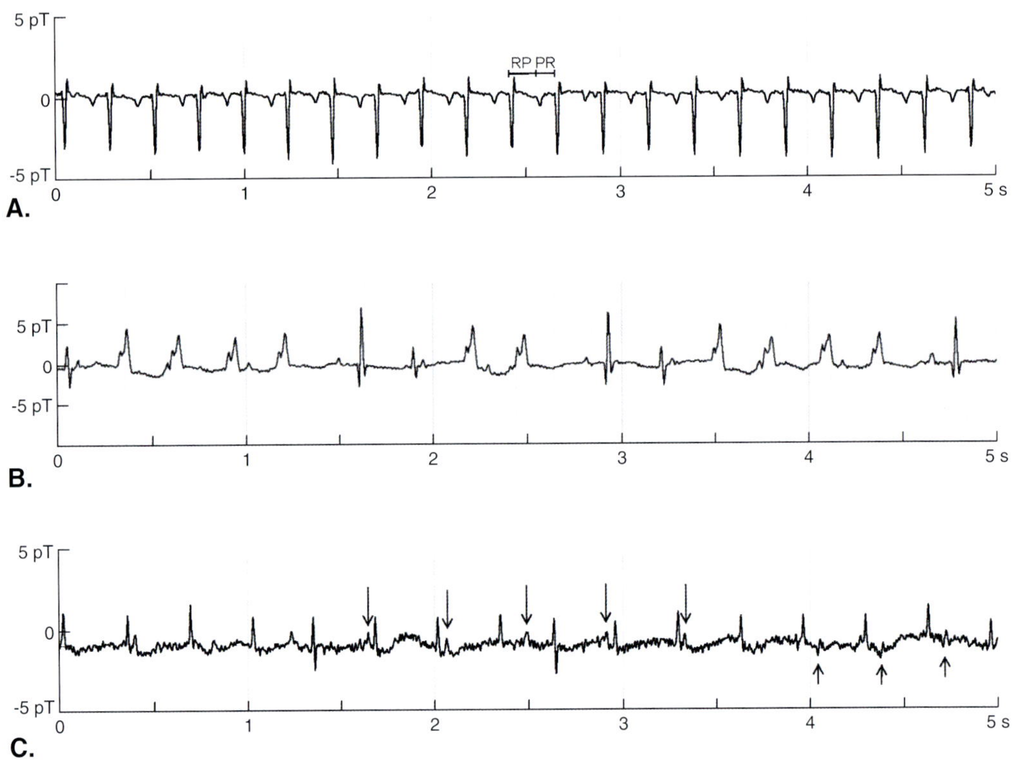

FIGURE 2.3.7 Fetal tachycardias. **A:** Atrioventricular reentrant tachycardia. This example shows a long RP tachycardia with RP > PR. **B:** Ventricular tachycardia (VT). The tracings of this hydropic fetus were dominated by salvos of VT. **C:** Junctional ectopic tachycardia (JET). JET is a narrow complex tachycardia arising from the atrioventricular (AV) node. The P-waves can be due to retrograde conduction or can arise from a dissociated sinus rhythm. This tracing shows a transition between these rhythms. The first 4 seconds shows the end of a brief period of AV dissociation. The dissociated P-waves are indicated by downward pointing arrows. The last second shows three retrograde P-waves indicated by upward pointing arrows.

fMCG can often provide a more precise differential diagnosis of SVT. The SVT shown in **FIG. 2.3.7A** is a long RP tachycardia; that is, the RP interval is longer than the PR interval. These tachycardias tend to be incessant and may call for more aggressive therapy. In addition, slow tachycardias (~180 bpm) are often difficult to diagnose because they are less common and are compatible with a number of etiologies, such as sinus tachycardia, atrial ectopic tachycardia, and VT. One example is junctional ectopic tachycardia (JET) **(FIG. 2.3.7C)**. Despite relatively low tachycardia rates, it is associated with a high incidence of hydrops fetalis, often resulting in premature delivery of a hydropic infant. Using fMCG to confirm a diagnosis of JET can result in successful treatment and improved outcome.[13]

Bradycardia

The most common fetal bradycardia is AV block. Fetal AV block is considered a simple rhythm but is often difficult to diagnose accurately because in many cases the rhythm is complicated by ectopy and/or tachycardia **(FIG. 2.3.8)**.[14] In these situations, fMCG is highly useful for identifying the rhythms and evaluating AV conduction. This can significantly influence management decisions. Therapy is more likely to be attempted in cases of incomplete AV block in order to prevent progression to complete block. It is also used to alleviate severe cases of complete block.

fMCG studies have shown that JET is commonly seen around the time of onset of AV block and that VT may occur as the disease progresses.[14] Fetuses that show tachycardia or that have flat heart rate tracings with rates ≤55 bpm usually require neonatal pacing. This knowledge is critical for proper anticipatory management of these fetuses at the time of delivery. In cases of complete AV block with fetal heart rate ≤55 bpm, some obstetricians consider delivering the baby as early as 32 weeks due to fears of fetal demise. We have used fMCG monitoring in these instances to convince the obstetrician to delay delivery by definitively ruling out the presence of a wide escape rhythm and PVCs. This saved the expense of several weeks in the neonatal ICU, allowed placement of permanent, versus temporary, pacemaker leads, and likely improved outcome.

The second most common bradycardia is blocked atrial bigeminy (BAB) **(FIG. 2.3.8D)**. BAB is usually due to reentrant premature atrial beats (PACs) that block at the AV node. The PACs are early so that the P-waves show a short-long pattern. With echocardiography, however, BAB is sometimes misdiagnosed as 2:1 AV block **(FIG. 2.3.8E)** because the time between the atrial contractions can be nearly uniform. Apparently, this occurs because the time to activate the atria is longer for PACs than sinus beats. fMCG can easily distinguish BAB from 2:1 AV block based on the timing of the P-waves.[2] It is critical to distinguish these arrhythmias because their prognosis and clinical management differ greatly. BAB is relatively benign and usually resolves spontaneously, whereas 2:1 AV block is associated with significant morbidity and often progresses to complete AV block even with treatment. Failure to diagnose BAB can lead to the unnecessary delivery of a premature infant.

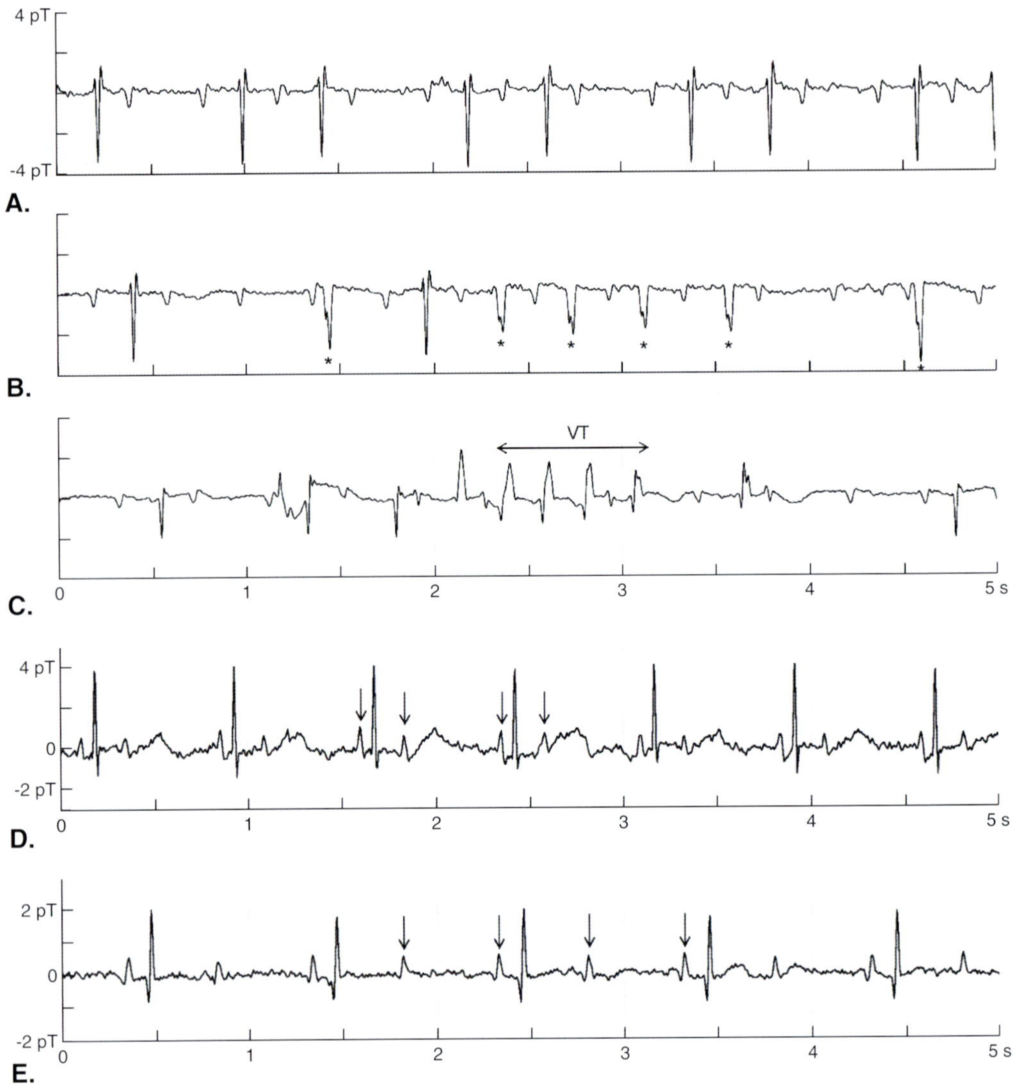

FIGURE 2.3.8 Fetal bradycardias: Panels A-C depict the diversity of rhythms present during the same session in a fetus with 2° atrioventricular (AV) block. **A:** The predominant rhythm shows a bigeminal pattern. Notice that the PR interval is marked prolonged and is longer for the second than for the first conducted beat due to Wenckebach phenomenon. **B:** The timing of some of the ectopic beats seen here can mimic that of conducted beats, but the waveform morphology allows conducted beats and premature ventricular contractions (asterisks) to be readily distinguished. **C:** A short run of ventricular tachycardia (VT) occurs at 2 to 3 seconds. **D:** The P-waves (arrows) in blocked atrial bigeminy show a short-long pattern. **E:** The P-waves in 2:1 AV block show a regular pattern.

Long QT Syndrome

LQTS is a leading cause of sudden death in early life, including during fetal development. It is believed to account for approximately 10% of sudden infant death syndrome deaths and unexplained intrauterine demise.[15] Recent fMCG data[16] suggest that the burden of fetal LQTS is significantly greater than is generally recognized due to the frequency and severity of cases resulting from spontaneous mutations, as exemplified by the case shown in FIG. 2.3.6.

fMCG is unrivaled in its ability to evaluate fetal LQTS. It is the only noninvasive technique that can diagnose fetal LQTS and other repolarization abnormalities. Not only can it detect QTc prolongation, it can diagnose the three characteristic LQTS rhythms—functional AV block, T-wave alternans, and TdP (FIG. 2.3.9A-C)—indicative of severe disease. The severity of QTc prolongation and the presence of T-wave alternans are important predictors of TdP,[17] but currently they can only be evaluated by fMCG. In the absence of fMCG, a low-for-gestational-age fetal heart rate (<3%), unexplained AV block, and/or tachycardia are potential indicators of LQTS; however, they are not specific.

TdP can be effectively treated in utero with drug therapy.[17,18] The ability of fMCG to definitively identify TdP versus other forms of tachycardia is crucial for guiding therapy. Furthermore, the initial diagnosis of TdP is often made by fMCG due to its superior ability to detect brief episodes of TdP.

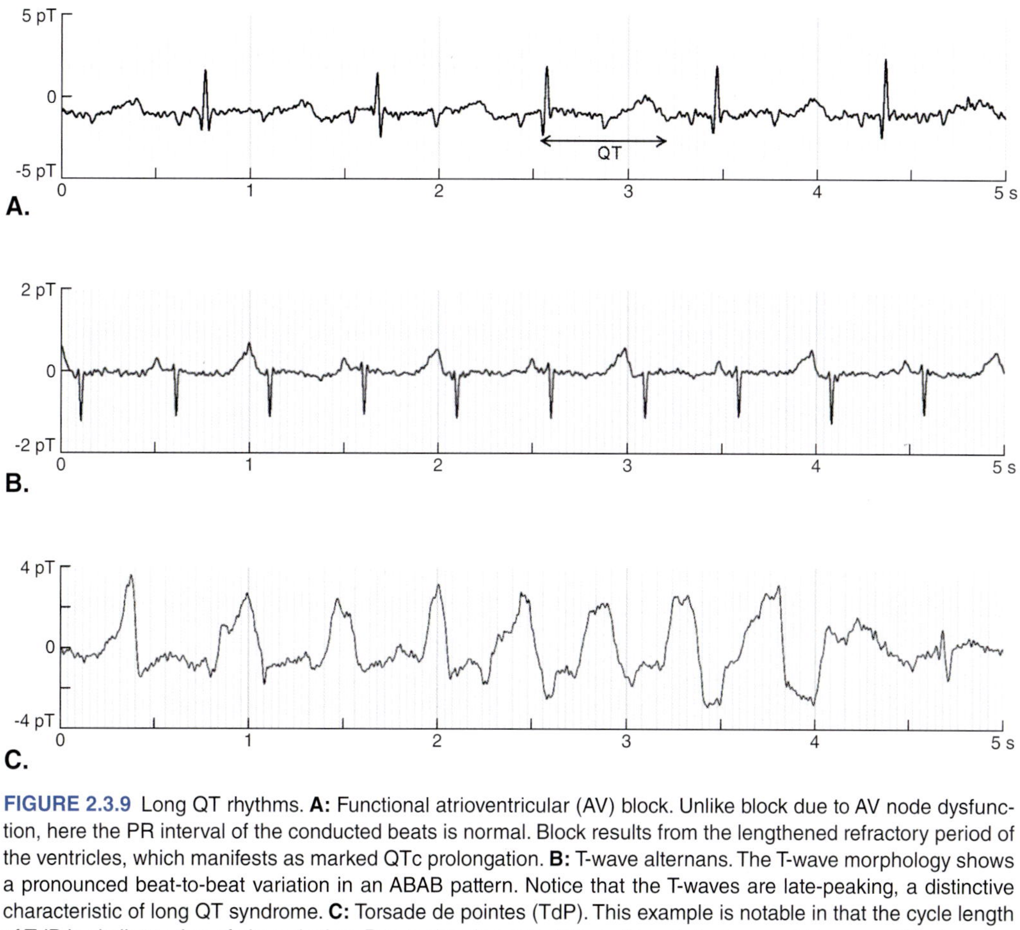

FIGURE 2.3.9 Long QT rhythms. **A:** Functional atrioventricular (AV) block. Unlike block due to AV node dysfunction, here the PR interval of the conducted beats is normal. Block results from the lengthened refractory period of the ventricles, which manifests as marked QTc prolongation. **B:** T-wave alternans. The T-wave morphology shows a pronounced beat-to-beat variation in an ABAB pattern. Notice that the T-waves are late-peaking, a distinctive characteristic of long QT syndrome. **C:** Torsade de pointes (TdP). This example is notable in that the cycle length of TdP is similar to that of sinus rhythm. Due to the slow rate, this malignant rhythm would be very difficult to recognize as TdP with echocardiography.

SUMMARY

Currently, fMCG is considered an investigational technique, but at some point in the foreseeable future it may become standard-of-care for assessment of complex fetal arrhythmia. The advantages of fMCG are especially compelling for evaluation of fetuses at risk of LQTS. Assessment of drug effect is also a promising application that has not been extensively investigated. This includes drugs for maternal conditions, as well as for fetal therapy. The main obstacle to widespread adoption has been the high cost and complexity of SQUID instrumentation; however, the development of OPMs will enable this obstacle to be overcome.

References

1. Donofrio MT, Moon-Grady AJ, Hornberger LK, et al. Diagnosis and treatment of fetal cardiac disease: a scientific statement from the american heart association. *Circulation.* 2014;129(21):2183-2242.
2. Wiggins DL, Strasburger JF, Gotteiner NL, Cuneo B, Wakai RT. Magnetophysiologic and echocardiographic comparison of blocked atrial bigeminy and 2:1 atrioventricular block in the fetus. *Heart Rhythm.* 2013;10(8):1192-1198.
3. Van Hare GF. Magnetocardiography in the diagnosis of fetal arrhythmias. *Heart Rhythm.* 2013;10(8):1199-1200.
4. Fagaly RL. Neuromagnetic instrumentation. *Adv Neurol.* 1990;54:11-32.
5. Shah VK, Wakai RT. A compact, high performance atomic magnetometer for biomedical applications. 2013;*Phys Med Biol.*58(22):8153-8161.
6. Chen ML, Wakai RT, Van Veen B. Eigenvector based spatial filtering of fetal biomagnetic signals. *J Perinat Med.* 2001;29(6):486-496.
7. Chen M, Van Veen BD, Wakai RT. Linear minimum mean-square error filtering for evoked responses: application to fetal MEG. *IEEE Trans Biomed Eng.* 2006;53(5):959-963.
8. Lutter WJ, Wakai RT. Indices and detectors for fetal MCG actography. *IEEE Trans Biomed Eng.* 2011;58(6):1874-1880.
9. Zhao H, Wakai RT. Simultaneity of foetal heart rate acceleration and foetal trunk movement determined by foetal magnetocardiogram actocardiography. *Phys Med Biol.* 2002;47(5):839-846.
10. Wakai RT, Strasburger JF, Li Z, Deal BJ, Gotteiner NL. Magnetocardiographic rhythm patterns at initiation and termination of fetal supraventricular tachycardia. *Circulation.* 2003;107(2):307-312.
11. Wakai RT. Assessment of fetal neurodevelopment via fetal magnetocardiography. *Exp Neurol.* 2004;190(suppl 1):S65-S71.
12. Wacker-Gussmann A, Strasburger JF, Cuneo B, Wiggins D, Gotteiner N, Wakai RT. Fetal arrhythmias associated with cardiac rhabdomyomas. *Heart Rhythm.* 2013;11(4):677-683.
13. Zaidi SJ, Siddiqui S, Cuneo BF, Strasburger JF, McDuffie R, Wakai RT. Prenatal diagnosis and management of junctional ectopic tachycardia. *HeartRhythm Case Rep.* 2017;3(11):503-508.
14. Zhao H, Cuneo BF, Strasburger JF, Huhta JC, Gotteiner NL, Wakai RT. Electrophysiological characteristics of fetal atrioventricular block. *J Am Coll Cardiol.* 2008;51(1):77-84.
15. Crotti L, Tester DJ, White WM, et al. Long QT syndrome-associated mutations in intrauterine fetal death. *J Am Med Assoc.* 2013;309(14):1473-1482.
16. Strand S, Strasburger JF, Cuneo BF, Wakai RT. Complex and novel arrhythmias precede stillbirth in fetuses with de Novo Long QT Syndrome. *Circ Arrhythm Electrophysiol.* In press.
17. Cuneo BF, Strasburger JF, Yu SH, et al. In utero diagnosis of long QT syndrome by magnetocardiography. *Circulation.* 2013;128(20):2183-2191.
18. Cuneo BF, Ovadia M, Strasburger JF, et al. Prenatal diagnosis and in utero treatment of torsaides de Pointes associated with congenital long QT syndrome. *Am J Cardiol.* 2003;91(11):1395-1398.

PART

3

Presentation and Diagnosis of Fetal Arrhythmias

Ectopy

Katherine Anne Kosiv • Anita J. Moon-Grady

OVERVIEW

Cardiac ectopy, composed of premature atrial (PACs) and ventricular contractions (PVCs), represents the most common fetal arrhythmia. Occurring in 1% to 2% of normal pregnancies,[1] fetal ectopy is typically benign and short-lived[2,3] with increasing incidence and frequency as gestation progresses.[4] Conversion to atrial tachyarrhythmia occurs rarely with PACs, in only ~0.5%, though increased risk is present in fetuses with atrial bigeminy or trigeminy and blocked PACs.[5,6] Atrioventricular reentrant tachycardia (AVRT; see Part 3, Chapter 2) is the most common tachyarrhythmia associated with PACs. AVRT is precipitated by a PAC and terminated by a blocked PAC; therefore, presence of atrial bigeminy, trigeminy, or blocked PACs suggests the potential presence of a reentrant pathway. The risk of developing ventricular tachycardia in the setting of PVCs in an otherwise normal fetal heart is unknown.

A baseline echocardiogram is recommended for the fetus with frequent ectopy to define the arrhythmia, assess heart function, and exclude significant structural heart disease.[7] The incidence of concomitant congenital heart disease is low at 0.3% (similar to baseline risk) though higher prevalence has been noted in some studies.[8] 1° and 2° atrioventricular (AV) block may also be present in 1% to 2% of these fetuses. Though most ectopy is isolated, occasional secondary causes include myocarditis, atrial septal aneurysm, or cardiac tumors. The fetus should be closely monitored if myocarditis is suspected or tumors diagnosed, since ventricular tachycardia can occur.

PREMATURE ATRIAL CONTRACTIONS

PACs are common, are present in 51% of healthy newborns,[9] and compromise 43% of fetal arrhythmias.[10] Occurring as early as 15 weeks, PACs increase in frequency in the last trimester when they are observed in 1% to 3% of pregnancies.[1] PACs typically originate in the atria from an automatic focus. Compared with a sinus beat, during a PAC, the atrial activation occurs early and the interval between the

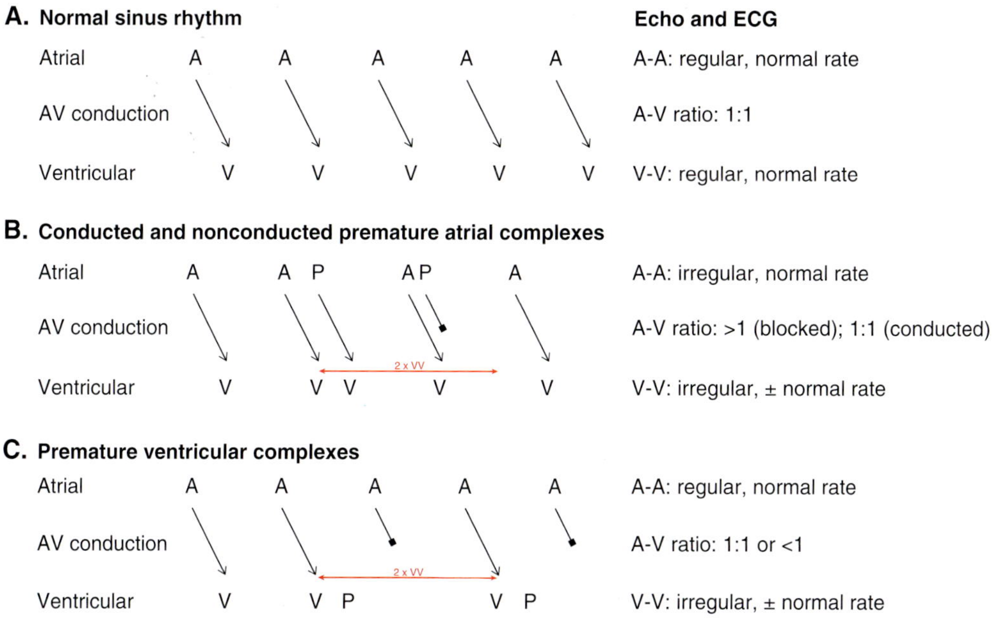

FIGURE 3.1.1 Diagrammatic representation of sequence of activation and echo and ECG correlations for **(A)** normal sinus rhythm, **(B)** premature atrial contractions, and **(C)** premature ventricular contractions. (Modified with permission from Jaeggi E, Öhman A. Fetal and Neonatal Arrhythmias. *Clin Perinatol*. 2016;43(1):99-112.)

atrial contraction before the PAC and the next normal atrial contraction is longer than the interval during normal sinus rhythm (**FIG. 3.1.1A** and **B**).[11] Premature atrial impulses can be conducted or blocked, or a combination of the two, depending on the refractoriness of the AV node (**FIG. 3.1.2**). They have a typical appearance on M-mode and spectral Doppler (**FIG. 3.1.3**). The etiology of PACs remains speculative, but some have suggested a prominent aneurysm of septum primum or redundancy of the foramen flap[1,8,12] may be causative; intracardiac tumors, for example, rhabdomyomas as seen in tuberous sclerosis, and congenital heart disease are also associated with PACs. In the setting of aneurysmal septum primum, fetal ectopy should resolve as the foramen ovale closes within the first few days of life.

The effects of atrial ectopy are reflected in the fetal venous system. There is exaggerated retrograde A-wave flow all the way to the ductus venosus (**FIG. 3.1.4A** and **B**). The irregular ventricular contractions secondary to PACs can be seen in the umbilical artery. The velocity arterial flow during PACs is higher than that of PVCs (**FIG. 3.1.4C** and **D**).

Blocked PACs occur when the AV node is refractory at the time of premature impulse arrival, such that the atrial impulse does not conduct to the ventricle and hence does not produce a ventricular contraction (**FIG. 3.1.5A**). The rhythm during blocked PACs can be irregular or regular. If every other atrial beat is a PAC that is not conducted, the rhythm is very regular, and referred to as blocked atrial bigeminy (BAB) (**FIG 3.1.5B**). BAB can be confused with 2° or 3° AV block because both

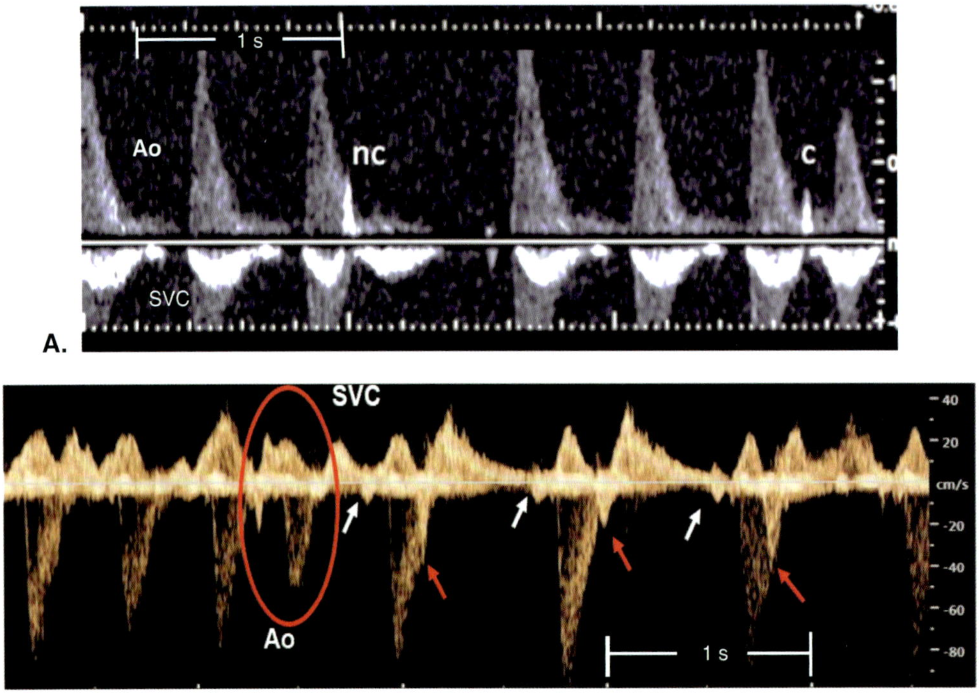

FIGURE 3.1.2 Spectral Doppler of the superior vena cava (SVC) and aorta (Ao) (above baseline) in a fetus with conducted and nonconducted premature atrial contractions (PACs). **A:** SVC flow is below baseline except for atrial contractions. The first PAC is not conducted (nc) to the ventricles, resulting in a *dropped* ventricular beat. The second PAC is conducted (c) resulting in an *early* ventricular beat. **B:** SVC flow is above baseline except for atrial contractions. Complex atrial ectopy. A conducted PAC results in an early ventricular beat (red circle). This is followed by a normal atrial contraction (white arrow), then a nonconducted atrial contraction (red arrow), and the pattern repeats. The last three complexes are an example of blocked atrial bigeminy (see Figs. 3.3.6 and 3.3.7).

result in ventricular bradycardia. Distinguishing BAB from AV block relies on the timing of atrial events. In BAB, the interval between the sinus beat (a) and the premature beat (a′) is shorter and the interval between the premature beat (a′) and subsequent sinus beat (a) is longer because a′ is premature. In contrast, the intervals between the conducted (a) and nonconducted atrial beats (a′) in AV block are constant (FIG. 3.1.6A). In other words, the a-a′ and a′-a intervals are the same and the atrial rate constants in AV block, including 2° AV block with 2:1 conduction (Part 3: Chapter 5) (FIG. 3.1.6B).

Another way to distinguish BAB from 2° AV block is by examining the isovolumic contraction time (IVCT), which is shorter in BAB than in 2° AV block with 2:1 conduction (FIG. 3.1.7).[13] Fetal magnetocardiography confirms that the interval between the sinus atrial beat (a) and the PAC (a′) is much shorter in BAB, compared to 2° AV block with 2:1 conduction (FIG. 3.1.8).[14] Distinguishing between the two rhythms is important since 2° AV block carries a more guarded prognosis and may represent evolving anti-Ro/SSA–mediated AV block or long QT syndrome (LQTS). On the other hand, BAB is almost always benign and usually resolves spontaneously.[1]

A.

B.

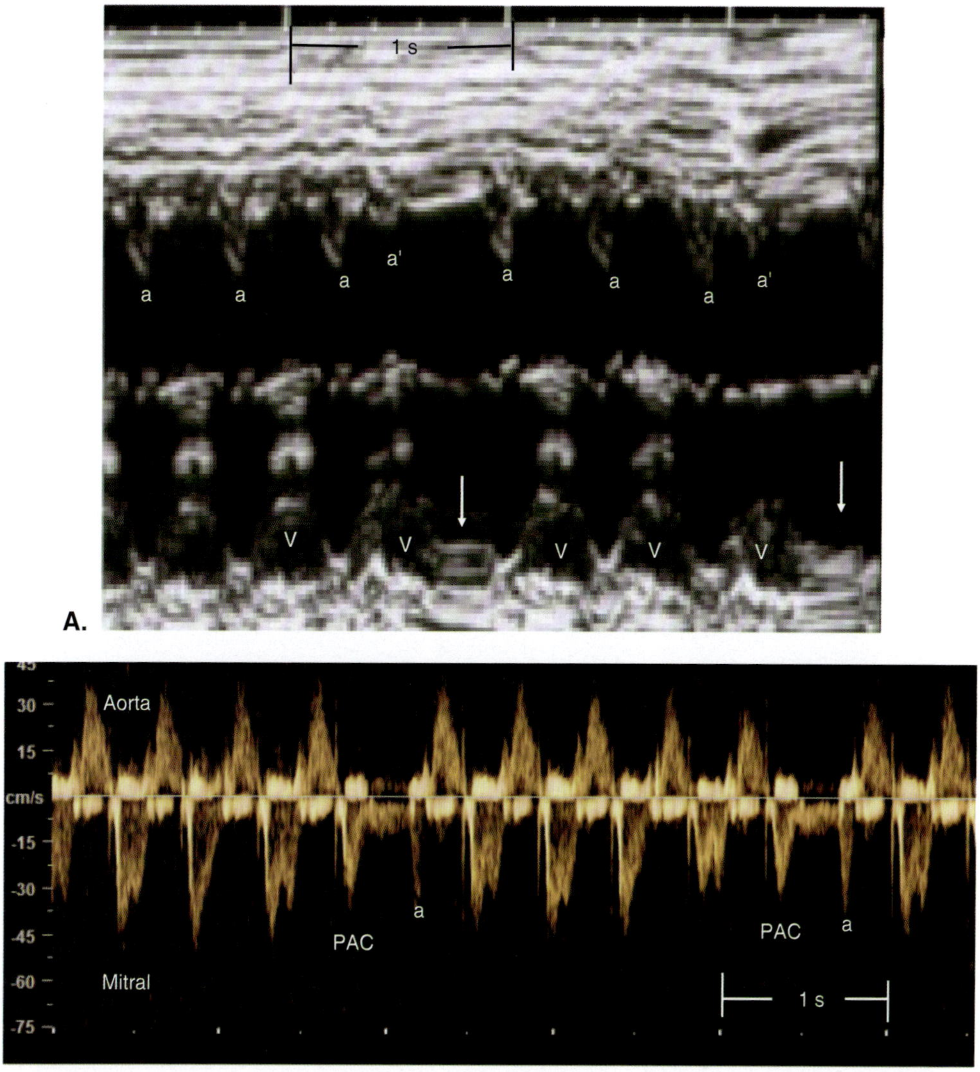

FIGURE 3.1.3 M-mode and spectral Doppler of premature atrial contractions (PACs). **A:** M-mode through the atrium (top) and ventricle (bottom). The normal atrial beats (a) are interrupted by a PAC (a′), which is not conducted to the ventricles (white arrow). **B:** Spectral Doppler. Biphasic mitral inflow is shown below baseline, and aortic outflow is above baseline. In the PAC, the mitral A-waves occur slightly before or simultaneously with the mitral E-wave; hence, there is a fused mitral A-wave. An atrial contraction (a) initiates the next ventricular contraction.

BAB can also be confused with type 1, 2° AV block (also known as Mobitz type 1 or Wenckebach). In type 1, 2° AV block, the interval between atrial and ventricular contraction consecutively lengthens until a sinus beat is nonconducted (see Part 3, Chapter 5). Distinguishing type 1, 2° AV block from BAB requires measurement of consecutive AV intervals until conduction blocks and ventricular activation fails. Type 1, 2° AV block can be diagnosed using SVC-Ao spectral Doppler or time velocity integral.[11,15]

(text continued on page 100)

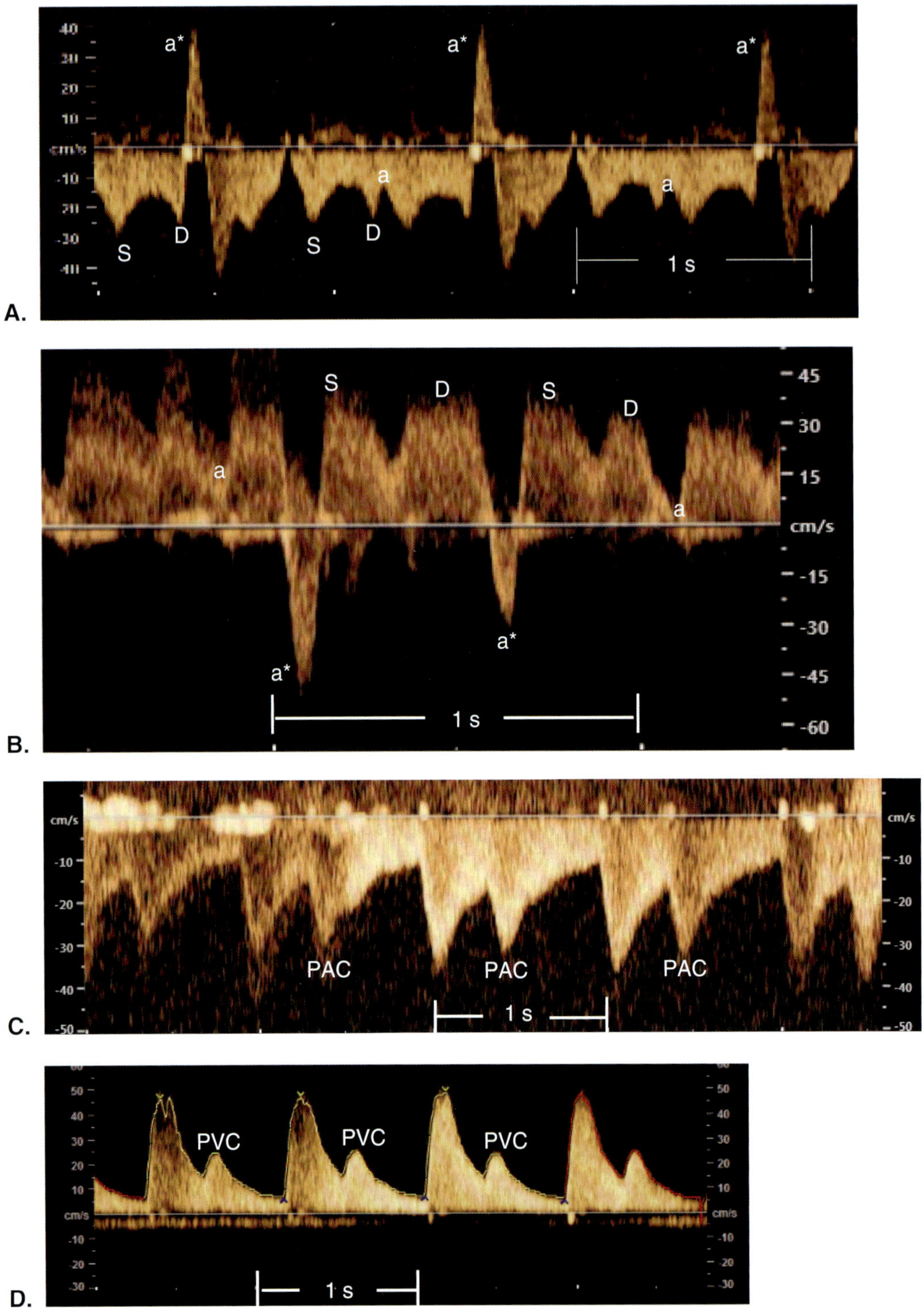

FIGURE 3.1.4 Spectral Doppler demonstrating the effects of ectopy on fetal veins and umbilical arterial (UA). **A:** Increased retrograde A-wave velocity (above baseline) in the pulmonary vein at the time of the premature atrial contraction (PAC) (a*), compared to the A-wave during sinus rhythm (a) (below baseline). **B:** Ductus venosus A-wave reversal (below baseline) during a PAC (a*) and sinus rhythm (a) (above baseline). **C:** Flow in the UA at the time of a PAC. **D:** Flow in the UA during a premature ventricular contraction (PVC). Note the difference in the peak flow velocity between the PAC and the PVC.

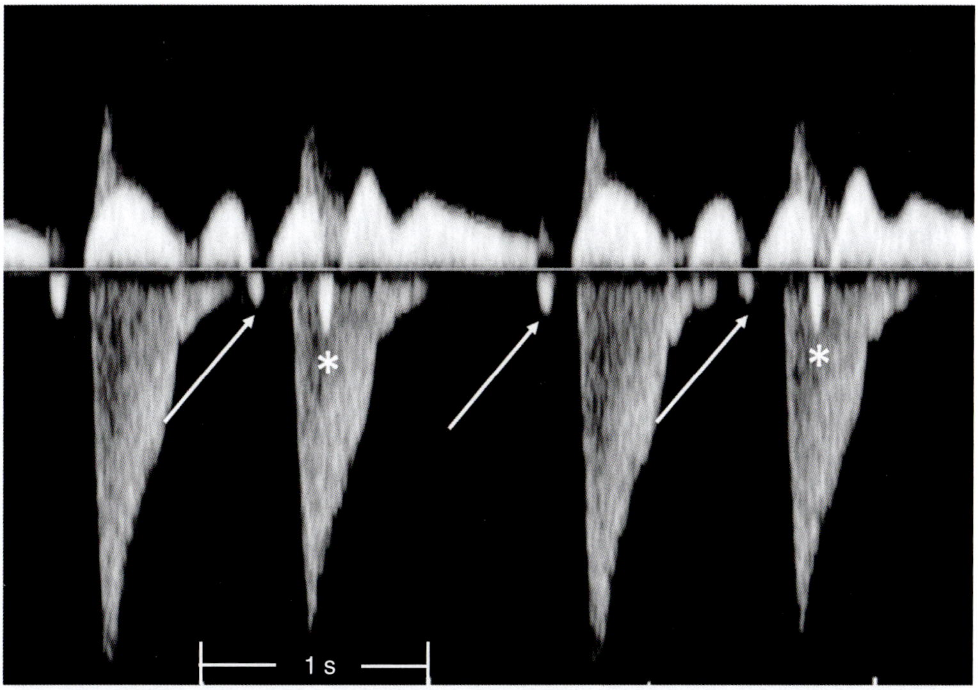

A.

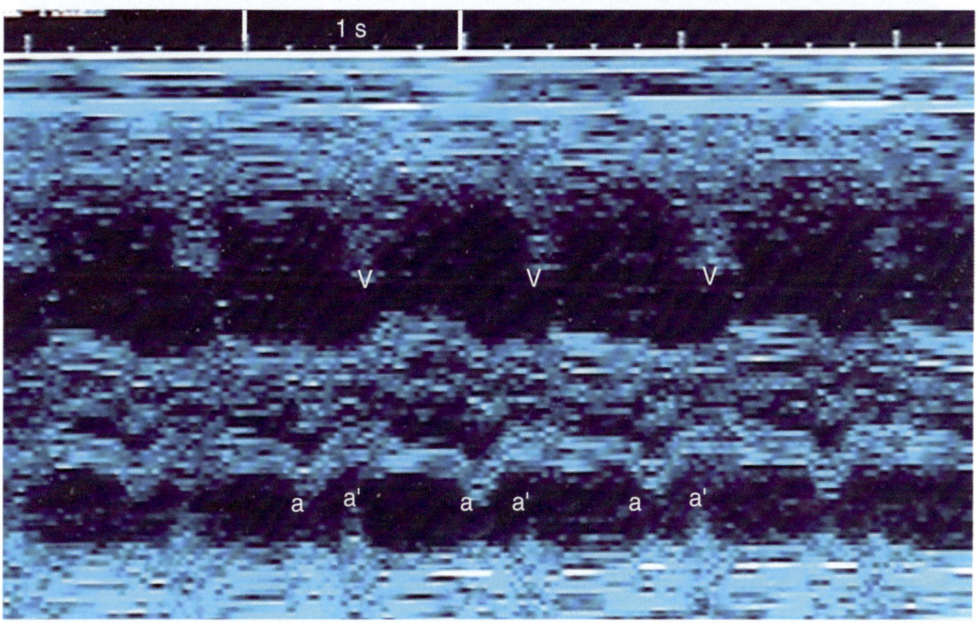

B.

FIGURE 3.1.5 Spectral Doppler and M-mode of conducted and nonconducted premature atrial contractions (PACs). **A:** Simultaneous superior vena cava (above baseline, except during atrial contractions) and aorta (below baseline) spectral Doppler. The first, second, fourth, and fifth (white arrows) atrial beats are conducted normally to the ventricles, but the third and sixth are very premature and not conducted (*). **B:** Simultaneous M-mode of atria (bottom panel) and ventricle (top panel). Note that the A-wave conducts to the ventricle (V) but the following premature atrial beat (a′) does not. This results in a ventricular bradycardia.

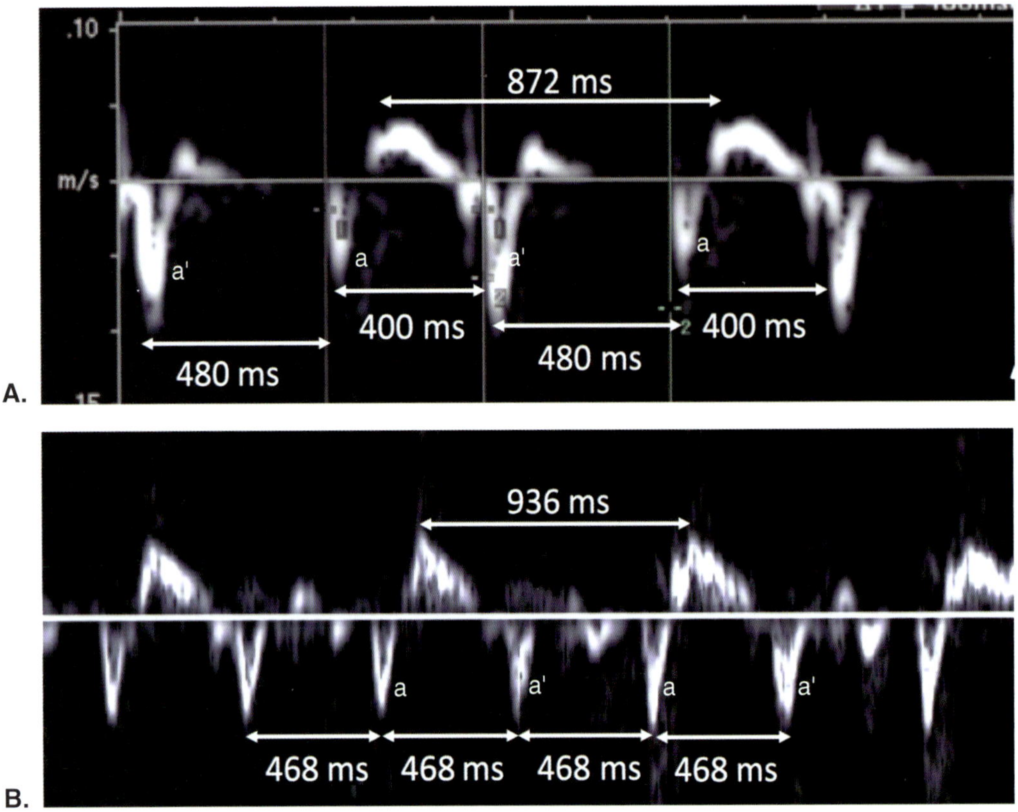

FIGURE 3.1.6 Tissue Doppler imaging (TDI) of lateral tricuspid annulus demonstrating blocked atrial bigeminy (BAB) and 2° atrioventricular (AV) block. Arial contractions are below baseline. (a), conducted atrial contraction; (a′), nonconducted atrial contraction. **A:** BAB. The cycle length is 872 ms. Note the variation in the atrial rate: a-a′ = 400 ms and a′-a = 480 ms. **B:** 2° AV block. The cycle length is 936 ms. The a-a′ and a′-a intervals are equal (468 ms).

The risk of developing a tachyarrhythmia (see Part 3, Chapter 2), most commonly AVRT, in the setting of atrial ectopy is <1%. The incidence is higher with complex atrial ectopy, including BAB.[1] Most reentrant tachyarrhythmias are initiated by a reentrant PAC and terminate with a blocked PAC[16] and require the presence of a pathway that will support tachycardia. Retrograde atrial activation occurs when an electrical impulse is transmitted from the ventricle up the fast pathway to the atria resulting in an early atrial contraction or "echo beat" that may not result in a sustained reentrant circuit if the AV node is still refractory. In the absence of a full electrocardiogram (ECG), an echo beat with subsequent block in the AV node looks very similar to a nonconducted PAC. Given the potential risk for tachyarrhythmia, the inability to exclude the presence of a pathway, and the fact that treatment can dramatically improve outcome for fetal tachycardias (see Part 4, Chapter 1), weekly follow-up with an obstetrician for fetal rhythm assessment has been recommended by consensus for frequent or complex ectopy until resolution.[7]

A. B.

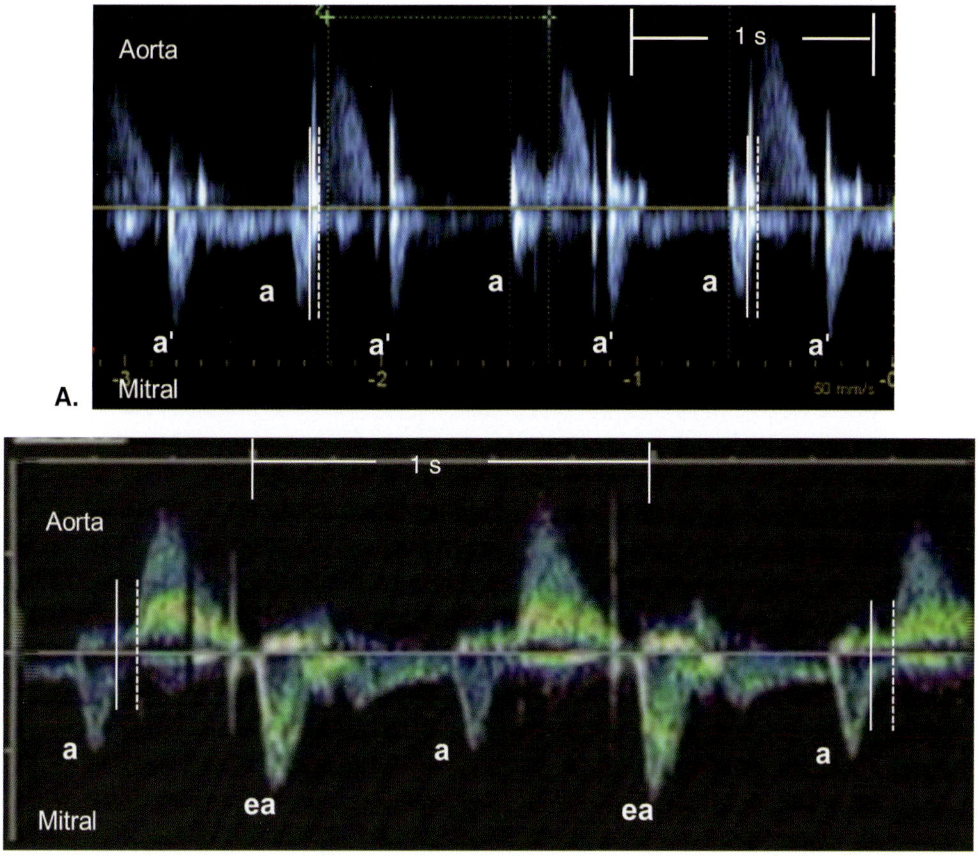

FIGURE 3.1.7 Spectral Doppler of mitral inflow (below baseline) and aortic outflow (above baseline) comparing isovolumic contraction time (IVCT) in blocked atrial bigeminy (BAB) and 2° atrioventricular (AV) block. The IVCT is measured from the end of atrial contraction to the beginning of ventricular contraction (from solid line to dotted line). **A:** In BAB, the IVCT is much shorter than in 2° AV block **(B)**. These findings help in differentiating these two rhythms.

If the fetal echocardiogram is otherwise normal, routine obstetric care can be resumed for the majority with no additional monitoring; reassurance should be provided to the expectant parents. In cases of frequent PACs (bigeminy, trigeminy, every fourth or fifth beat), weekly heart rhythm checks by the obstetrician are recommended until resolution of the arrhythmia.[7] Avoidance of maternal ingestion of cardiac stimulants is suggested if possible.[16] Treatment with antiarrhythmic medications is generally unnecessary and prognosis is good.

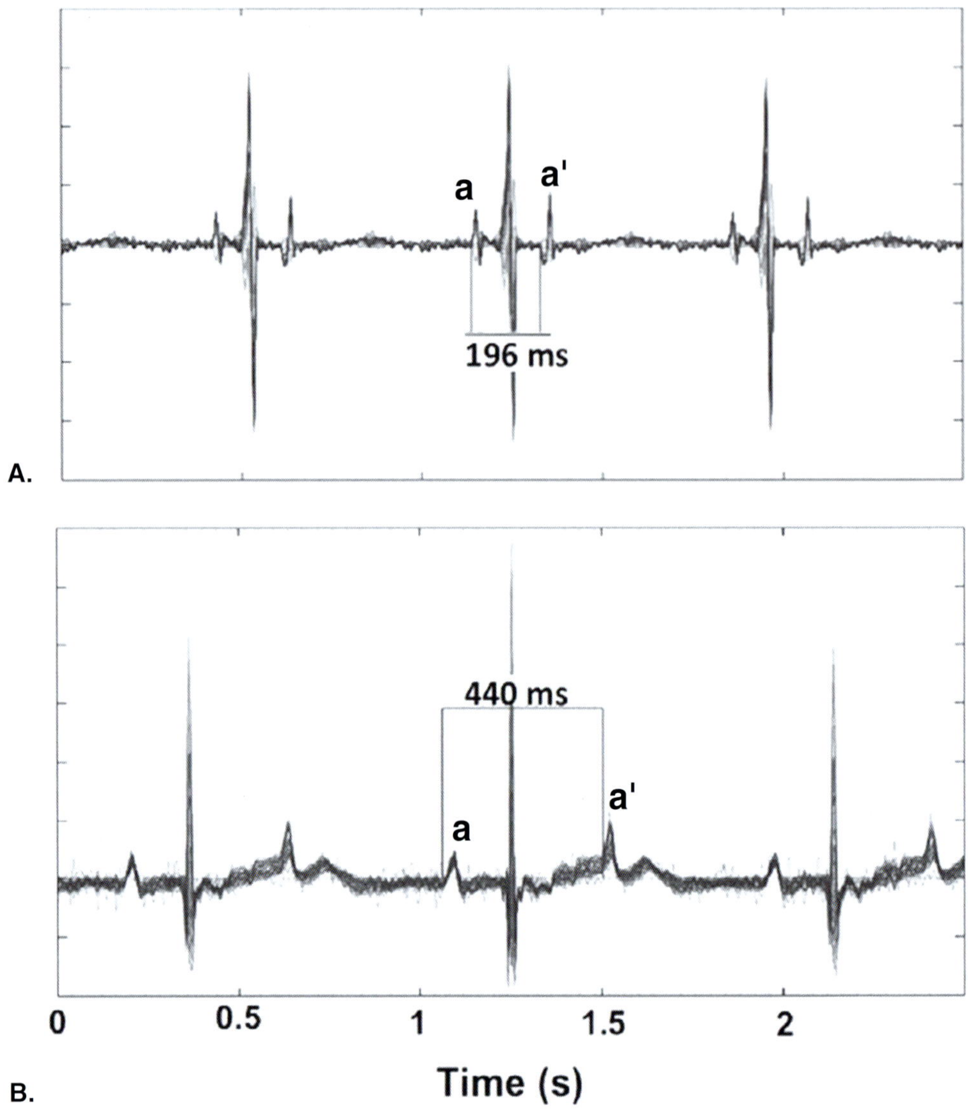

FIGURE 3.1.8 Signal-averaged magnetocardiograms of two fetuses with bradycardia. **A:** Blocked atrial bigeminy. The a-a′ interval is 196 ms and the a′-a interval is 504 ms. **B:** 2° atrioventricular block. The a-a′ and a′-a intervals are 440 ms. (Reprinted from Wiggins DL, Strasburger JF, Gotteiner NL, Cuneo B, Wakai RT. Magnetophysiologic and echocardiographic comparison of blocked atrial bigeminy and 2:1 atrioventricular block in the fetus. *Heart Rhythm*. 2013;10(8):1192-1198.)

PREMATURE VENTRICULAR CONTRACTIONS

PVCs originate from His-Purkinje system within the ventricles. Though seen in the newborn period,[10] PVCs are relatively uncommon in the fetus.[5] Although isolated PVCs are generally benign, evaluation is necessary to confirm the arrhythmia and distinguish it from PACs, assess heart function, and evaluate cardiac anatomy to exclude significant structural or functional pathology.

Diagnosis of PVCs proceeds in a similar manner as described for PACs. Using M-mode or spectral Doppler, atrial contractions will be seen to be entirely regular, while the PVC occurs without a preceding atrial contraction (FIG. 3.1.9). On M-mode, the ventricular free wall may show a distorted thickening pattern.[1] In the absence of AV node disease, normal ventricular contractions following the atrial beats may continue at the same rate (with an "interpolated" PVC) or the ventricle may remain refractory for a time until the next atrial contraction producing a noncompensatory pause—the basis for distinguishing PVCs from PACs based on arterial traces alone (FIG. 3.1.1B and C). Diagnosis of PVCs in the presence of AV dissociation and a regular ventricular escape rate may be more difficult.

In ventricular bigeminy, the ventricular rate is irregular, subsequent to the compensatory pause, but the atrial rate is regular (FIG. 3.1.10).[8]

Comorbidities are more likely to be present with PVCs in comparison to PACs. When accompanied by AV block, ventricular dysfunction or dilation, PVCs may be a harbinger of more concerning cardiac disease including LQTS,[17] myocarditis, or anti-Ro/SSA–mediated or infectious cardiomyopathy (FIG. 3.1.11).[5] Congenital ventricular wall aneurysms and diverticula are rare but can present with PVCs in the fetus, including bigeminy and trigeminy (FIG. 3.1.12).[18] Weekly heart rate monitoring has been recommended for fetuses with PVCs. However, if the fetal evaluation is otherwise normal, treatment is not necessary, and the prognosis is also good.

(text continued on page 106)

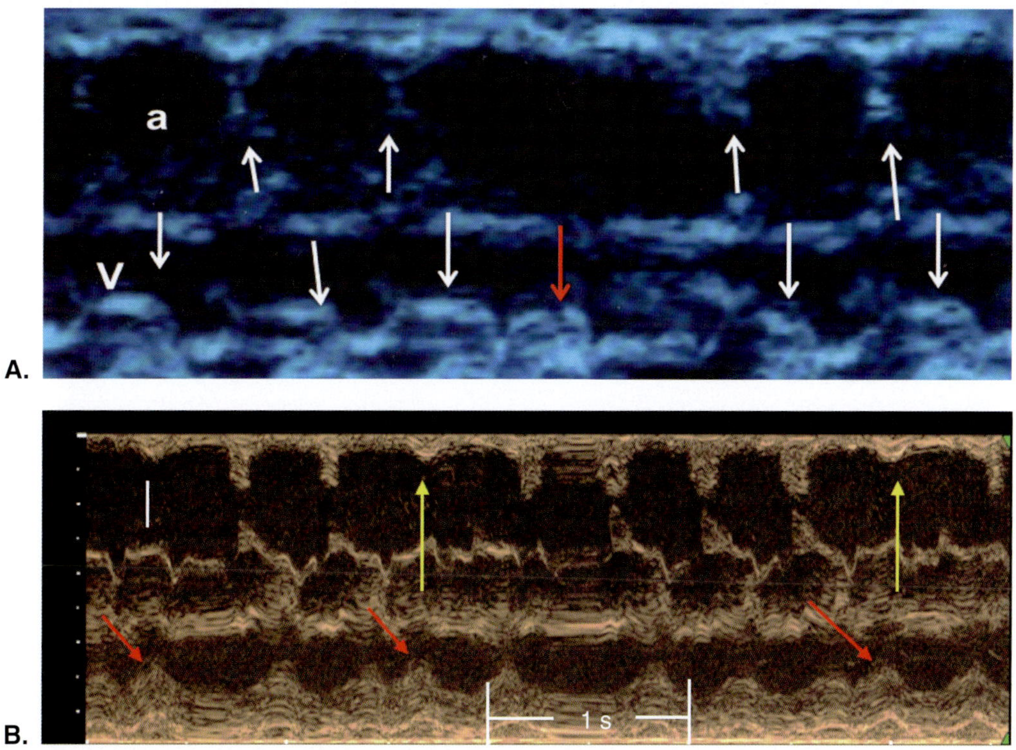

FIGURE 3.1.9 Simultaneous atrial (a) and ventricular (V) M-modes of isolated premature ventricular contraction (PVC). **A:** PVC (bottom panel, red arrow) with no retrograde conduction to the atrium (top panel, a). **B:** PVC (bottom panel, red arrows) with retrograde conduction to the atrium (top panel). Note the atrial contraction after the PVC is of different size and morphology than the other atrial beats.

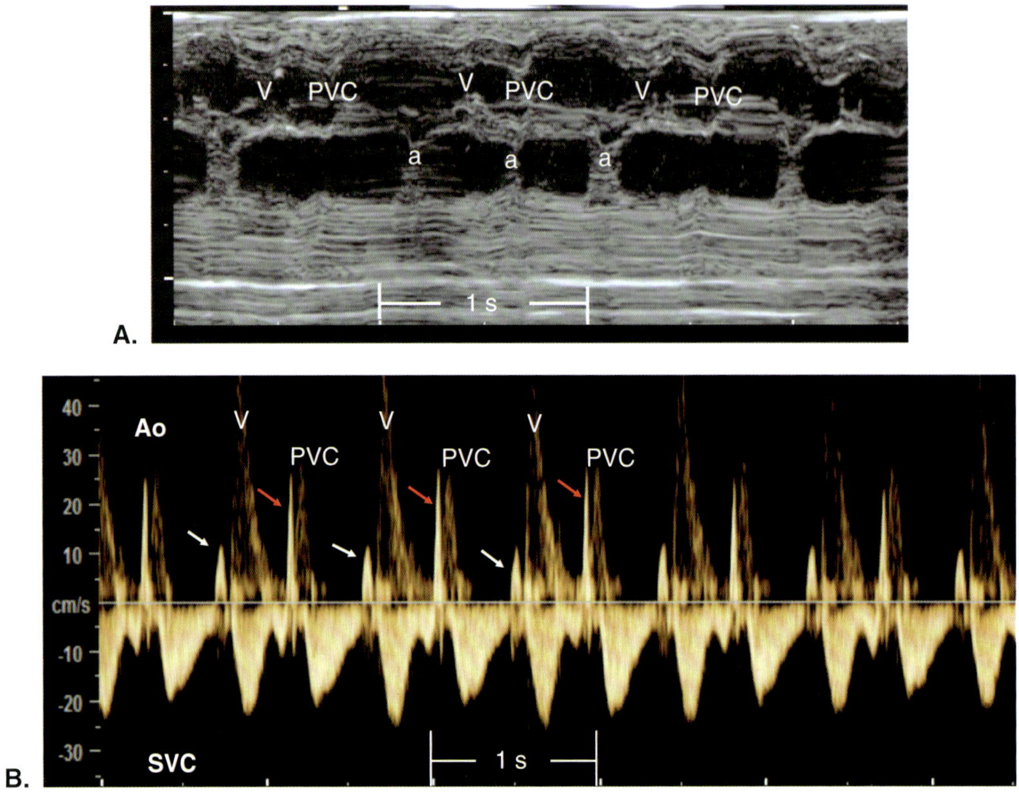

FIGURE 3.1.10 M-mode and spectral Doppler demonstrating ventricular bigeminy. **A:** M-mode showing normal ventricular beats (V) and premature ventricular contractions (PVCs) (top panel). Note the regular atrial rate (a). **B:** Simultaneous superior vena cava (SVC) (below baseline, except for atrial contractions) and aorta (Ao) (above baseline) spectral Doppler. The atrial rate is regular (arrows). The atrial contractions and the PVCs are almost simultaneous (PVC and red arrows), but it is the ventricular, not the atrial beats that are premature.

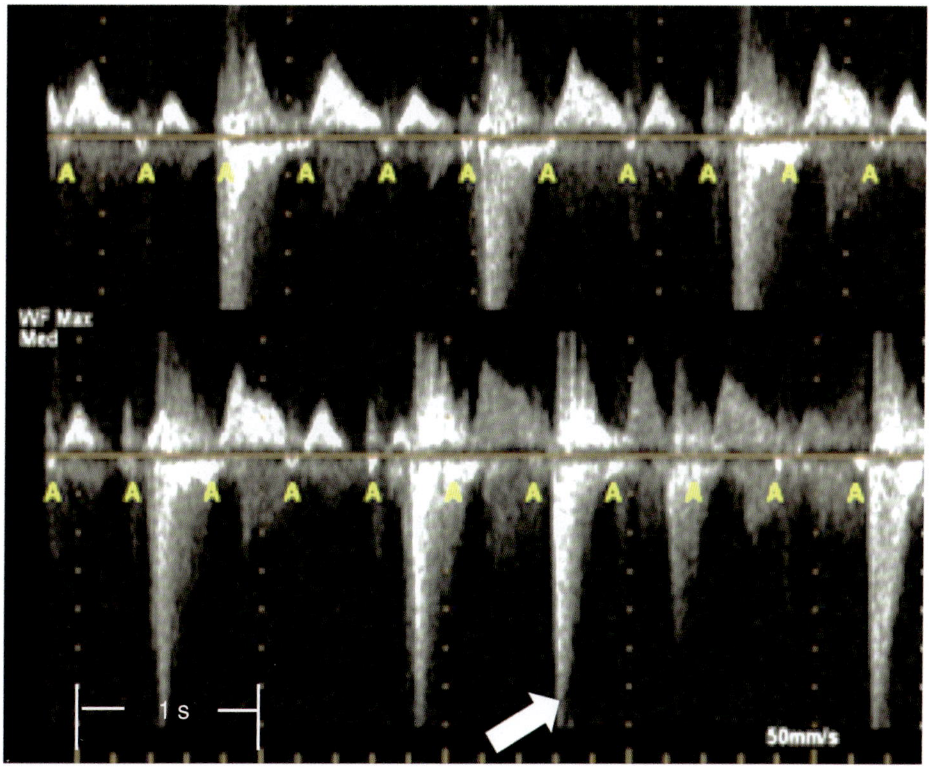

A.

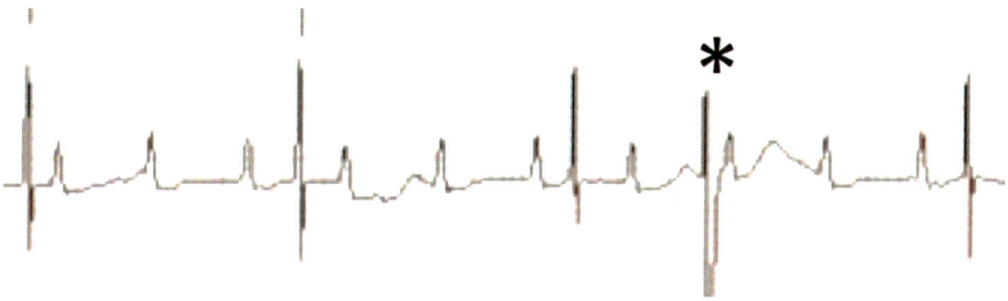

B.

FIGURE 3.1.11 Spectral Doppler and postnatal rhythm tracing of a fetus with anti-Ro/SSA antibody–mediated cardiomyopathy and 3° atrioventricular (AV) block. **A:** Superior vena cava-aorta Doppler demonstrating regular ventricular escape rate in the presence of AV dissociation. A ventricular ectopic beat (white arrow). The atrial rate in both Doppler images is 135 bpm and regular, and the ventricular rate is 42 bpm. The rhythm subsequently deteriorated to ventricular tachycardia and the fetus was urgently delivered preterm at 32 weeks, defibrillated, and stabilized with temporary pacing wires until a permanent pacing system could be placed. She ultimately survived with a permanent pacing system. **B:** The single premature ventricular contraction (*) in the presence of 3° AV block.

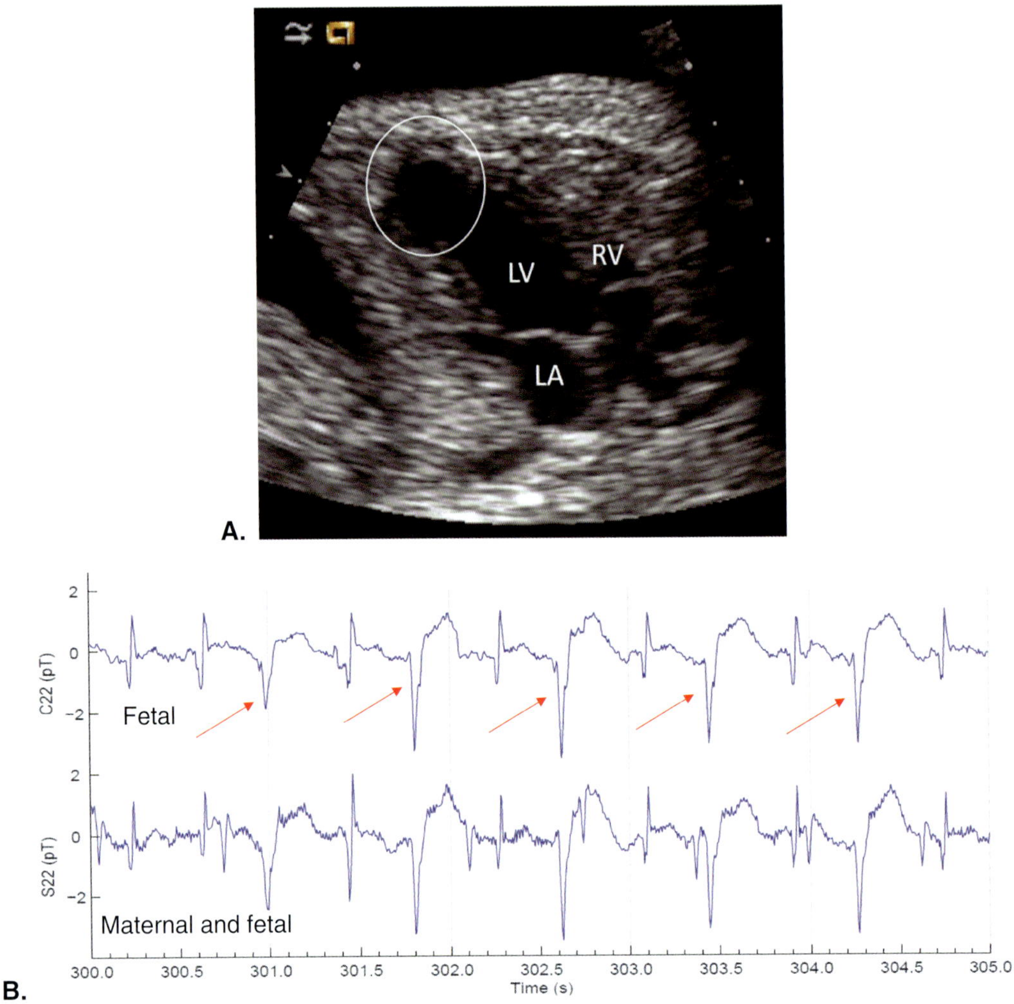

FIGURE 3.1.12 Two-dimensional image and fetal magnetocardiography (fMCG) tracing of a 32-week fetus with a small left ventricular aneurysm and an irregular rhythm. **A:** The small apical LV aneurysm (circle) (LA, left atrium; LV, left ventricle; RV, right ventricle). **B:** fMCG (top tracing: of fetal rhythm; bottom tracing fetal and maternal rhythm) demonstrating the monomorphic premature ventricular contractions (red arrows).

SUMMARY

Fetal ectopy, comprising PACs and PVCs, occurs in up to 3% of pregnancies and is a frequent reason for referral for fetal echocardiography. PACs are more common toward the end of pregnancy. PACs are at least 10 times more common than PVCs. Atrial bigeminy, trigeminy, or blocked PACs pose a higher likelihood of associated initiation of fetal SVT. Fetal cardiac evaluation is recommended for PACs and PVCs to evaluate the underlying arrhythmia and exclude the presence of concomitant congenital heart disease. However, medical treatment is rarely needed. A fetal echo should also be considered if the ectopy occurs between 18 and 24 weeks of gestation, as it is not possible by auscultation to differentiate ectopy (needs no treatment) from type 1 or intermittent type 2, 2° AV block (treatment may prevent progression to 3° AV block). In the setting of AV block, ventricular dysfunction, or dilation, PVCs can be a marker of cardiomyopathy, LQTS, or myocarditis.

Simple atrial ectopy can be followed by weekly auscultation of heart to be sure fetal SVT has not developed (TABLE 3.1.1). The parents should be reassured the fetus does not have a "heart problem" and if the ectopy persists, it almost always resolves in the newborn period.

TABLE 3.1.1 FETAL ECTOPY: APPROXIMATE FREQUENCY, ASSOCIATIONS, AND RECOMMENDATIONS FOR FOLLOW-UP AND MANAGEMENT

	Frequency	Association	Recommendation
PAC	1%-3% of pregnancies More common in third trimester	Usually benign Foramen ovale aneurysm, congenital heart disease, and rhabdomyomas ~0.5% associated with SVT, higher with BAB	• Fetal heart assessment for anatomy, function, rhythm • Weekly FHR checks with OB/MFM if frequent PACs, until arrhythmia resolves • Prompt referral to fetal cardiologist if tachycardia develops • Avoidance of cardiac stimulants • Postnatal ECG if persists
PVC	Relatively uncommon True prevalence unknown	Long QT syndrome (including spontaneous mutations) In setting of AV block, ventricular dysfunction, or dilation, consider myocarditis, infectious or immune-mediated cardiomyopathy Rarely congenital ventricular aneurysm or diverticula	• Fetal echocardiogram for anatomy, function, rhythm • Consider fetal magnetocardiogram to assess for long QT • Weekly FHR checks with OB/MFM until resolves • Prompt referral to fetal cardiologist if tachycardia develops • Avoidance of cardiac stimulants • Postnatal ECG
BAB	Prevalence unknown	Usually benign Increased risk of co-occurring SVT May be misinterpreted as fetal bradycardia Important to distinguish from 2:1 AV block and Wenckebach	• Fetal echocardiogram to assess anatomy, function, and rhythm • Weekly FHR checks with OB/MFM until resolves • Prompt referral for fetal echocardiogram if tachycardia develops • Avoidance of cardiac stimulants • Postnatal ECG if persists

AV, atrioventricular; BAB, blocked atrial bigeminy; ECG, electrocardiogram; FHR, fetal heart rate; OB/MFM, obstetrician/maternal-fetal medicine physician; PAC, premature atrial contraction; PVC, premature ventricular contraction; SVT, supraventricular tachycardia.

References

1. Strasburger JF. Fetal arrhythmia. *Prog Pediatr Cardiol.* 2000;11:1-17.
2. Matta M, Cuneo B. Doppler echocardiography for managing fetal arrhythmia. *Clin Obstet Gynecol.* 2010;53(4):899-914.
3. Kleinman C. Prenatal diagnosis and management of intrauterine arrhythmias. *Fetal Ther.* 1986;1:92-95.
4. Southall DP, Richards J, Hardwick RA, et al. Prospective study of fetal heart rate and rhythm patterns. *Arch Dis Child.* 1980;55:506-511.
5. Strasburger J, Cheulkar B, Whichman H. Fetal arrhythmia: diagnosis and management. *Clin Perinatol.* 2007;34(4):627-652.
6. Naheed ZJ, Strasburger JF, Deal BJ, Benson DW Jr, Gidding SS. Fetal tachycardia: mechanisms and predictors of hydrops fetalis. *J Am Coll Cardiol.* 1996;27(7):1736-1740.
7. Donofrio M, Moon-Grady AJ, Hornberger LK, et al. Diagnosis and treatment of fetal cardiac disease: a scientific statement for the American Heart Association. *Circulation.* 2014;129:2183-2242.
8. Fouron JC, Proulx C, Miro J, Gosselin J. Doppler and M-mode ultrasonography to time fetal atrial and ventricular contractions. *Obstet Gynecol.* 2000;96(5):732-736.
9. Nagashima M, Matsushima M, Ogawa A, et al. Cardiac arrhythmias in healthy children revealed by 24-hour ambulatory ECG monitoring. *Pediatr Cardiol.* 1987;8:103-108.
10. Copel JA, Liang RI, Demasio K, Ozeren S, Kleinman CS. The clinical significance of the irregular fetal heart rhythm. *Am J Obstet Gynecol.* 2000;182(4):813-819.
11. Tutschek B, Schmidt KG. Pulsed-wave tissue Doppler echocardiography for the analysis of fetal cardiac arrhythmias. *Ultrasound Obstet Gynecol.* 2011;38:406-412.
12. Toro L, Weintraub RG, Shiota T, et al. Relation between persistent atrial arrhythmias and redundant septum primum flap (atrial septal aneurysm) in fetuses. *Am J Cardiol.* 1994;73:711-713.
13. Sonesson SE, Eliasson H, Conner P, Wahren-Herlenius. Doppler echocardiographic isovolumetric time intervals in diagnosis of fetal blocked atrial bigeminy and 2:1 atrioventricular block. *Ultrasound Obstet Gyencol.* 2014;44:171-175.
14. Wiggens DL. Magnetophysiologic and echocardiographic comparison of blocked atrial bigeminy and 2:1 atrioventricular block in the fetus. *Heart Rhythm.* 2013;10(8):1192-1198.
15. Raboisson MJ. Fetal Doppler echocardiographic diagnosis and successful steroid therapy of Luciani-Wenckebach phenomenon and endocardial fibroelastosis related to maternal anti-Ro and anti-La antibodies. *J Am Soc Echocardiogr.* 2005;18:375-380.
16. Wakai RT, Strasburger JF, Li Z, Deal BJ, Gotteiner NL. Magnetocardiographic rhythm patterns at initiation and termination of fetal supraventricular tachycardia. *Circulation.* 2003;107:307-312.
17. Cuneo BF, Strasburger JE, Wakai RT. The natural history of fetal long QT syndrome. *J Electrocardiol.* 2016;49:807-813.
18. Peters C, Wacker-Gussmann A, Strasburger JF, et al. Electrophysiologic features of fetal ventricular aneurysms and diverticula. *Prenat Diagn.* 2015;35:129-136.

Supraventricular Tachyarrhythmias

Stacy Ann Stratemann Killen • Frank A. Fish

INTRODUCTION

The supraventricular tachyarrhythmias (SVT) include incessant and/or paroxysmal episodes of increased fetal heart rates ≥180 beats per minute (bpm). SVT may be confined to the atria as seen in atrial ectopic tachycardia (AET) or atrial flutter (AF). Alternatively, SVT may be due to a reciprocating rhythm involving both the atria and ventricles utilizing the atrioventricular (AV) node and an accessory connection, as exemplified by atrioventricular reentrant tachycardia (AVRT) and permanent junctional reciprocating tachycardia (PJRT). In this chapter, the abbreviation "SVT" refers to all the supraventricular tachyarrhythmias. This chapter will describe the mechanism, presentation, and assessment of fetal SVT, which complicate 0.5% of pregnancies and is associated with morbidity and mortality.[1-3]

TACHYCARDIA EVALUATION

Echocardiographic evaluation of fetal tachycardias, using M-mode (through atria and ventricles) and spectral Doppler (left ventricular inflow and outflow, superior vena cava and ascending aorta/innominate vein and transverse aorta, pulmonary artery and pulmonary vein), should seek to determine the atrial and ventricular rates, the relationship of atrial and ventricular contractions, and the onset and termination of tachycardia.[4-9] Atrial and ventricular M-mode or spectral Doppler venous and atrial flow signals infer atrial (A) and ventricular (V) contractions[5] and are analogous to P-wave and R-wave seen on an electrocardiogram (ECG).

Fetal position, activity, and image resolution can limit echocardiographic assessment of fetal rhythm. When simultaneous assessment of atrial and ventricular motion cannot be made by traditional M-mode, color M-mode allows the aortic outflow Doppler signal to overlie the M-mode atrial signal; mechanical and flow events are displayed simultaneously[9] (FIG. 3.2.1). This technique can be especially helpful in understanding atrial and ventricular relationships during tachycardia.

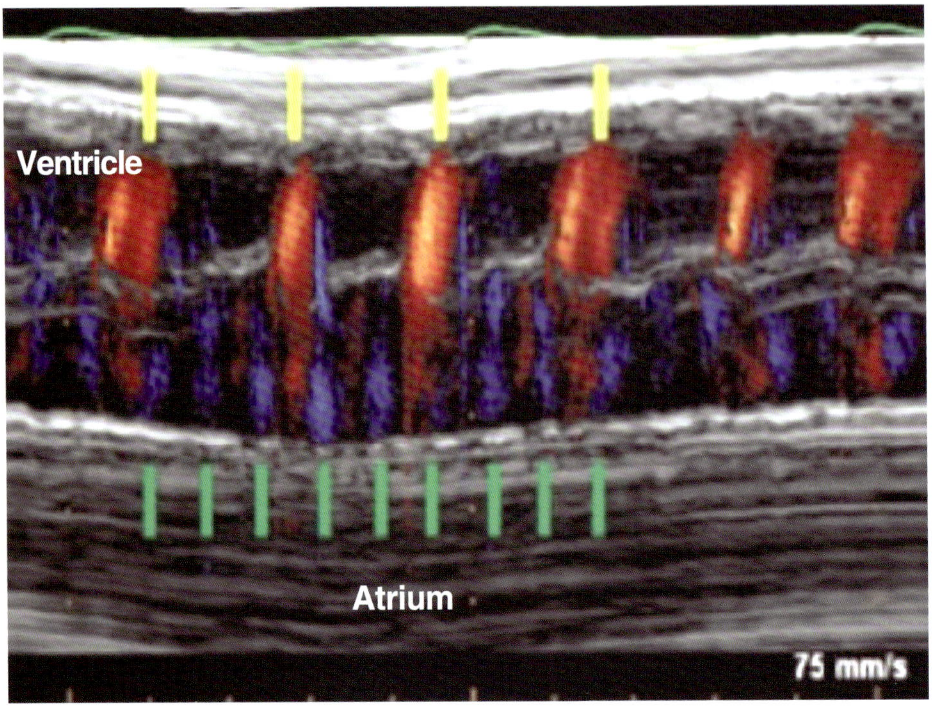

FIGURE 3.2.1 Color M-mode during atrial flutter. The atrial contractions (bottom line, green arrows) occur at twice the rate of the ventricular contractions (top line, yellow arrows). (Reprinted from Detterich JA, Pruetz J, Sklansky MS. Color M-mode sonography for evaluation of fetal arrhythmias. *J Ultrasound Med*. 2012;31(10):1681-1688.)

Echocardiography can also assess the effects of tachycardia on hemodynamics. Notching in the umbilical vein, hydrops, and atrioventricular valve insufficiency are all signs of a compromised fetus. Even after sinus rhythm has been restored, Doppler waveforms may take several days to normalize (FIG. 3.2.2).

Other techniques to assess fetal tachycardia include fetal magnetocardiography and fetal electrocardiography, which are described in Part 2, Chapter 3 and Part 6, Chapter 1, respectively.

A.

B.

C.

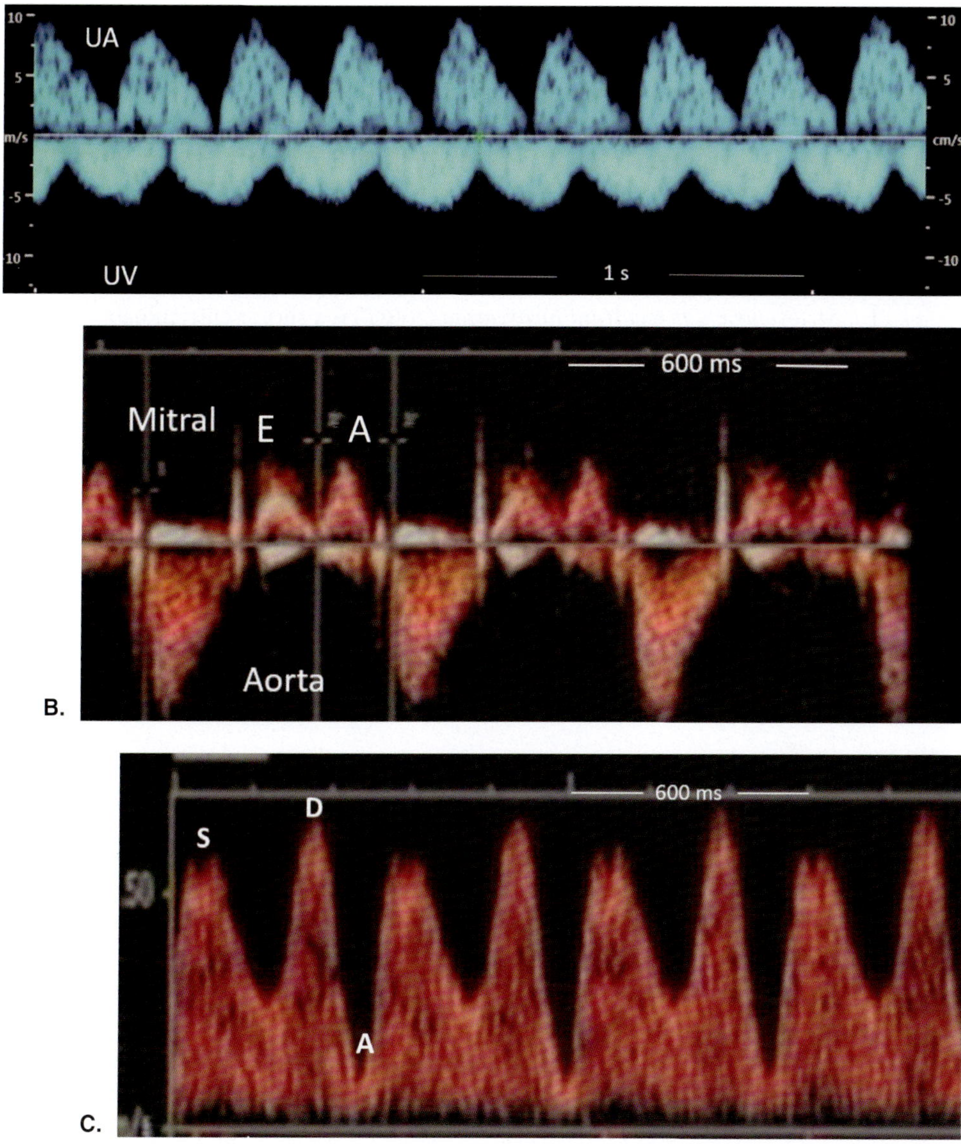

FIGURE 3.2.2 Spectral Doppler findings during and immediately after supraventricular tachyarrhythmia (SVT). **A:** Umbilical artery (UA) (top) and umbilical vein (UV) in a severely hydropic fetus during SVT. Note the notching in the vein and the reduced end-diastolic flow in the artery. **B:** Mitral inflow (above baseline)/aortic outflow (below baseline) in a fetus with recently converted atrial flutter. The velocity of the mitral A-wave, which normally should be higher than the velocity of the E-wave, is diminished, probably due to atrial fatigue after prolonged atrial flutter. A-wave velocity increased after several weeks in sinus rhythm. The AV interval in this fetus is prolonged (~180 ms) secondary to antiarrhythmic treatment. **C:** Ductus venosus in the same fetus. The A-wave is very close to baseline. This finding improved in several days after tachycardia conversion.

TACHYCARDIA MECHANISMS

Fetal SVT represents about 10% of fetal arrhythmias.[1,10] Associated congenital heart disease occurs in ~5% to 10% of fetuses with SVT.[1,10] Morbidity is a function of fetal gestational age and the proportion of time in tachycardia. Interestingly, AVRT has a longer cycle length (slower heart rate) in the fetus than in the neonate.[11] AVRT (60%-70%) and AF (30%) are the most commonly observed SVT types.[12,13]

This chapter will focus on four primary mechanisms that produce SVT (TABLE 3.2.1):

1. *Atrioventricular reentrant tachycardia (AVRT)* is a short ventriculoatrial (VA) tachycardia that involves the AV node for antegrade conduction and a retrograde-conducting accessory AV connection.
2. *Permanent junctional reciprocating tachycardia (PJRT)*, a long VA tachycardia, is a variant of AVRT with reentry across a concealed slow retrograde-conducting accessory connection.
3. *Atrial ectopic tachycardia (AET)*, another long VA tachycardia, is due to enhanced automaticity of atrial tissue rather than reentry.
4. *Atrial flutter (AF)*, which is due to macro-reentry within the atrial myocardium and is characteristically associated with AV block of varying degree.

These mechanisms are identified in the fetus by the respective heart rates and timing relationships of the atria and ventricles (TABLE 3.2.2).

Atrioventricular Reentrant Tachycardia (Figs. 3.2.3 and 3.2.4)

AVRT, the most common type of fetal SVT, may demonstrate sudden onset (paroxysmal) and termination of tachycardia. AVRT is a reentrant or reciprocating (the terms can be used interchangeably) tachycardia involving the atria, ventricles, AV node, and an accessory connection.[14] AVRT has a fixed 1:1 relationship between atrial and ventricular contraction with rates of 210 to 320 bpm. Typically, there is little heart rate variability. Onset is most commonly between 18- and 32-weeks gestation. The typical form of AVRT involves ventricular activation occurring through the normal conduction system and atrial re-activation initiated via an accessory AV connection. The accessory connection completes a reentrant circuit, and reciprocating antegrade-retrograde conduction perpetuates the circuit.[13] Characteristically, the VA interval is shorter than the AV interval ("short VA" tachycardia). Thus, the VA interval is less than half of the cardiac cycle length and the VA/AV ratio is <1. The tachycardia rate is related to the rel-

TABLE 3.2.1 ETIOLOGIES OF FETAL SUPRAVENTRICULAR TACHYARRHYTHMIA

Supraventricular tachycardia	• Accessory connections
	  • Atrioventricular reentrant tachycardia/orthodromic reciprocating tachycardia
	  • Permanent junctional reciprocating tachycardia
	  • Atrioventricular nodal reentrant tachycardia
	• Atrial foci
	  • Atrial ectopic tachycardia
	  • Atrial flutter

TABLE 3.2.2 CHARACTERISTICS OF FETAL SUPRAVENTRICULAR TACHYCARDIAS

SVT Category	Gestational Age	Typical Rates	AV Relationship	Onset/Termination
Short VA AVRT/ORT AVNRT (faster and later)	>18 wk	>180 bpm (200-320 bpm)	1:1 VA interval < half of the VV interval VA/AV ratio <1	Sudden onset/offset Blocks in the AV node and terminates with a nonconducted atrial beat
Long VA AET PJRT (slower and earlier)	>12 wk	170-220 bpm	1:1 but may be variable (AET) VA interval > half of the VV interval VA/AV ratio >1	Gradual onset and offset (AET) Terminates with a nonconducted ventricular beat (AET)
Atrial flutter (variable AV conduction)	>28 wk	Atrial rate 300-550 bpm Ventricular rate 180-240 bpm	Variable degrees of AV block (primarily 2:1 or 3:1); fixed/unvarying ventricular rate	

AET, atrial ectopic tachycardia; AV, atrioventricular; AVNRT, atrioventricular nodal reentrant tachycardia; AVRT, atrioventricular reentrant tachycardia; ORT, orthodromic reciprocating tachycardia; PJRT, permanent junctional reciprocating tachycardia; SVT, supraventricular tachyarrhythmia; VA, ventriculoatrial.

ative conduction properties of the accessory connection and the AV node. Tachycardia onset is triggered by an initiating event, usually a PAC,[15,16] and begins abruptly. There may be repeated self-limited episodes or tachycardia may remain incessant. If either the AV node or the accessory connection fails to transmit a single impulse, reentry terminates, which is the reason that antiarrhythmic agents that slow conduction across the AV node often successfully terminate reentrant SVT.

(text continued on page 116)

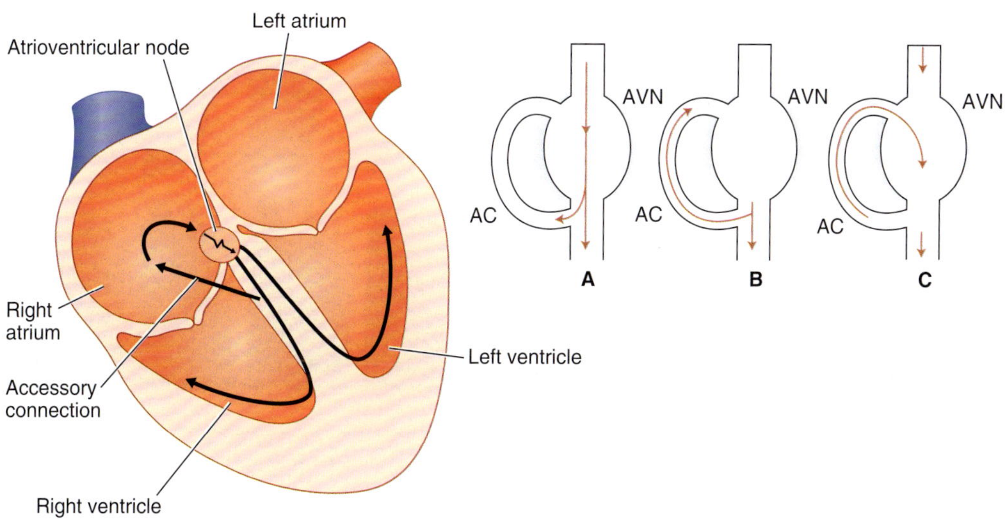

FIGURE 3.2.3 Diagram of atrioventricular reentrant tachycardia. *A,* Antegrade conduction down the AVN. *B,* Retrograde conduction up the accessory connection (AC). *C,* Circuit of rapid conduction maintained by conduction from the AC down the AVN and back up the AC. AVN, atrioventricular node. (Modified from Jones RM. *Patient Assessment in Pharmacy Practice*. 3rd ed. Philadelphia, PA: Wolters Kluwer; 2015 and Gant L, Lebowitz D, Rosario J, Vera A. *Step-Up to USMLE Step 2 CK*. 5th ed. Philadelphia, PA: Wolters Kluwer; 2019.)

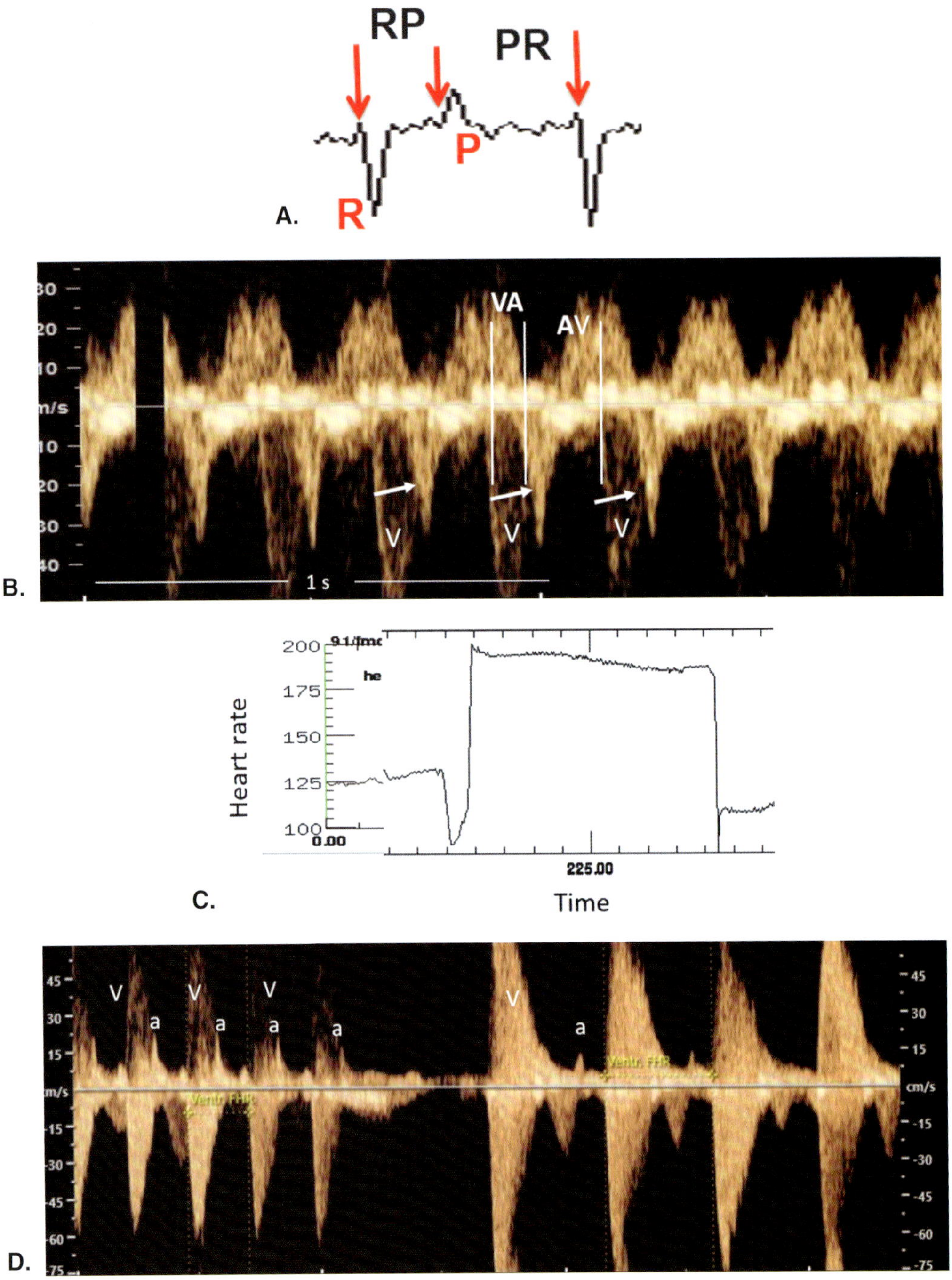
RP
PR
P
R
A.
VA
AV
V
V
V
1 s
B.
200
175
150
125
100
0.00
Heart rate
225.00
Time
C.
V
a
V
a
V
a
a
V
a
Ventr. FHR
cm/s
D.

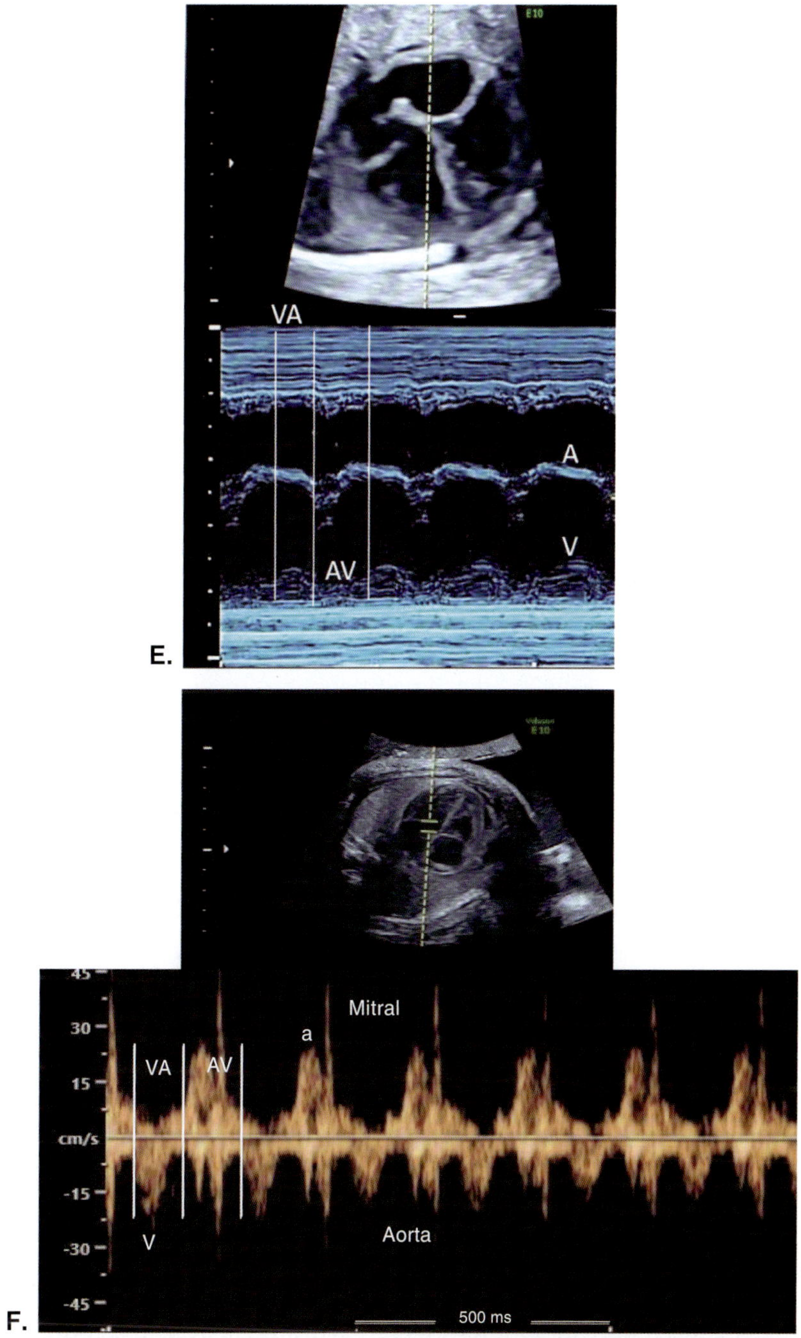

FIGURE 3.2.4 Rhythm tracing and Doppler findings in short RP (ventriculoatrial, VA) tachycardia. **A:** The (electrical) R-P interval on the ECG corresponds to the (mechanical) V-A interval on the spectral Doppler **(B)**. **B:** Superior vena cava/aorta (SVC/Ao) spectral Doppler. Atrial events are represented by reverse flow in the SVC (arrows, below baseline) and ventricular events are demonstrated by aortic outflow (V, below baseline). Note the V-A interval is shorter than the A-V interval. **C:** Characteristics of a reentrant tachycardia mechanism. There are paroxysms of tachycardia which begin and end abruptly. **D:** SVC/Ao spectral Doppler tracing showing termination of AVRT with resumption of sinus rhythm. The last beat is a nonconducted atrial beat (a), indicating that the tachycardia blocks in the atrioventricular (AV) node. This observation excludes the possibility of automatic atrial tachycardia (atrial ectopic tachycardia). **E:** M-mode of short VA tachycardia with VA and AV intervals demonstrated. **F:** Mitral inflow/aortic outflow of short VA tachycardia with VA and AV intervals calculated.

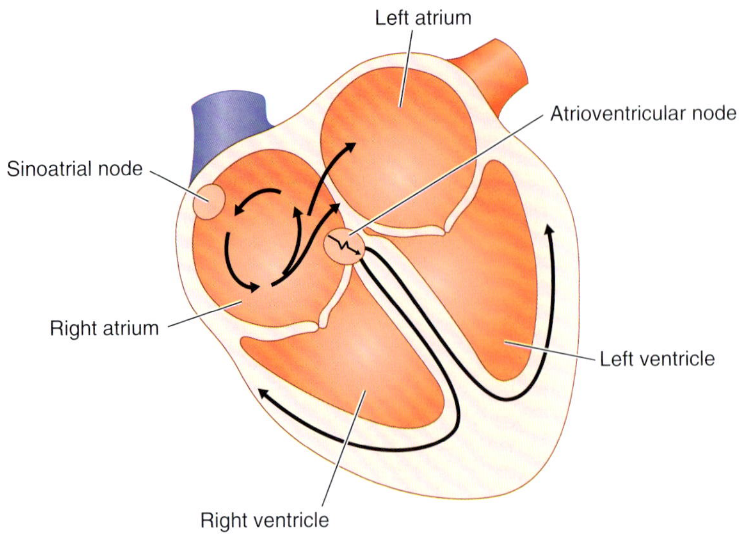

FIGURE 3.2.5 Diagram of atrial flutter. The circle in the right atrium indicates reentry within the atrium. (Modified from Jones RM. *Patient Assessment in Pharmacy Practice*. 3rd ed. Philadelphia, PA: Wolters Kluwer; 2015.)

Atrial Flutter (Figs. 3.2.5 and 3.2.6)

AF is the second most common type of SVT[17] and usually presents after 28 weeks gestation.[16,17] In the fetus, AF is thought to be caused by intra-atrial reentry. About 70% of fetuses with AF also have accessory connections.[17-21] The mechanism for the alternation between AVRT and AF is not well understood, but in the absence of underlying intrinsic heart disease, it is thought to result from premature atrial depolarization, presumably during increased atrial vulnerability in tachycardia.[19] This explains why, in some cases, medications that block the AV node may prevent recurrences of AF.

Episodes of AF are often initiated and terminated by premature atrial contractions.[20] Atrial rates typically range from 300 to 500 bpm with slower ventricular rates of 150 to 250 bpm due to variable degrees of block (primarily 2:1 AV conduction) within the AV node.[22] AF can also be associated with myocarditis, congenital heart disease (20%-30%), and immune-mediated heart block/carditis.[23,24]

Permanent Junctional Reciprocating Tachycardia (Fig. 3.2.7)

PJRT is a much rarer form of reentrant SVT that occurs via an accessory connection, with slow retrograde conductive properties.[25,26] PJRT is one of the long VA tachycardias with a VA interval that is more than half of the cardiac cycle length and a VA/AV ratio >1 (FIG. 3.2.8). PJRT differs from the other long VA tachycardias, for example, AET (FIG. 3.2.9), because the latter has an automatic, not a reentrant, mechanism. The relatively slow tachycardia rates (170-220 bpm) of PJRT favor both the perpetuation of reentry and the reinitiation of tachycardia. PJRT initiates with an atrial beat and terminates with an atrial beat, as the AV node is involved in the reentry circuit (FIG. 3.2.8E). Long VA SVT may occur as early as 12 weeks gestation.[27] Because long VA tachycardias have slower rates and atrial contraction during ventricular diastole, they are less likely to cause hydrops. Even so, they are usually incessant and, thus, predispose to depressed ventricular function.

Atrial Ectopic Tachycardia (Figs. 3.2.9 and 3.2.10)

AET is usually due to abnormal atrial automaticity arising from a nonsinus atrial pacemaker that surpasses the rate of the sinus node.[26] Atrial rates may vary but over short periods of time, tend to display perpetual, monotonous behavior. This type of SVT may demonstrate variable AV conduction, depending upon the atrial rate and conduction properties of the AV node. Ventricular rates typically range from 170 to 220 bpm and gradually increase and decrease at initiation and cessation of tachycardia, respectively.[26] Since the AV node is not involved in the tachycardia circuit, AET usually terminates with a ventricular contraction (**FIGS. 3.2.8E** and **3.2.10B**).

It can be difficult to distinguish AET from PJRT. Gozar and colleagues[28] described mildly increasing abdominal pressure during the fetal echo to initiate a vagal response. In AET, this maneuver resulted in a progressively decreasing heart rate or blocked atrial contractions. In fetuses with PJRT, this did not occur.

FIG. 3.2.11 describes a question and answer approach to diagnose the fetus with SVT.

(text continued on page 123)

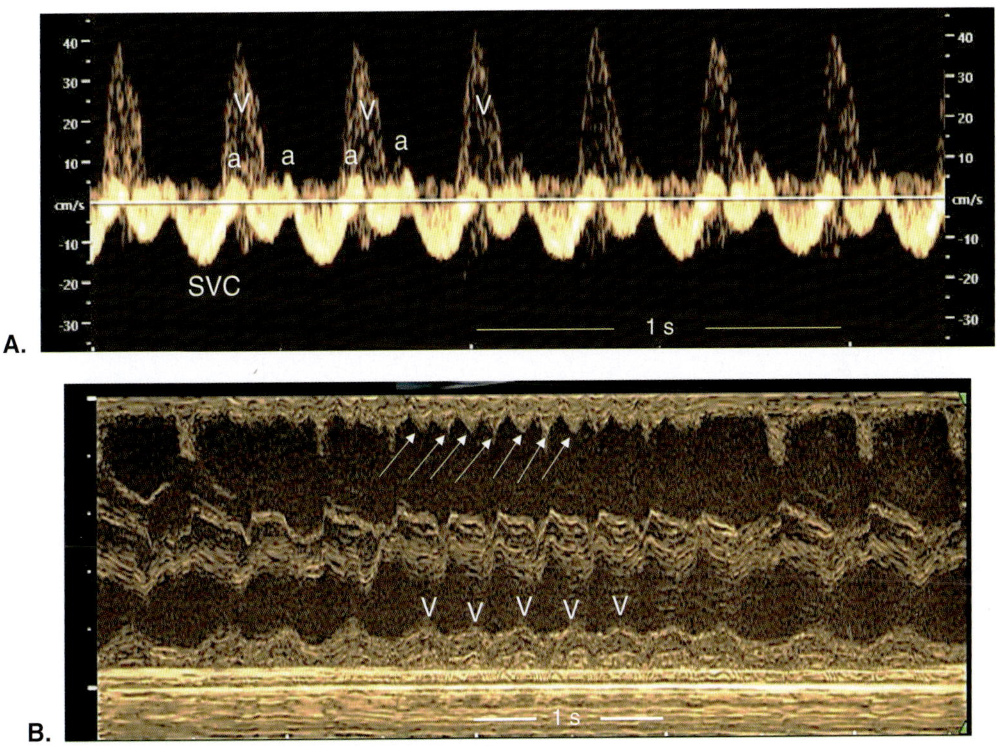

FIGURE 3.2.6 Atrial flutter. **A:** Superior vena cava/aorta (SVC/Ao) spectral Doppler of atrial flutter with 2:1 conduction. Atrial contractions (a) are seen as reverse flow above baseline and ventricular contractions (V) are represented by aortic outflow, also above baseline. **B:** Simultaneous atrial and ventricular M-mode of a fetus with intermittent atrial flutter. Rapid atrial contractions occur at about twice the ventricular rate (V). **C:** Signal-averaged fetal magnetocardiography of atrial flutter. **D:** Continuous rhythm tracing of a fetus with both atrial flutter and atrioventricular reentrant tachycardia. In **B-D**, arrows show atrial contractions (or P-waves on fMCG). SVT, supraventricular tachyarrhythmia.

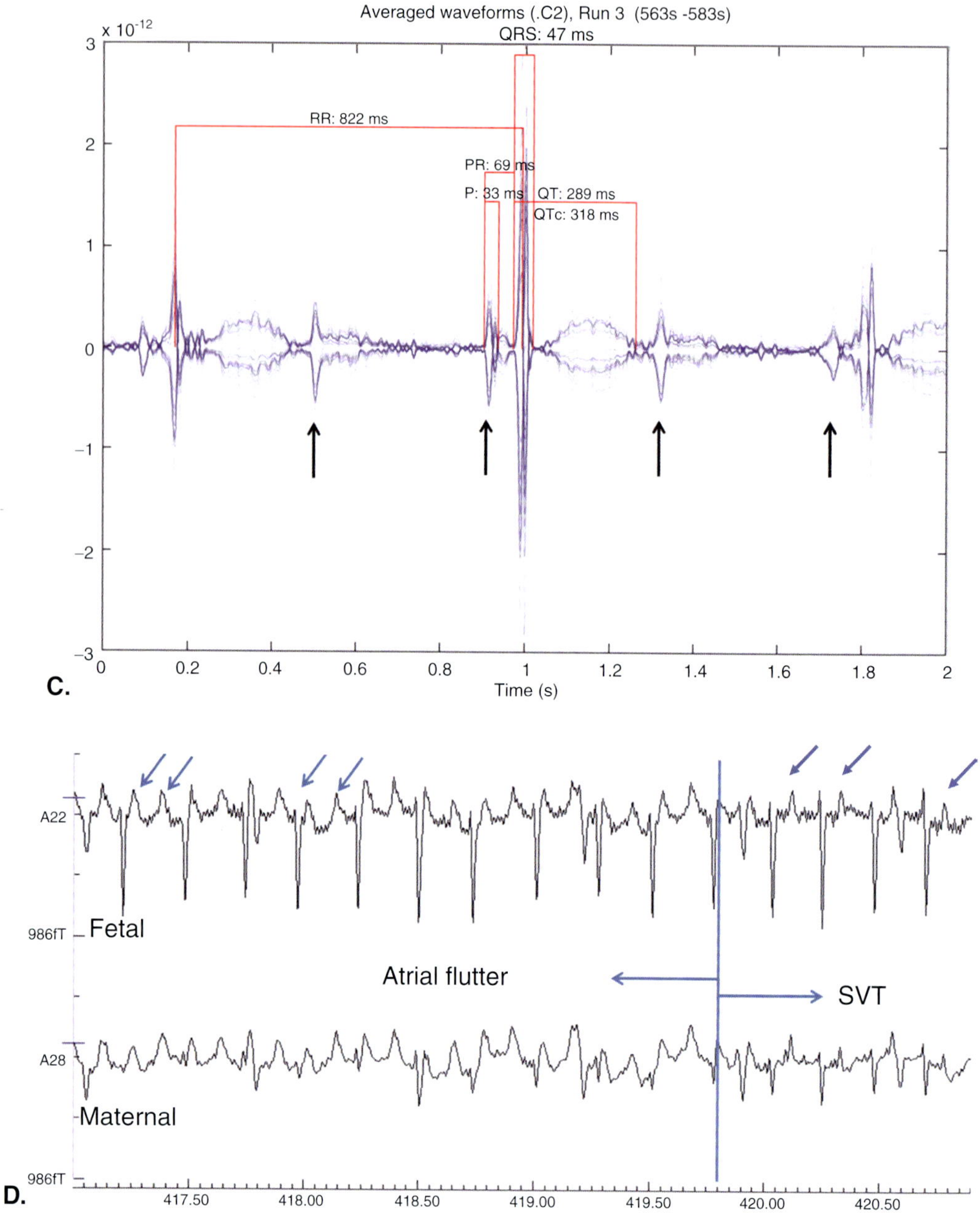

FIGURE 3.2.6 Cont'd

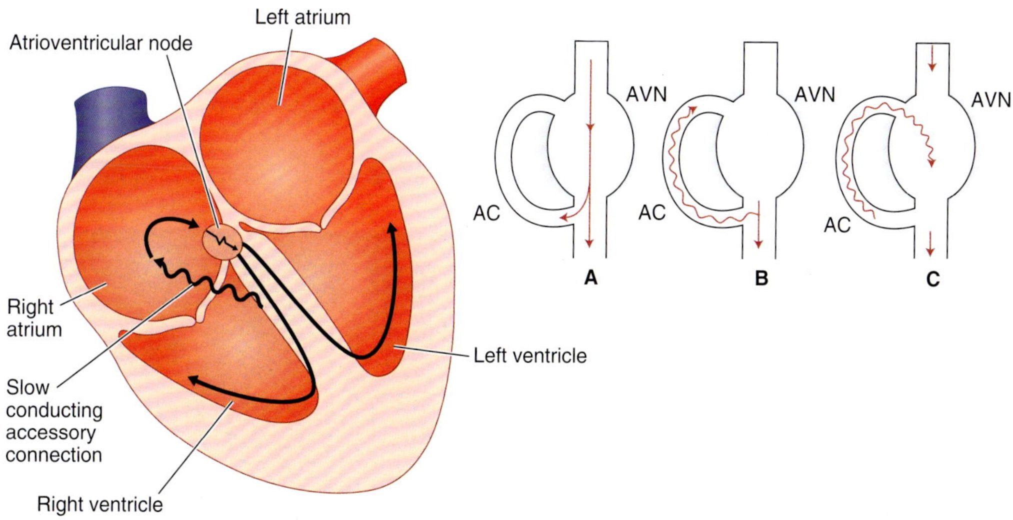

FIGURE 3.2.7 Diagram of permanent junctional reciprocating tachycardia. *A,* Antegrade conduction down the AVN. *B,* Retrograde conduction up the accessory connection (AC). *C,* Circuit of rapid conduction maintained by conduction from the AC down the AVN and back up the AV. AVN, atrioventricular node. (Modified from Jones RM. *Patient Assessment in Pharmacy Practice*. 3rd ed. Philadelphia, PA: Wolters Kluwer; 2015 and Gant L, Lebowitz D, Rosario J, Vera A. *Step-Up to USMLE Step 2 CK*. 5th ed. Philadelphia, PA: Wolters Kluwer; 2019.)

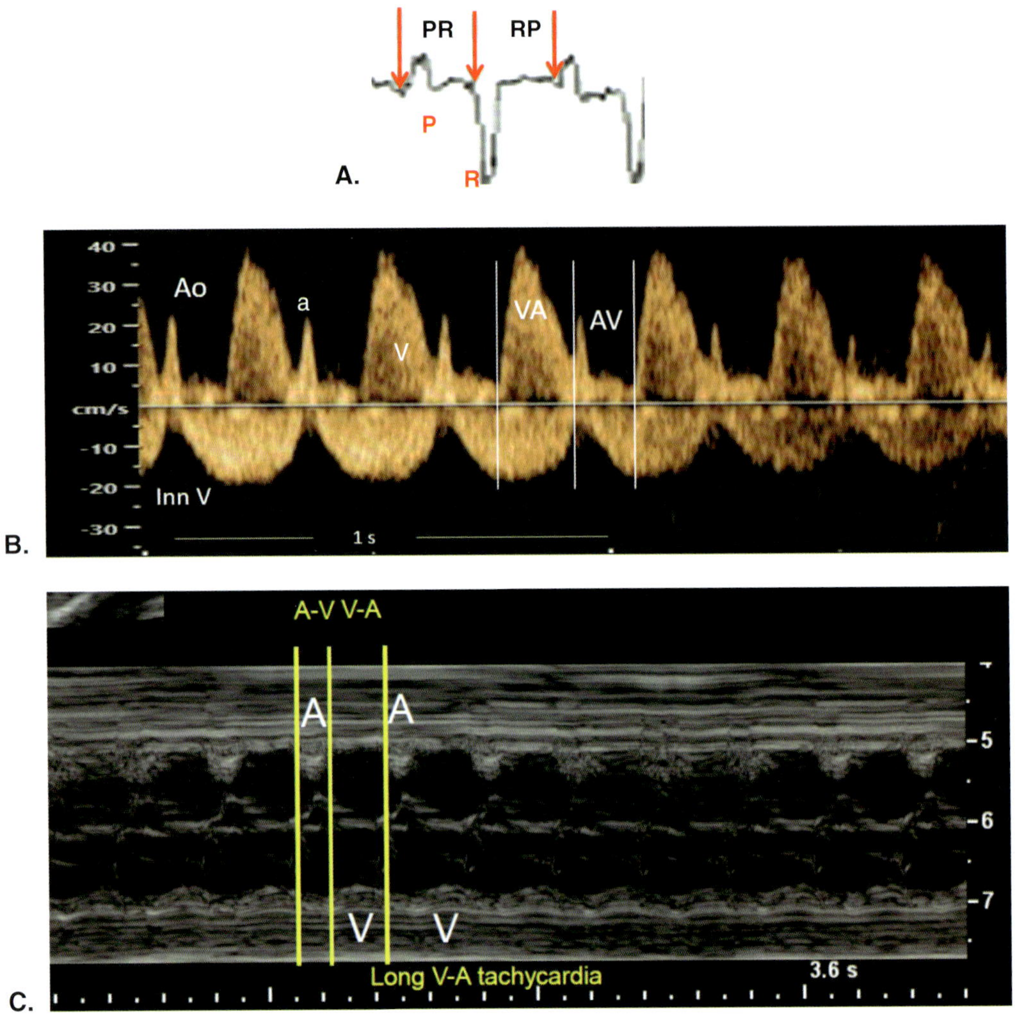

FIGURE 3.2.8 ECG and echo findings in long VA tachycardia. **A:** The RP interval on the ECG corresponds to the Doppler VA interval. **B:** Innominate vein/Aorta (Ao) spectral Doppler. Atrial events are represented by reverse flow in the innominate vein (A, above baseline) and ventricular events demonstrated by aortic outflow (V above baseline). Note the VA interval is longer than the AV interval. **C:** M-mode of a long VA tachycardia with VA and AV intervals. **D:** Typical fetal heart rate tracing of a long VA tachycardia. **E:** Tachycardia (first seven beats on the left) terminates with an atrial contraction, then sinus rhythm resumes. This is typical of a tachycardia which requires the AV node.

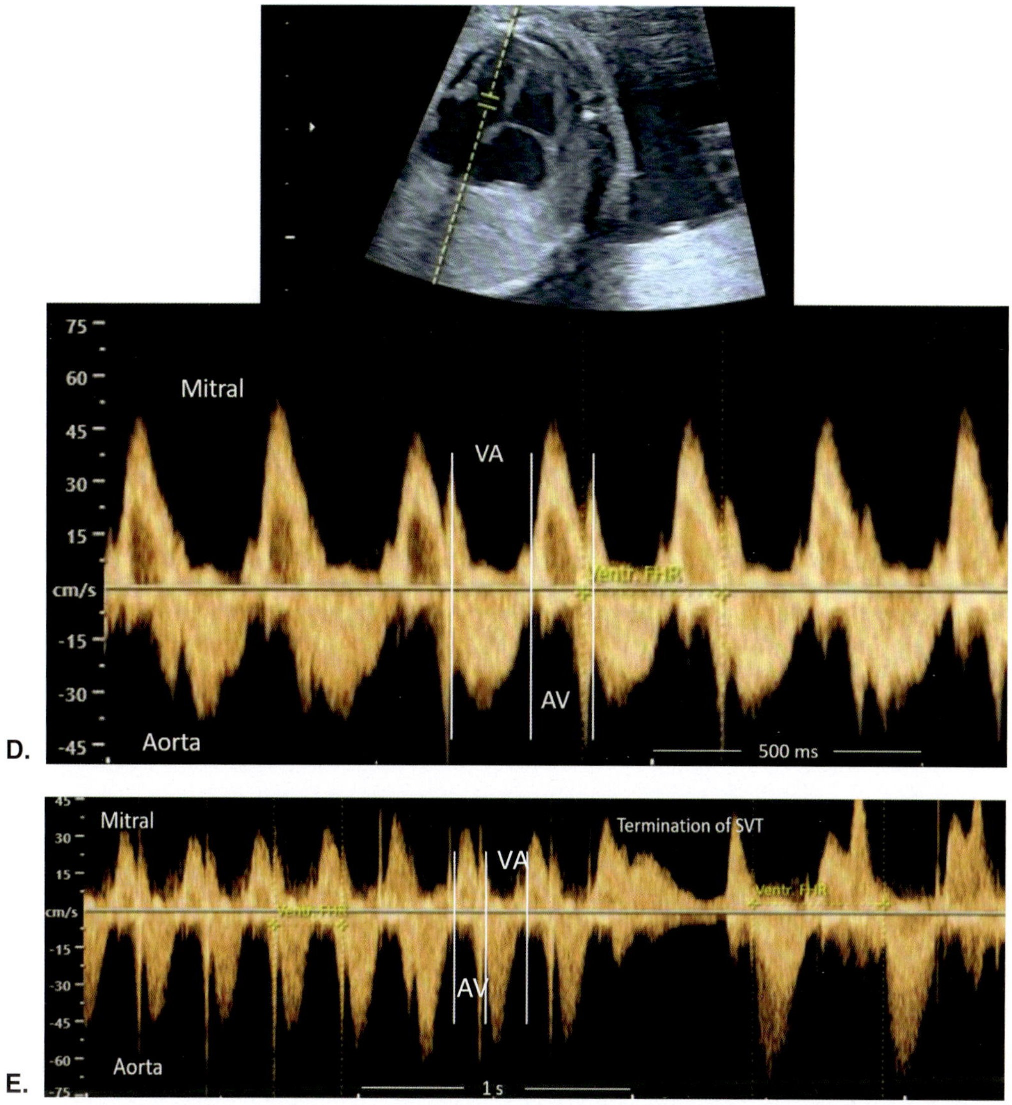

FIGURE 3.2.8 Cont'd

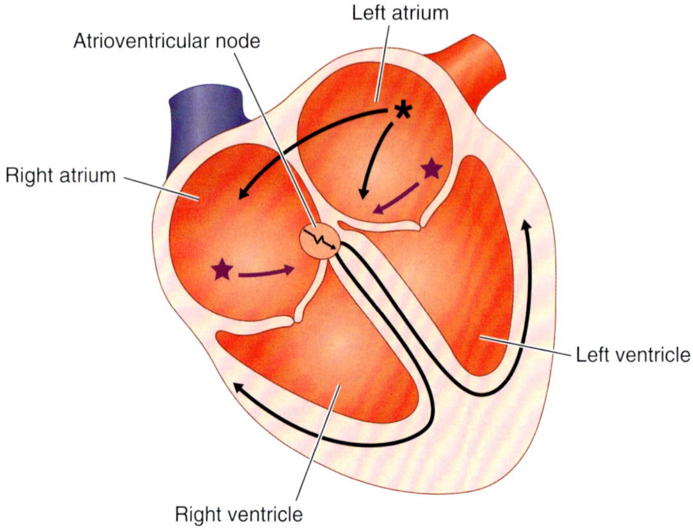

FIGURE 3.2.9 Diagram of atrial ectopic tachycardia. Stars indicated ectopic atrial foci in the left and right atrium which initiate the tachycardia. (Modified from Jones RM. *Patient Assessment in Pharmacy Practice*. 3rd ed. Philadelphia, PA: Wolters Kluwer; 2015.)

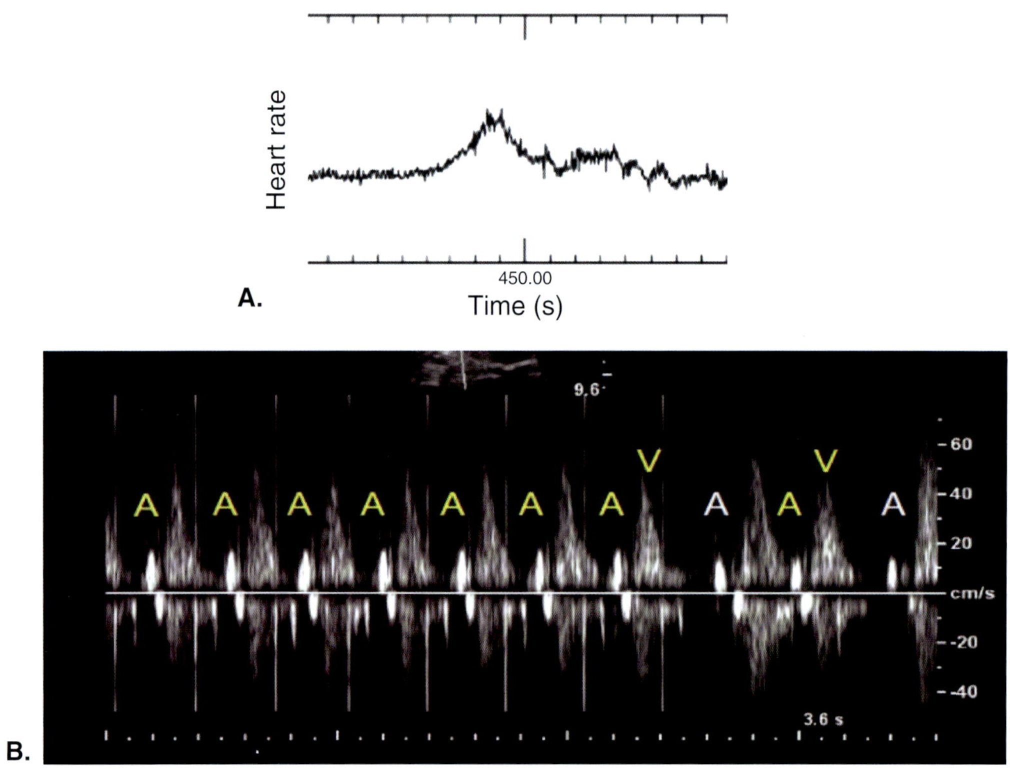

FIGURE 3.2.10 Atrial ectopic tachycardia (AET) characteristics. **A:** Fetal heart rate tracing at initiation and termination of an automatic tachycardia mechanism. In contrast to a reentrant mechanism, the tachycardia slowly starts and stops. This mechanism is typical for AET, a long ventriculoatrial (VA) tachycardia. **B:** Typical termination of AET. The last beat of the tachycardia is a ventricular beat (V); thus, the tachycardia does not require the atrioventricular node in the tachycardia circuit as does atrioventricular reentrant tachycardia.

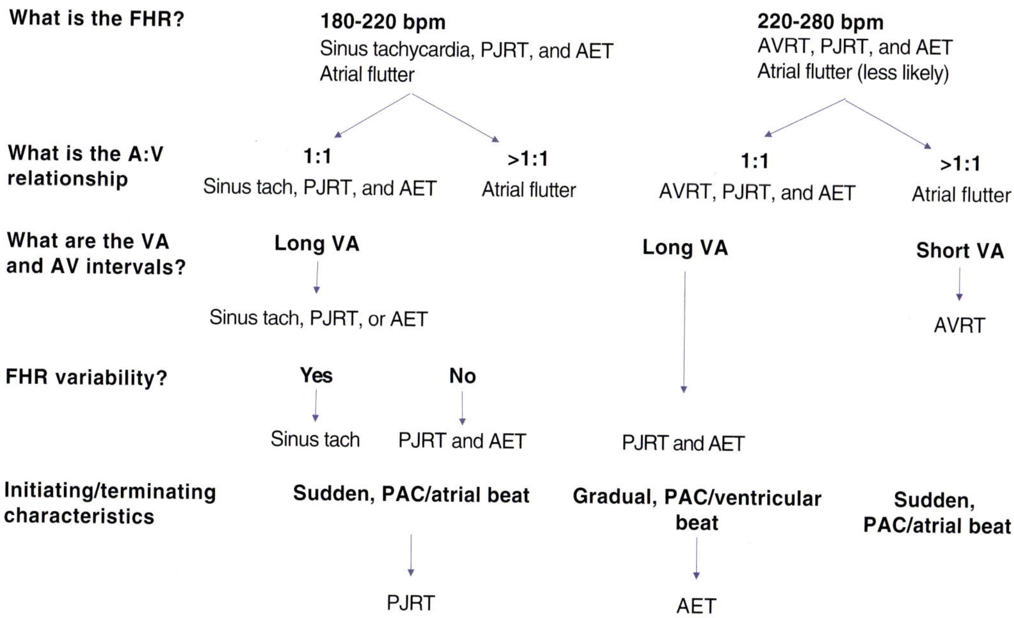

FIGURE 3.2.11 Approach to the fetus with supraventricular tachyarrhythmia.

TACHYCARDIA OUTCOMES

Successful conversion of fetal SVT (described in Part 4, Chapter 1) can facilitate term, vaginal delivery, which should be the goal in the current era. However, it is important to remember that SVT can recur postnatally even when in utero control is achieved. There appear to be few prenatal predictive factors for postnatal recurrence of SVT. In a study by Moodley et al, ~2/3 of fetuses with SVT demonstrated postnatal tachycardia usually within the first 48 hours.[29] Forty-four percent of those who converted to sinus rhythm prenatally demonstrated SVT postnatally.[29] Hinkle et al found a 61% postnatal recurrence rate of SVT in their cohort, with a strong correlation between postnatal SVT and a later gestational age at fetal SVT diagnosis (median EGA 30 vs 27.5 weeks, $P = .006$).[30] Strasburger et al reported that 50% of infants with fetal SVT require no antiarrhythmic treatment postnatally; encouragingly, even more outgrow the need for medications by 1 year of age.[3] The loss of susceptibility to SVT recurrence appears to be due in part to observed developmental changes in electrophysiologic properties of accessory AV connections.[14]

AF is less likely to occur postnatally than reentrant SVT; once sinus rhythm has been established, recurrence of AF is uncommon in the absence of congenital heart disease.[33] However, some children who have AVRT postnatally had AF in utero. Only a small percentage of children (~10%) with fetal tachycardia are found to have Wolff-Parkinson-White syndrome/pre-excitation postnatally.[11]

After delivery of a fetus who has been treated for SVT in utero, it is important to reassess tachycardia mechanism based upon electrocardiographic and telemetry/Holter monitoring data. Fetuses who develop congestive heart failure (CHF) secondary to SVT appear to develop CHF from multiple SVT episodes recurring at relatively long cycle lengths (slow heart rates), whereas neonates with postnatal CHF appear to develop symptoms during a sustained tachycardia episode with relatively short cycle lengths (fast heart rates).[11] This may have important implications for need for therapy and therapy type if the child is delivered in sinus rhythm and on selection of agents. Considerations include presence or absence of pre-excitation, feasibility of enteral therapies, and ability to directly monitor the neonate for adverse or excessive drug effects. Finally, if sinus rhythm is present at birth, observation with continuous cardiac monitoring for arrhythmia recurrence should be of an ample duration for clearance of transplacental antiarrhythmics (usually about 3 to 4 days). Parents can be taught to assess their infant's heart rate and identify tachycardia recurrence. Ambulatory ECG can be helpful in assessing short periods of SVT unappreciated by auscultation. When postnatal assessment with transesophageal pacing can aid in making these determinations, as well as, in identifying infants with fetal or postnatal AF who may also be at risk for AVRT.[11,14,17,30]

SUMMARY

Although fetal SVT can be a cause of in utero fetal demise and perinatal morbidity, outcomes are improving in the current era due to accurate arrhythmia detection, correct and timely diagnosis, and increased utilization of therapy. Even a hydropic fetus has a >80% chance of a successful outcome with current approaches to transplacental antiarrhythmic therapy, described in Part 4, Chapter 1.

References

1. Simpson LL. Fetal supraventricular tachycardias: diagnosis and management. *Semin Perinatol.* 2000;24(5):360-372.
2. Southall DP, Richards J, Hardwick RA, et al. Prospective study of fetal heart rate and rhythm patterns. *Arch Dis Child.* 1980;55(7):506-511.
3. Strasburger JF. Fetal arrhythmias. *Prog Pediat Cardiol.* 2000;11(1):1-17.
4. Wacker-Gussmann A, Strasburger JF, Cueno BF, Wakai RT. Diagnosis and treatment of fetal arrhythmia. *Am J Perinatol.* 2014;31(7):617-628.
5. Jaeggi E, Ohman A. Fetal and neonatal arrhythmias. *Clin Perinatol.* 2016;43(1):99-112.
6. Fouron JC. Fetal arrhythmias: the Saint-Justine hospital experience. *Prenat Diagn.* 2004;24:1068-1080.
7. Carvalho JS, Prefumo F, Ciardelli V, Sairam S, Bhide A, Shinebourne EA. Evaluation of fetal arrhythmias from simultaneous pulsed wave Doppler in pulmonary artery and vein. *Heart.* 2007;93(11):1448-1453.
8. Howley LW, Schuchardt E, Park D, Gilber L, Gruenwald J, Cuneo BF. Simultaneous recording of pulsed-wave Doppler signals in innominate vein and transverse aortic arch: new technique to evaluate atrioventricular conduction and fetal heart rhythm. *Ultrasound Obstet Gynecol.* 2018;52(4):544-545.
9. Detterich JA, Pruetz J, Sklansky MS. Color M-mode sonography for evaluation of fetal arrhythmias. *J Ultrasound Med.* 2012;31(10):1681-1688.
10. Hornberger LK, Sahn DJ. Rhythm abnormalities of the fetus. *Heart.* 2007;93:1294-1300.
11. Zales V, Dunnigan A, Benson DW. Clinical and electrophysiologic features of fetal and neonatal paroxysmal atrial tachycardia resulting in congestive heart failure.*Am J Cardiol.* 1988;62(4):225-228.
12. Simpson JM, Sharland GK. Fetal tachycardias: management and outcome of 127 consecutive cases. *Heart.* 1998;79(6):576-581.
13. Carvalho JS. Fetal dysrhythmias. *Best Pract Res Clin Obstet Gynaecol* 2019;58:28-41.

14. Benson DW, Dunnigan A, Benditt DS. Follow-up evaluation of infant paroxysmal atrial tachycardias: a transesophageal study. *Circulation*. 1987;75:542-549.
15. Dunnigan A, Benditt DG, Benson DW. Modes of onset ("initiating events") for paroxysmal atrial tachycardia in infants and children. *Am J Cardiol*. 1986;57:1280-1287.
16. Wakai RT, Strasburger JF, Li Z, Deal BJ Gotteiner NL. Magnetocardiographic rhythm patterns at initiation and termination of fetal tachycardia. *Circulation*. 2003;107;307-312.
17. Dunnigan A, Benson DW Jr, Benditt DG. Atrial flutter in infancy: diagnosis, clinical features and treatment. *Pediatrics*. 1985;75:725-729.
18. Till J, Wren C. Atrial flutter in the fetus and young infant: an association with accessory connections. *Br Heart J*. 1992;67(1):80-83.
19. Johnson WH Jr, Dunnigan A, Fehr P, Benson DW Jr. Association of atrial flutter with orthodromic reciprocating fetal tachycardia. *Am J Cardiol*. 1987;59(4):374-375.
20. Wacker-Gussmann A, Strasburger JF, Srinivasan S, Cuneo BF, Lutter W, Wakai RT. Fetal atrial flutter: electrophysiology and associations with rhythms involving an accessory pathway. *J Am Heart Assoc*. 2016;5(6):e003673.
21. Naheed ZJ, Strasburger JF, Deal BJ, Benson DW Jr, Gidding SS. Fetal tachycardia: mechanisms and predictors of hydrops fetalis. *J Am Coll Cardiol*. 1996;27(7):1736-1740.
22. Jaeggi E, Fouron JC, Drblik SP. Fetal atrial flutter: diagnosis, clinical features, treatment, and outcome. *J Pediatr*. 1998;132:335-339.
23. Cuneo B, Strasburger JF, Niksch A, Ovadia M, Wakai RT. An expanded phenotype of maternal SSA/SSB antibody-associated fetal cardiac disease. *J Matern Fetal Neonatal Med*. 2009;22(3):233-238.
24. Donofrio MT, Moon-Grady AJ, Hornberger LK, et al. Diagnosis and treatment of fetal cardiac disease: a scientific statement from the American Heart Association. *Circulation*. 2014;129(21):2183-2242.
25. Oudijk MA, Stoutenbeek P, Sreeram N, Visser GH, Meijboom EJ. Persistent junctional reciprocating tachycardia in the fetus. *J Matern Fetal Neonatal Med*. 2003;13(3):191-196.
26. Srinivasan S, Strasburger J. Overview of fetal arrhythmias. *Curr Opin Pediatr*. 2008;20(5):522-531.
27. Bravo-Valenzuela NJ, Peixoto AB, Araujo Júnior E, Tonni G. Fetal supraventricular tachycardia at 12 weeks of gestation: diagnosis and follow up. A case report. *Med Ultrason*. 2019;21(1):93-95.
28. Gozar L, Marginean C, Toganel R, Muntean I. The role of echocardiography in fetal tachyarrhythmia diagnosis. A burden for the pediatric cardiologist and a review of the literature. *Med Ultrason*. 2017;19(2):232-235.
29. Moodley S, Sanatani S, Potts JE, Sandor GG. Postnatal outcome in patients with fetal tachycardia. *Pediatr Cardiol*. 2013;34(1):81-87.
30. Hinkle KA, Peyvandi S, Stiver C, et al. Postnatal outcomes of fetal supraventricular tachycardia: a multicenter study. *Pediatr Cardiol*. 2017;38(7):1317-1323.

Ventricular Tachycardias

Sally-Ann Barker Clur • Lisa K. Hornberger • Arja Suzanne Vink • Nico A. Blom

INTRODUCTION

Ventricular tachycardia (VT) is a rare condition responsible for only 1% to 8% of fetal arrhythmias and only 1% to 2% of fetal tachycardias.[1,2] VT is diagnosed when three or more successive ventricular ectopic (VE) beats occur and the ventricular rate is increased to the range of 170 to 300 bpm.[3-11] When VT occurs, there may also be atrioventricular (A-V) dissociation resulting in a slower atrial rate than ventricular rate, but there may be V-A association due to retrograde conduction from the ventricle to the atrium resulting in equal ventricular and atrial rates (FIG. 3.3.1).

Although fetal VT is rare, it is important to recognize it and treat it appropriately for several reasons. First, if persistent, VT can lead to intrauterine cardiac dysfunction, nonimmune hydrops fetalis, and fetal demise.[5] Second, misdiagnosing VT as supraventricular tachycardia (SVT) may lead to inappropriate drug therapy, resulting in an exacerbation of the arrhythmia with worsening of cardiac function, and fetal loss.[12-19] On the other hand, appropriate therapy can restore sinus rhythm, resolve fetal hydrops, and prolong the pregnancy until maturity.[1,7,11,14] Finally, the prognosis, etiology, and outcome of VT differ from those of SVT.

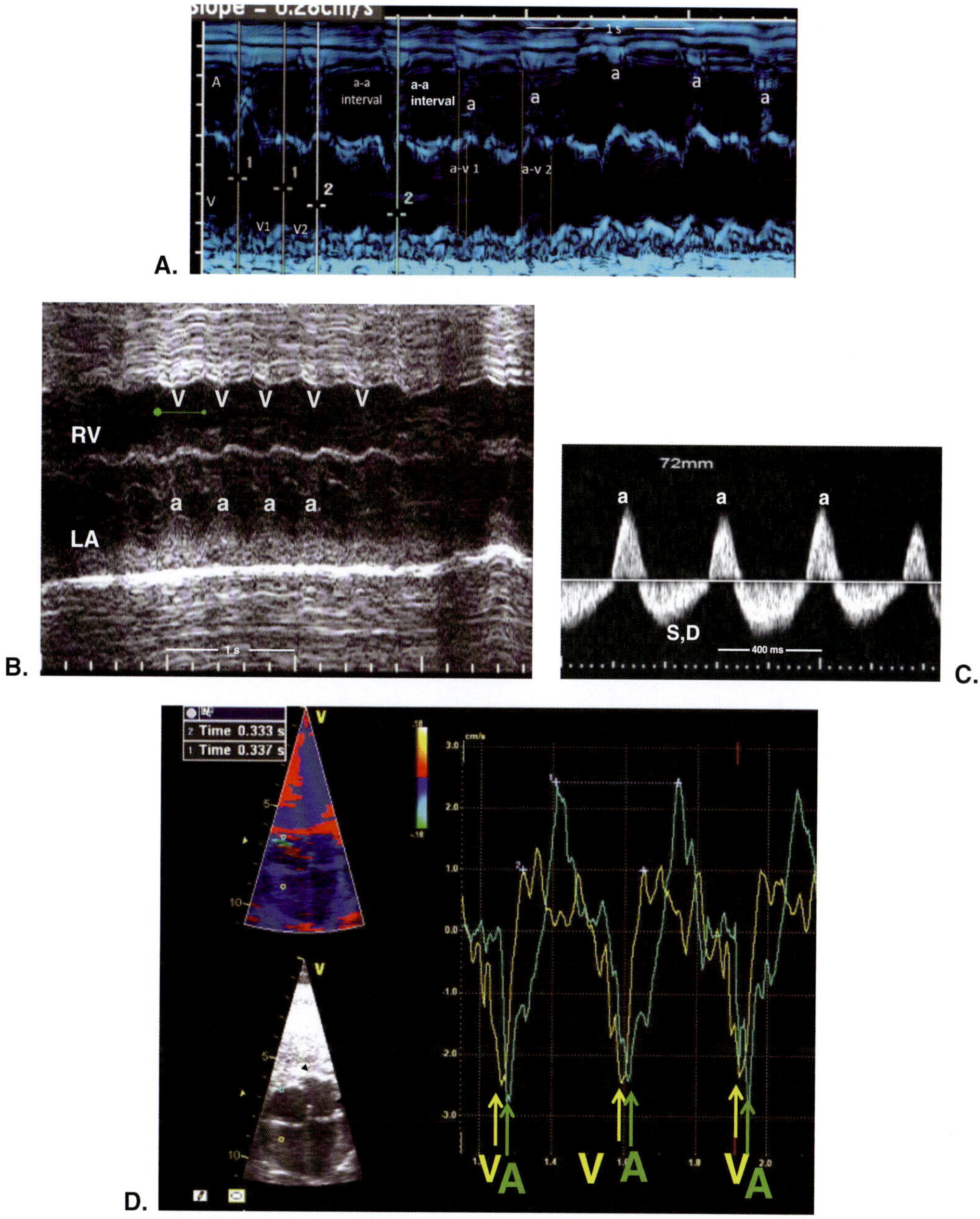

FIGURE 3.3.1 Fetal ventricular tachycardia (VT) tracings highlighting atrioventricular (A-V) relationships during VT. A: M-mode of a 32-week fetus with VT of 260 to 280 bpm. Simultaneous atrial (a, top tracing) and ventricular (V, bottom tracing) M-mode. The ventricular rate is ~260 bpm and the atrial rate is ~120 bpm. Note at times the V-V (V1, V2) and a-a intervals are irregular as are the a-v (a-v1, a-v2, yellow lines) intervals. This variation is typical of VT with V-A dissociation. **B-D:** 37-week fetus with VT of 170 to 180 bpm. **B:** M-mode shows 1:1 A-V relationship. At this point, one cannot distinguish VT from supraventricular tachycardia. **C:** Inferior vena cava Doppler tracings at this rate demonstrated a large and consistent A-wave reversal (above baseline). This was due to the retrograde V-A conduction with atrial systole occurring at the end of ventricular systole resulting in the atria contracting against a closed AV valve. These findings suggest a diagnosis of VT. **D:** Tissue Doppler imaging shows a retrograde V-A conduction.

ETIOLOGY AND MECHANISMS

Most of our current knowledge about fetal VT is derived from prenatal case reports and small case series or extrapolated from neonatal data. The mechanism of VT includes prolonged ventricular repolarization, an abnormally irritable focus, or a reentry circuit. Based on 12-lead ECG characteristics, there are two broad categories of VT: monomorphic and polymorphic (FIG. 3.3.2). The signature rhythm of long QT syndrome (LQTS), an inherited ion channelopathy, is a polymorphic VT called torsades de pointes (TdP). VT may occur in the absence of structural or functional heart disease. It may also be associated with myocardial disease (including myocarditis, cardiomyopathy, and aneurysms), with intracardiac tumors such as fibromas and rhabdomyomas, with myocardial ischemia or with inherited channelopathies other than LQTS, discussed in Part 1, Chapter 3 and Part 3, Chapter 6. VT can also be idiopathic.

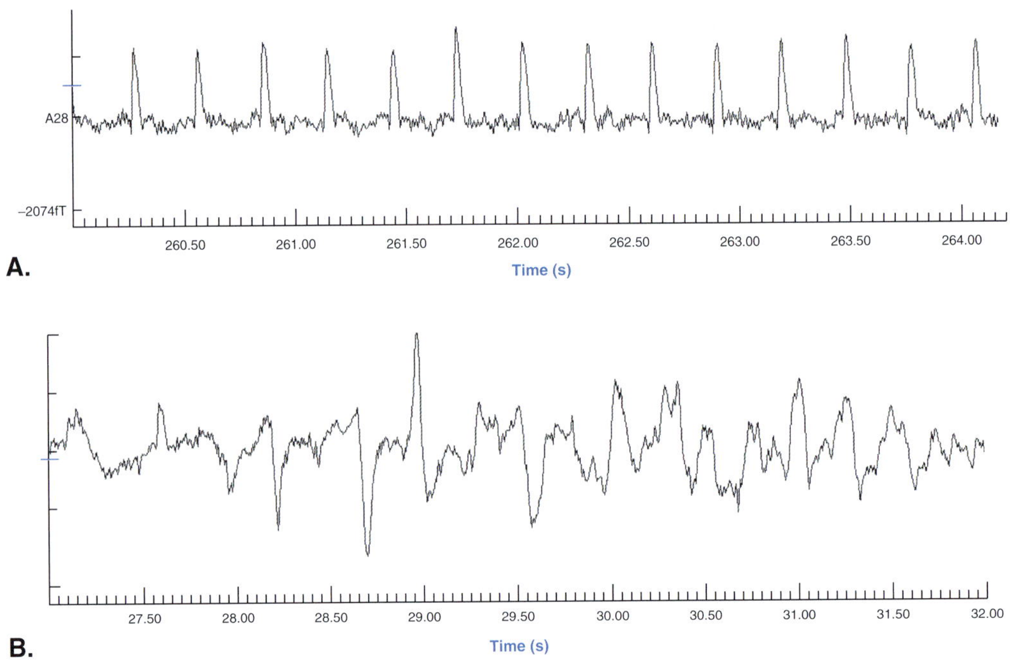

FIGURE 3.3.2 **Fetal magnetocardiogram rhythm tracings of ventricular tachycardia (VT). A:** 25-week fetus with monomorphic VT at a rate of about 212 bpm. The wide complex (prolonged QRS duration) is typical of VT, but can also be seen with antidromic supraventricular tachycardia. **B:** 32-week fetus with torsades de pointes, a polymorphic VT that "twists around the points."

DIAGNOSIS OF FETAL VT

In addition to excluding an obvious primary structural or functional cardiac defect by fetal echo, initial steps in the evaluation of fetal VT should include soliciting a family history suggestive of an inherited arrhythmia or myocardial disease, including unexpected losses in utero or in infancy. Acquisition of a 12-lead ECG from both parents may be informative. Additional testing for maternal infection, particularly viral etiologies, and maternal autoantibodies (anti-SSA/Ro and SSB/La) should be considered to assess for possible myocarditis including, in the latter, autoimmune-mediated fetal myocardial disease.

The diagnosis of fetal VT relies on identifying unique characteristics as seen by M-mode, tissue Doppler,[20] and spectral Doppler. These characteristics include (1) variable A-V and V-A intervals; (2) A-V dissociation with a slower atrial rate than ventricular rate; (3) ventricular asynchrony; and (4) in cases of slow VT (<200 bpm), intermittent retrograde V-A conduction. These characteristics are described below.

The variable A-V and V-A intervals, which occur because of A-V dissociation, can be seen by M-mode and spectral Doppler (FIG. 3.3.1A). These variable intervals contrast with the very regular A-V and V-A intervals characteristic of SVT. In VT, the atrial rates may be slower than the ventricular rates as seen in FIG. 3.3.3 in a fetus with both ventricular bigeminy and VT. As seen in FIG. 3.3.4, A-V dissociation can be also be in-

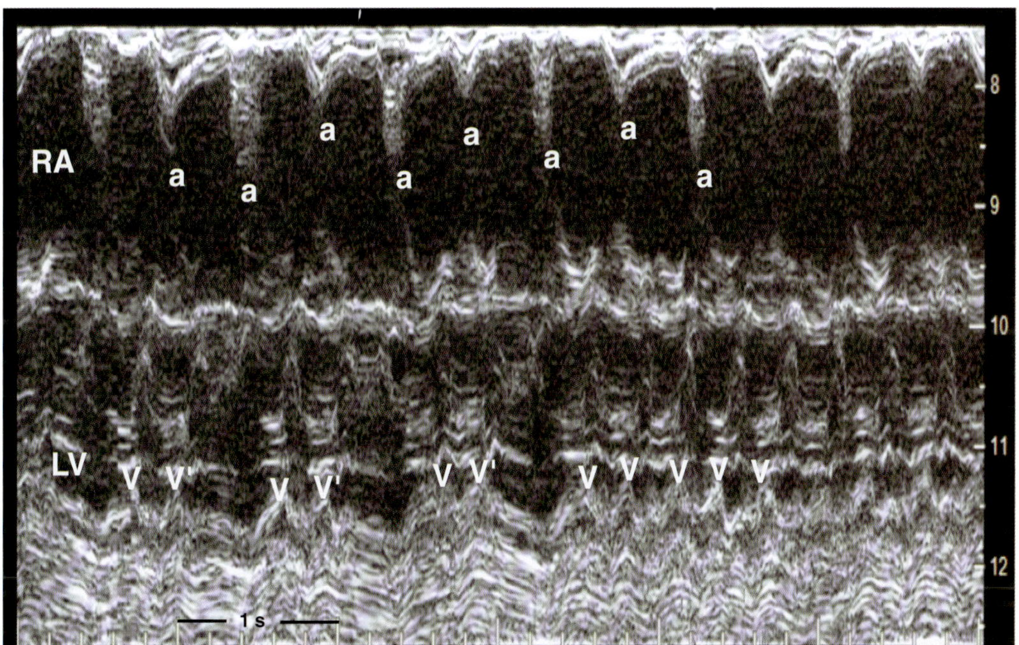

FIGURE 3.3.3 32-week fetus with idiopathic ventricular tachycardia. By M-mode, the atrial (a) rates were found to be constant at 140 to 150 bpm. Initially there was ventricular bigeminy (V′) followed by a run of ventricular tachycardia with ventricular rates > 200 bpm and atrioventricular dissociation. V, ventricular contraction.

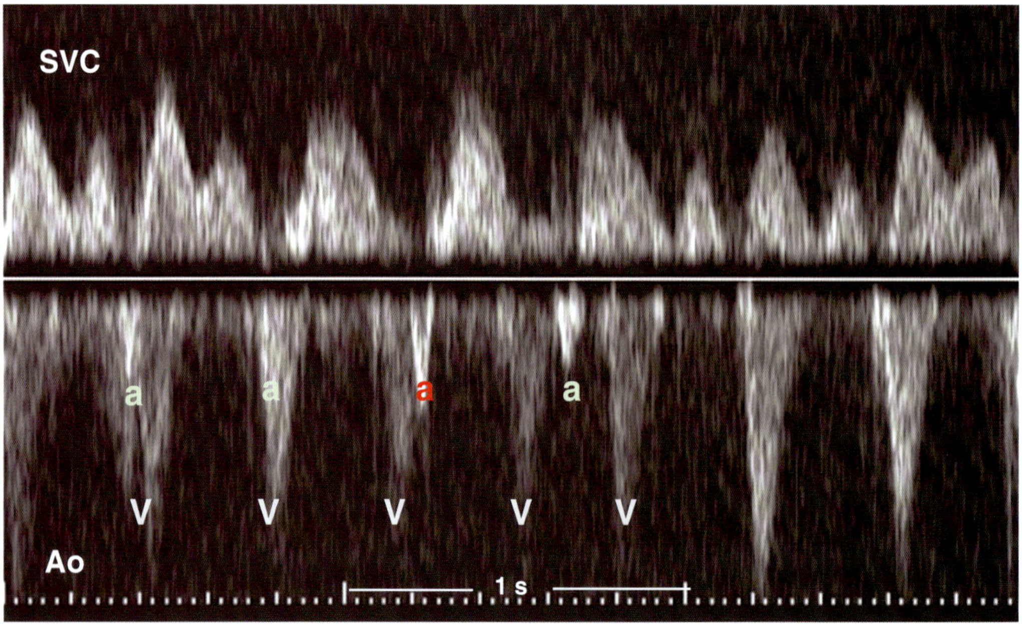

FIGURE 3.3.4 Spectral Doppler tracings from fetus with slow ventricular tachycardia (180-200 bpm). Tracing from superior vena cava (SVC, top tracing) and aorta (V, bottom tracing). Reverse flow in the SVC denotes atrial contractions which are seen below the baseline (a). The ventricular rate is slightly faster than the atrial rate, and atrio-ventricular dissociation is seen by the varying atrioventricular relationship and the prominent A-wave reversal (red "a") seen when the atrium contracts during ventricular systole.

ferred from pulsed Doppler tracings in the systemic veins, and the retrograde A-waves of the fetus with VT occur without a clear pattern.

Ventricular asynchrony refers to the finding that rather than virtually simultaneous ventricular contraction (which occurs during sinus rhythm), one of the ventricles will contract before the other. Ventricular asynchrony can be detected by simultaneous spectral Doppler interrogation in the aortic isthmus (AoI) and the arterial duct (AD) (FIG. 3.3.5). If the right ventricle begins contraction before the left ventricle, the AD waveform will occur before the AoI waveform. There may also be a pulsation and a brief period of retrograde flow in the AoI (FIG. 3.3.5A). On the other hand, if contraction initiates in left ventricle, the AoI waveform will be seen before the AD waveform (FIG. 3.3.5B).[21]

A unique feature of "slow" VT (≤ ~200 bpm) is episodes of retrograde V-A conduction. During retrograde V-A conduction, the atrial and ventricular rates are the same and flow reversal in the ductus venosus is prominent and regular (FIG. 3.3.1B-D). This finding can make it difficult to distinguish VT with retrograde V-A conduction from SVT, but in general SVT rates are faster.

In summary, VT will frequently have A-V dissociation. When the VT rate is "slow," retrograde V-A conduction may result in equal atrial and ventricular rates. Because polymorphic VT is usually faster than monomorphic VT, A-V dissociation is usually present.

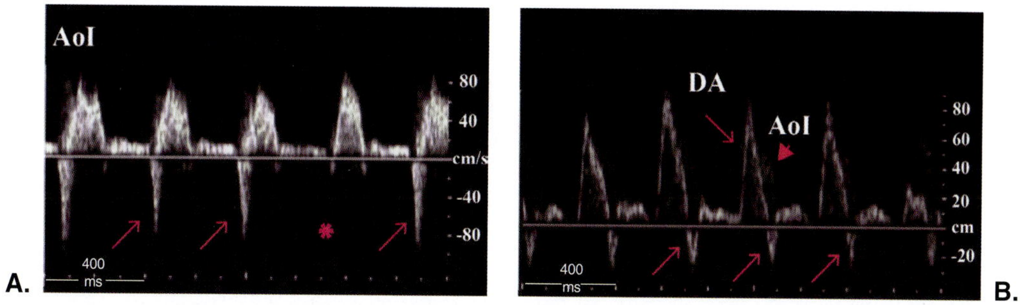

FIGURE 3.3.5 Fetal accelerated ventricular rhythm ventricular asynchrony. A: Flow velocity profile in aortic isthmus (AoI). Deep retrograde waves (arrows) precede forward systolic waveforms, illustrating earlier contraction of right ventricle responsible for wider systolic wave (180 ms). During the fourth cycle, "*" indicates the hemodynamic effect of a fusion beat, in which right and left ventricular contraction is synchronous and the early-systolic retrograde wave is absent. **B:** Flow velocity profile in ductus arteriosus (DA) showing deep end-systolic reversed waves (lower arrows); in background of third cycle, a forward Doppler wave is recorded from AoI (arrowhead) in late systole, a consequence of delayed left ventricular depolarization causing late-retrograde reversed wave in the DA. (Modified from Fouron JC, McNeal-Davidson A, Abadir S, et al. Prenatal diagnosis and prognosis of accelerated idioventricular rhythm. *Ultrasound Obstet Gynecol.* 2017;50(5):624-631.)

Echocardiography can differentiate polymorphic from monomorphic VT based on the findings in polymorphic VT: (1) concurrence with functional 2° AV block with 2:1 conduction and (2) irregularity of ventricular rates and gradually tapering peak systolic flow velocities (FIG. 3.3.6). Monomorphic VT is regular with a consistent ventricular rate and peak systolic flow velocities (FIG. 3.3.7A), while bursts of an irregular tachycardia with varying peak velocities (FIG. 3.3.7B) suggest polymorphic VT.

Cardiac dysfunction may be a sequela of VT and can also be assessed by echocardiography. Specifically, mitral and tricuspid valve insufficiency, cardiomegaly, decreased ventricular shortening or abnormal strain, pericardial or pleural fluid collections, ascites, skin and placental edema all indicate severe cardiac dysfunction secondary to prolonged VT.

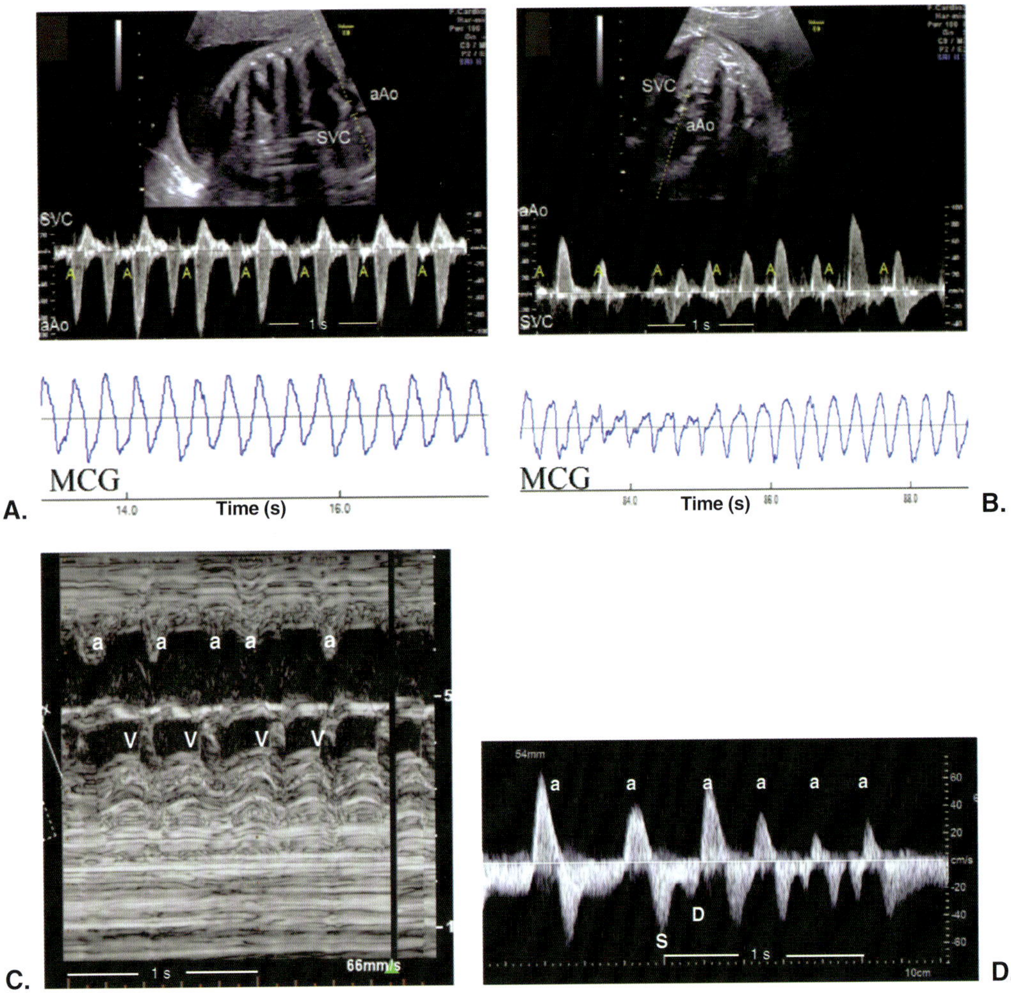

FIGURE 3.3.6 Doppler and magnetocardiography (MCG) tracings from 28-week fetus with ventricular tachycardia associated with LQT2. A: Monomorphic ventricular tachycardia (VT) with relatively uniform ejection waves and a ventricular rate of 220 bpm. Atrioventricular (A-V) dissociation is seen with an atrial rate of 130 bpm. **B:** Torsade de pointes with irregular ascending aorta (aAo) Doppler signals with unequal and extremely low-amplitude ejection waves. The ventricular rate is 190 to 220 bpm. A-V dissociation is seen with an atrial rate of 130 bpm. SVC, superior vena cava. **C:** Another example of polymorphic VT seen by the irregular ventricular contractions (v). Note also the slower and irregular atrial contractions. **D:** Hepatic vein spectral Doppler showing irregular a-a intervals and variable retrograde flow during atrial systole. D, diastole; S, systole. (A and B, Modified from Miyoshi T, Sakaguchi H, Shiraishi I, Yoshimatsu J, Ikeda T. Potential utility of pulsed-wave Doppler for prenatal diagnosis of fetal ventricular tachycardia secondary to long QT syndrome. *Ultrasound Obstet Gynecol*. 2018;51(5):697-699.)

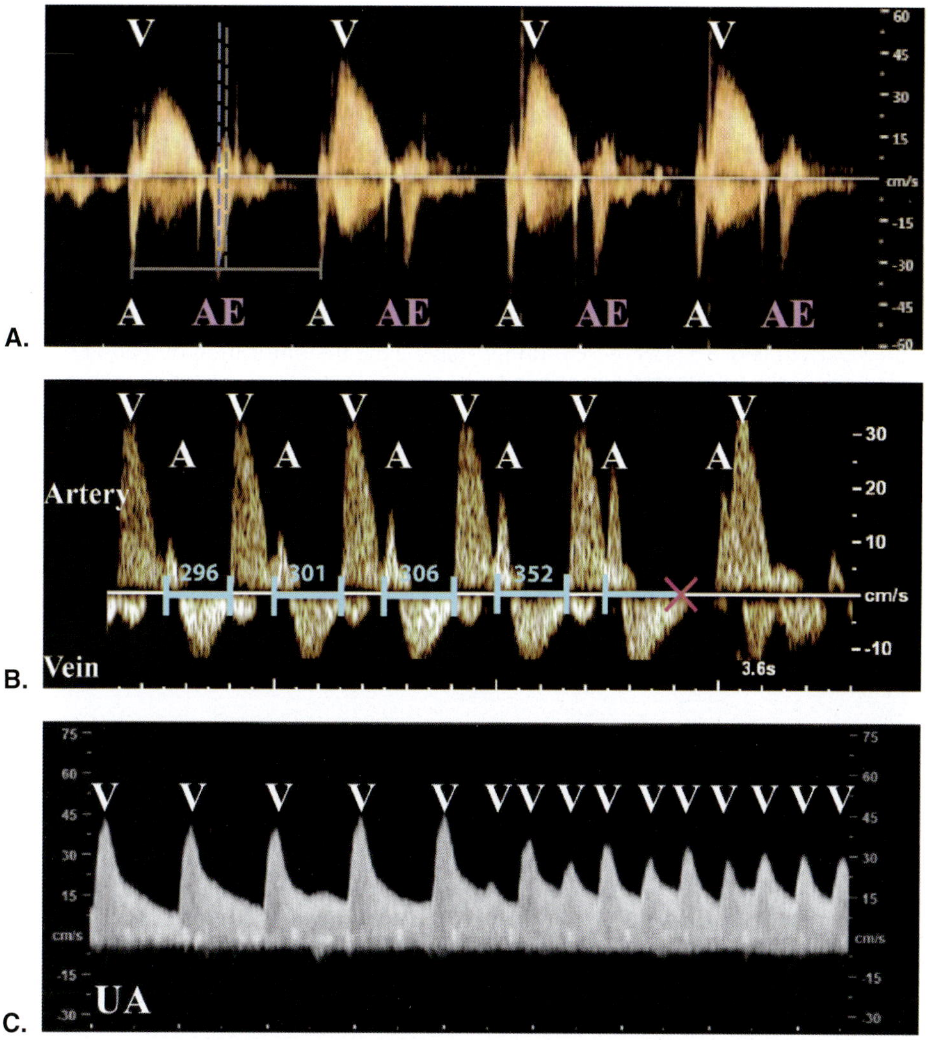

FIGURE 3.3.7 Arrhythmias seen in fetuses with long QT syndrome (LQTS). A: Blocked atrial ectopic (AE) contractions in bigeminy in a fetus with LQT1. Note that this can easily be misinterpreted as 2:1 AV block as the AE contractions (blue dotted line) fall just before the sinus beat would have (gray dotted line). **B:** Simultaneous Dopplers of an artery and vein in a fetus with LQT2 and type 1, 2° AV block. The atrial rate is 120 bpm. The time between the atrial and ventricular activities gets successively longer until an unconducted atrial activity is seen. This is called a Wenkebach block. The usual type of AV block seen in LQTS is a functional 2° AV block with 2:1 conduction. **C:** Umbilical artery (UA) Doppler during sinus rhythm (first 5 beats) and ventricular tachycardia (VT). Note the decrease in amplitude during the VT.

DIAGNOSIS OF VT IN SPECIFIC CLINICAL SETTINGS

Long QT Syndrome

Most the cases of fetal VT due to LQTS reported in the literature had the genotype of LQT type 2 or a specific LQT3 variant (R1623Q).[22,23] In such cases, the symptomatic fetus was often the proband in the family and would thus not have come to attention due to a family history. In addition to VT, a high index of suspicion of fetal LQTS may occur when the fetal heart rate is less than the third percentile for gestational age, especially when associated with a prolonged left ventricular isovolumetric relaxation time (LVIRT) (FIG. 3.3.8) as these findings may be the first indication of fetal LQTS.[24,25] If suspicion for fetal LQTS is high, 12-lead electrocardiograms of the parents may be helpful, but if the parent's QTc interval is not prolonged, a fetal de novo pathogenic variant is still possible.

The VT seen in LQTS may be monomorphic or polymorphic (FIGS. 3.3.6 and 3.3.9).[26] Bradycardia in the presence of QT-interval prolongation corrected for the heart rate (QTc) increases the tendency to develop ventricular arrhythmias owing to inhomogeneous ventricular refractoriness. The functional AV block that occurs with LQTS can be type 1 or type 2, 2° AV block (FIGS. 3.3.7B and 3.3.9C). Generally, the cardiac

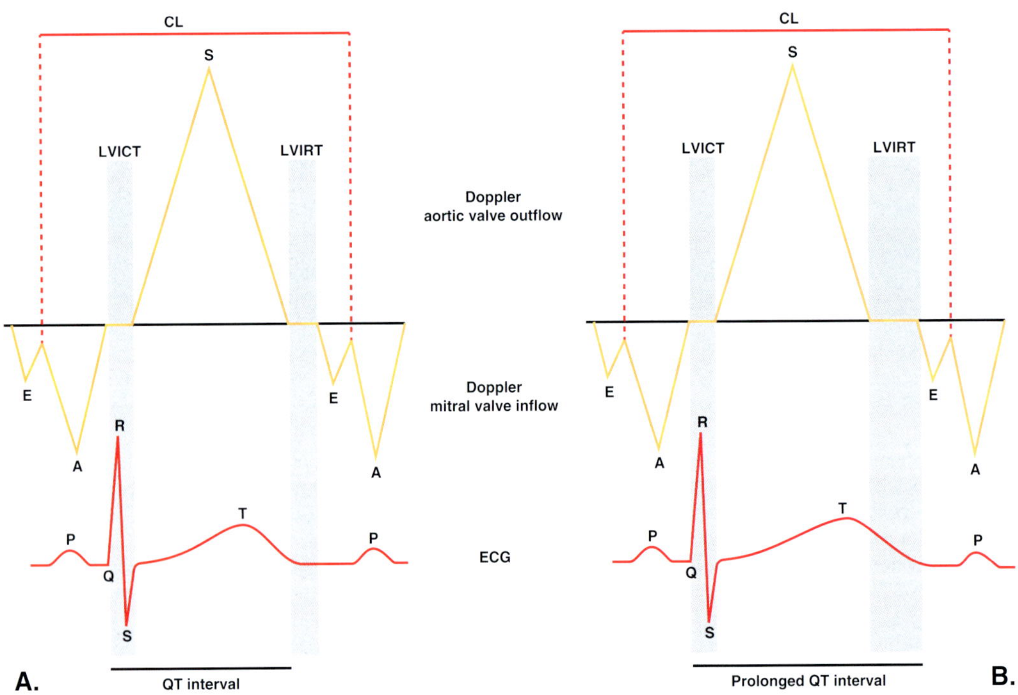

FIGURE 3.3.8 Cartoon showing the relationship between the left ventricular isovolumic contraction and relaxation times (LVICT and LVIRT) in the left ventricle as measured from simultaneous mitral inflow and aortic outflow Doppler time compared to the electrocardiogram. A: Normal fetus; **B:** fetus with long QT syndrome. CL, cardiac cycle length. (Reprinted from Clur SB, Vink AS, Etheridge SP, et al. Left ventricular isovolumetric relaxation time is prolonged in fetal long-QT syndrome. *Circ Arrhythm Electrophysiol*. 2018;11(4):e005797.)

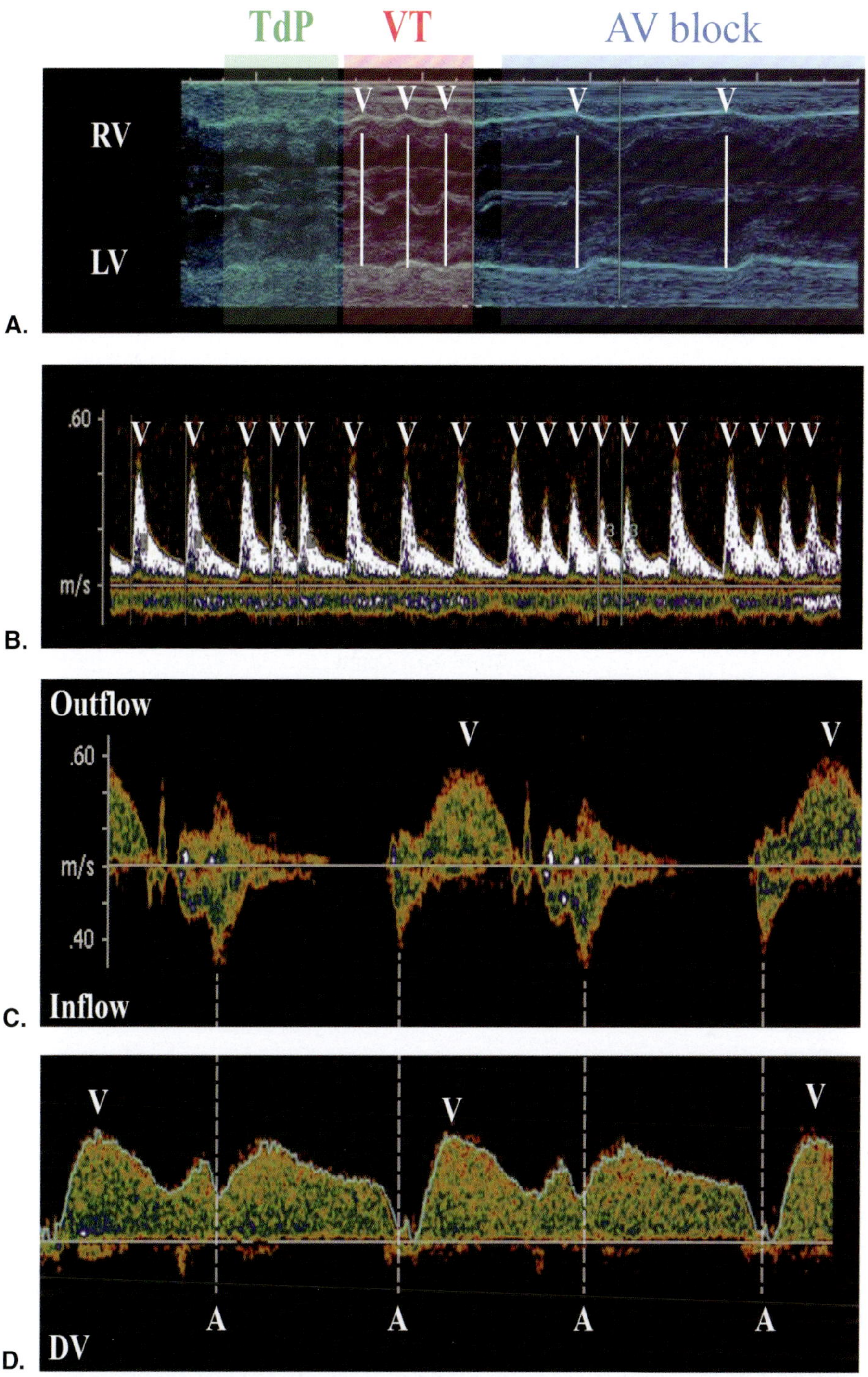

FIGURE 3.3.9 Signature fetal and neonatal rhythms in long QT syndrome. A: M-mode registration through the right and left ventricles (RV, LV) showing a short burst of torsade de pointes (TdP) followed by four beats of a more regular ventricular tachycardia (VT) with a ventricular rate of 260 bpm. Immediately thereafter 2:1 AV block occurs with a ventricular rate of 60 bpm. **B:** Umbilical artery Doppler tracing showing runs of polymorphic VT. Note the variable velocities of the arterial pulsations. **C:** Doppler of mitral inflow (below baseline) and aortic outflow (above baseline). Atrial contractions are shown by dotted lines. The rhythm is functional 2° AV block with 2:1 conduction. **D:** Ductus venosus (DV) Doppler tracing corresponding to the arrhythmia in panel **C**. Note the second atrial contraction occurs nearly simultaneous with onset of ventricular contraction. **E:** TdP registered on the monitor postnatally. **F:** Postnatal monitor recording showing functional 2:1 AV block due to a very long QT-interval.

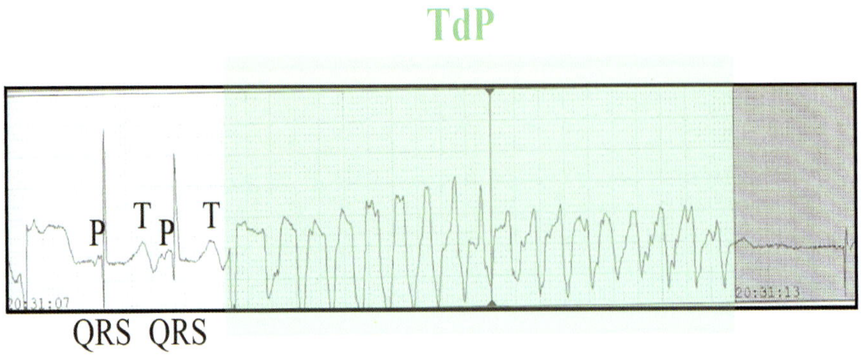

E.

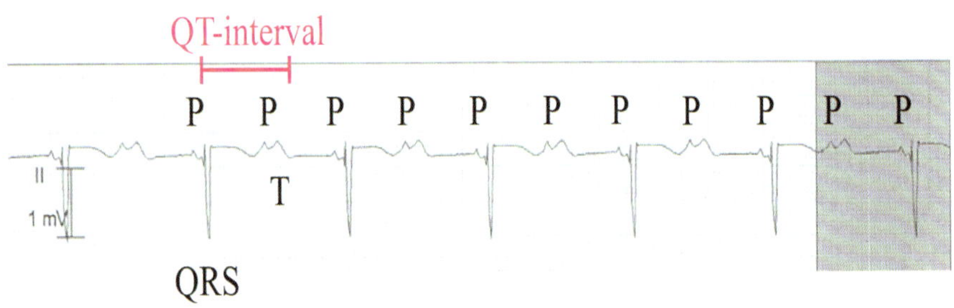

F.

FIGURE 3.3.9 Cont'd

output during TdP can be related to the amplitude of the aortic ejection wave. Variable velocities on the umbilical artery Doppler are seen during runs of TdP (FIGS. 3.3.7C and 3.3.9B).[26] It is not surprising then that these fetuses may rapidly develop hydrops fetalis if untreated. A more extensive discourse on LQTS is found in Part 3, Chapter 7 of this book.

Fetal Cardiomyopathy

Fetuses with a cardiomyopathy including those with cardiomyopathy secondary to maternal anti-Ro/SSA antibodies may also present with AV block and VT.[5,27,28] Some cases of anti-Ro/SSA–mediated cardiomyopathy can present with a prolonged QT-interval, which theoretically increases susceptibility to TdP. The differentiation between LQTS and anti-Ro/SSA antibody–mediated AV block is important, because anti-inflammatory agents such as dexamethasone and intravenous immune globulin may be helpful if anti-Ro/SSA antibodies are present. During periods of bradycardia, complete AV block suggests anti-Ro/SSA antibody disease while functional 2:1 AV block (due to the extremely long QT-interval) or blocked AE in bigeminy suggests LQTS.[24]

PROGNOSIS OF FETAL VT

Fetal VT associated with structural or functional myocardial disease has a guarded prognosis. In the absence of heart disease and LQTS, the clinical outcome associated with idiopathic fetal VT is benign with spontaneous resolution in late gestation or within a few months after birth.[29] Those with only intermittent and short-lived runs of VT may not require prenatal therapy, whereas persistent VT may cause cardiovascular compromise and warrants initiation of transplacental therapy.

DIAGNOSIS OF ACCELERATED VENTRICULAR RHYTHM

Accelerated ventricular rhythm (AVR) is an arrhythmia with some electrocardiographic characteristics of VT, that is, V-A dissociation and a ventricular rate faster than the atrial rate, but the ventricular rate is just slightly faster (15%-25%) than the atrial rate in sinus rhythm.[4,21,30,31] This results in an occurrence of almost simultaneous atrial and ventricular contractions.[21] The true incidence of AVR is unknown. Fouron et al[21] found three cases in 27,912 fetuses. Of the few fetal cases reported, a third had evidence of a pericardial effusion or hydrops,[21] raising concerns that AVR might be less well tolerated by the fetus than in postnatal life when it is usually self-limiting and benign. As the almost simultaneous atrial and ventricular contractions occurring during AVR elevate the fetal central venous pressure, increasing the risk of heart failure, it has been suggested that AVR might be an underappreciated and unrecognized cause of hydrops fetalis.[30]

SUMMARY

VT in the fetus is rare. Making the correct diagnosis using echocardiography can be challenging but is possible with the careful use of techniques that record the ventricular and atrial activity simultaneously, such as the superior vena cava (SVC) and ascending aorta (aAo) approach. Hydrops may occur depending on the duration and rate of the tachycardia. Polymorphic VT is recognized by variable systolic velocities in the aAo or umbilical artery Doppler. When short bursts of (polymorphic) VT are seen, especially when associated with 2:1 AV block or sinus bradycardia, fetal LQTS should be suspected. In AVR the basic findings of a VT are also present with A-V dissociation, but the ventricular rate is typically slower and periods of 1:1 VA-association and almost simultaneous ventricular and atrial activity are frequently seen. This results in cannon A waves in the DV Doppler and elevation of fetal central venous pressure, predisposing to hydrops even in the absence of a fast ventricular rate.

A conservative approach can be justified for intermittent VT without signs of heart failure in view of reports of spontaneous resolution. Pharmacological treatment discussed in Part 4, Chapter 4 should be tailored to the type of VT and the presumed cause. Delivery considerations for the fetus with VT are discussed in Part 5, Chapter 3.

ACKNOWLEDGMENTS

In addition to the authors, the following individuals contributed images to this chapter: Annika Rydberg, MD, PhD, University of Umea, Sweden; Ulrike Herberg, MD, PhD, University of Bonn, Bonn, Germany; Stacy Killen, MD, Vanderbilt University, Nashville, TN, USA; and RT Wakai, PhD, University of Wisconsin-Madison, Madison, WI, USA.

References

1. Hornberger LK, Sahn DJ. Rhythm abnormalities of the fetus. *Heart*. 2007;93(10):1294-1300.
2. Jaeggi ET, Nii M. Fetal brady- and tachyarrhythmias: new and accepted diagnostic and treatment methods. *Semin Fetal Neonatal Med*. 2005;10(6):504-514.
3. Brugada J, Blom N, Sarquella-Brugada G, et al. Pharmacological and non-pharmacological therapy for arrhythmias in the pediatric population: EHRA and AEPC-Arrhythmia Working Group joint consensus statement. *Europace*. 2013;15(9):1337-1382.
4. Fouron JC. Fetal arrhythmias: the Saint-Justine hospital experience. *Prenat Diagn*. 2004;24(13):1068-1080.
5. Duke C, Stuart G, Simpson JM. Ventricular tachycardia secondary to prolongation of the QT interval in a fetus with autoimmune mediated congenital complete heart block. *Cardiol Young*. 2005;15(3):319-321.
6. Stevens DC, Schreiner RL, Hurwitz RA, Gresham EL. Fetal and neonatal ventricular arrhythmia. *Pediatrics*. 1979;63(5):771-777.
7. Schleich JM, Bernard Du Haut Cilly F, Laurent MC, Almange C. Early prenatal management of a fetal ventricular tachycardia treated in utero by amiodarone with long term follow-up. *Prenat Diagn*. 2000;20(6):449-452.
8. Simpson JM, Sharland GK. Fetal tachycardias: management and outcome of 127 consecutive cases. *Heart*. 1998;79(6):576-581.
9. Lulic Jurjevic R, Podnar T, Vesel S. Diagnosis, clinical features, management, and post-natal follow-up of fetal tachycardias. *Cardiol Young*. 2009;19(5):486-493.
10. van Engelen AD, Weijtens O, Brenner JI, et al. Management outcome and follow-up of fetal tachycardia. *J Am Coll Cardiol*. 1994;24(5):1371-1375.
11. Ueda K, Maeno Y, Miyoshi T, et al. The impact of intrauterine treatment on fetal tachycardia: a nationwide survey in Japan. *J Matern Fetal Neonatal Med*. 2018;31(19):2605-2610.
12. Strasburger JF, Cheulkar B, Wichman HJ. Perinatal arrhythmias: diagnosis and management. *Clin Perinatol*. 2007;34(4):627-652.
13. Cuneo BF, Ovadia M, Strasburger JF, et al. Prenatal diagnosis and in utero treatment of torsades de pointes associated with congenital long QT syndrome. *Am J Cardiol*. 2003;91(11):1395-1398.
14. Simpson JM, Maxwell D, Rosenthal E, et al. Fetal ventricular tachycardia secondary to long QT syndrome treated with maternal intravenous magnesium: case report and review of the literature. *Ultrasound Obstet Gynecol*. 2009;34(4):475-480.
15. Hofbeck M, Ulmer H, Beinder E, Sieber E, Singer H. Prenatal findings in patients with prolonged QT interval in the neonatal period. *Heart*. 1997;77(3):198-204.
16. Miller TE, Estrella E, Myerburg RJ, et al. Recurrent third-trimester fetal loss and maternal mosaicism for long-QT syndrome. *Circulation*. 2004;109(24):3029-3034.
17. Oudijk MA, Gooskens RH, Stoutenbeek P, De Vries LS, Visser GH, Meijboom EJ. Neurological outcome of children who were treated for fetal tachycardia complicated by hydrops. *Ultrasound Obstet Gynecol*. 2004;24(2):154-158.
18. Bhuiyan ZA, Momenah TS, Gong Q, et al. Recurrent intrauterine fetal loss due to near absence of HERG: clinical and functional characterization of a homozygous nonsense HERG Q1070X mutation. *Heart Rhythm*. 2008;5(4):553-561.
19. Sherer DM, Sadovksy E, Menashe M, Mordel N, Rein AJ. Fetal ventricular tachycardia associated with nonimmunologic hydrops fetalis. A case report. *J Reprod Med*. 1990;35(3):292-294.
20. Rein AJ, Levine JC, Nir A. Use of high-frame rate imaging and Doppler tissue echocardiography in the diagnosis of fetal ventricular tachycardia. *J Am Soc Echocardiogr*. 2001;14(2):149-151.

21. Fouron JC, McNeal-Davidson A, Abadir S, et al. Prenatal diagnosis and prognosis of accelerated idioventricular rhythm. *Ultrasound Obstet Gynecol.* 2017;50(5):624-631.
22. Cuneo BF, Strasburger JF, Yu S, et al. In utero diagnosis of long QT syndrome by magnetocardiography. *Circulation.* 2013;128(20):2183-2191.
23. Cuneo BF, Etheridge SP, Horigome H, et al. Arrhythmia phenotype during fetal life suggests long-QT syndrome genotype: risk stratification of perinatal long-QT syndrome. *Circ Arrhythm Electrophysiol.* 2013;6(5):946-951.
24. Clur SB, Vink AS, Etheridge SP, et al. Left ventricular isovolumetric relaxation time is prolonged in fetal long-QT syndrome. *Circ Arrhythm Electrophysiol.* 2018;11(4):e005797.
25. Mitchell JL, Cuneo BF, Etheridge SP, Horigome H, Weng HY, Benson DW. Fetal heart rate predictors of long QT syndrome. *Circulation.* 2012;126(23):2688-2695.
26. Miyoshi T, Sakaguchi H, Shiraishi I, Yoshimatsu J, Ikeda T. Potential utility of pulsed-wave Doppler for prenatal diagnosis of fetal ventricular tachycardia secondary to long QT syndrome. *Ultrasound Obstet Gynecol.* 2018;51(5):697-699.
27. Walls J, Dipchand A, Sanatani S. Dilated cardiomyopathy masquerading as long QT syndrome. *Pediatr Cardiol.* 2006;27(1):156-159.
28. Zhao H, Cuneo BF, Strasburger JF, Huhta JC, Gotteiner NL, Wakai RT. Electrophysiological characteristics of fetal AV block. *J Am Coll Cardiol.* 2008;51:77-84.
29. Yumoto Y, Satoh S, Koga T, Nagata H, Nagamatsu R, Nakano H. Prenatal diagnosis of slow-rate ventricular tachycardia using fetal electrocardiography. *Prenat Diagn.* 2004;24(6):463-467.
30. Lopes L, Cha S, Scanavacca M, Tuma-Calil VM, Zugaib M. Fetal idiopathic ventricular tachycadia with non-immune hydrops: benign course. *Pediatr Cardiol.* 1996;17:192-193.
31. Wren C. Cardiac arrhythmias in the fetus and newborn. *Semin Fetal Neonatal Med.* 2006;11(3):182-190.

Atrioventricular Block and Structural Cardiac Defects

Fayeza Alrais • Anita J. Moon-Grady

INTRODUCTION

Although the obstetrical definition of fetal bradycardia is a fetal heart rate (FHR) < 110 beats per minute at any time during gestation,[1] recent studies suggest that an FHR < third percentile for gestational age[2] may have superior sensitivity and specificity. Bradycardia may be either sinus bradycardia with 1:1 atrioventricular (AV) conduction, AV block, or blocked atrial bigeminy (see Part 3, Chapter 1). Bradycardia may also occur with congenital (structural) heart abnormalities (ie, congenital heart disease [CHD]). In these cases, the sinoatrial (SA) node or AV node is usually displaced, duplicated, or even absent. For the fetal cardiologist, the distinction between the anti-Ro/SSA–mediated AV block (discussed in Part 3, Chapter 5) and AV block associated with CHD is important due to the differences in pre- and postnatal outcome (FIG. 3.4.1).

Approximately 30% of newborns with 3° (or complete) AV block have associated CHD.[3-6] The fetal presentation is much more common than 30%, suggesting many die in utero. Thus, the prognosis for a fetus with 3° AV block and CHD is extremely poor. Review of several larger series identified that fewer than 15% were alive at the end of the neonatal period (TABLE 3.4.1). Fetuses at highest risk for a poor outcome are those with hydrops and a ventricular rate of <50 to 55 beats per minute (bpm). If the fetus is liveborn, the infant many succumb during the neonatal period even if they receive a pacemaker.

Pathophysiology of AV Block and CHD

Why does bradycardia and AV block have such a profound effect on fetal survival in the presence of CHD? Fetal cardiac output primarily increases by heart rate,[7] which is not possible with an abnormal conduction system. Inability to increase heart rate leads to a decline in cardiac output, impaired cardiac filling, and venous congestion,[4,8] which is particularly poorly tolerated in the presence of concomitant CHD. Impairments in myocardial oxygen delivery translate clinically into fetal myocardial diastolic dysfunction, cardiomyopathy, and eventually may lead to fetal nonimmune hydrops; all of which either separately or collectively negatively affect prognosis and increase perinatal mortality risk in affected fetuses.

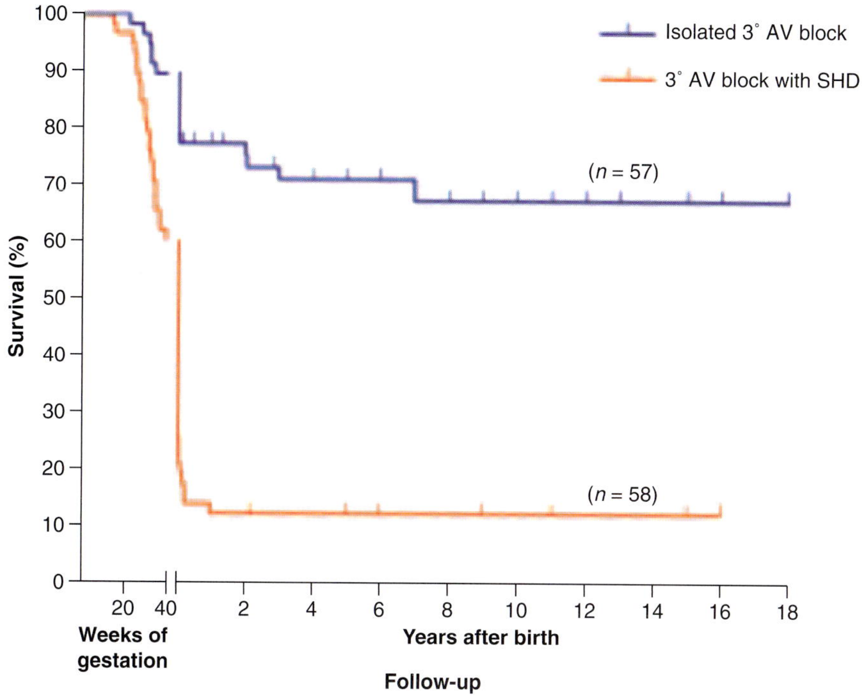

FIGURE 3.4.1 Kaplan-Meier survival curves for isolated complete heart block (3° AV block, purple line) and complete heart block associated with structural (congenital) heart disease (SHD, orange line) before and after birth. (Reprinted from Lopes LM, Tavares GM, Damiano AP, et al. Perinatal outcome of fetal atrioventricular block: one-hundred-sixteen cases from a single institution. *Circulation*. 2008;118(12):1268-1275.)

TABLE 3.4.1 PRESENTATION AND OUTCOME OF FETAL AV BLOCK AND LEFT ATRIAL ISOMERISM OR CONGENITALLY CORRECTED TRANSPOSITION OF THE GREAT VESSELS

Reference (y)	AV Block + CHD	LAI (Hydrops)	Fetal/ Neonatal Mortality	cc-TGA (Hydrops)	Fetal/ Neonatal Mortality
Machado[29] (1988)	21	21 (10)	86%	0	–
Gembruch[30] (1989)	18	5 (5)	77%	4 (0)	0%
Schmidt[6] (1991)	24	17 (14)	100%	7 (0)	43%
Jaeggi[27] (2005)	24	18 (8)	94%	3 (0)	100%
Berg[23] (2005)	32	31	97%	1 (0)	0%
Lim[31] (2005)	13	52 (ND)	85%	0	–
Lopes[3] (2008)	48	40 (ND)	88%	8 (0)	25%
Escobar-Diaz[18] (2014)	8	8 (4)	–	0	50%
Vigneswaran[19] (2019)	4	0	–	4 (0)	0%
Sharland[20] (2005)	2	0	–	2 (0)	50%
Paladini[21] (2006)	3	0	–	3(0)	0%
Wan[22] (2009)	1	0	–	1(0)	0%
Miyoshi[27] (2015)	26	22 (11)	41%	4	0%

AV, atrioventricular; cc-TGA, congenitally corrected transposition of the great vessels; CHD, congenital heart disease; LAI, left atrial isomerism; ND, no data.

CONGENITAL HEART DEFECTS ASSOCIATED WITH BRADYCARDIA AND AV BLOCK

In most published studies, a majority of affected fetuses with sinus bradycardia or 3° AV block had either heterotaxy (an abnormality where the internal thoracoabdominal organs demonstrate abnormal arrangement across the left-right axis of the body)[9] (FIG. 3.4.2A and B) or discordant AV connection (also known as congenitally corrected transposition of the great arteries [cc-TGA]) (FIG. 3.4.2C). In heterotaxy, abnormal cardiac development often leads to atrial appendage isomerism, resulting in either bilateral paired right atria (right atrial isomerism, RAI) or paired left atria (left atrial isomerism, LAI). Fetuses with RAI often have dual SA nodes (because they are right-sided structures) resulting in an ectopic atrial rhythm with a slower beat rate than normal (FIG. 3.4.3). On the other hand, fetuses with LAI have bilateral left atrial morphology and frequently lack a normal SA node. Bradycardia in this setting may result in a nonsinus atrial pacemaker from a left atrial focus, or they may have AV block (FIG. 3.4.4). The exact pathophysiology of AV block in LAI lies in the discontinuity between the AV node and the conduction axis.[10] This discontinuity is found to be distal to the AV node, in contrast to the pattern of atrial-axis discontinuity found in anti-Ro/SSA AV block caused mainly by replacement of the SA node and AV node by a loose fibrous tissue.

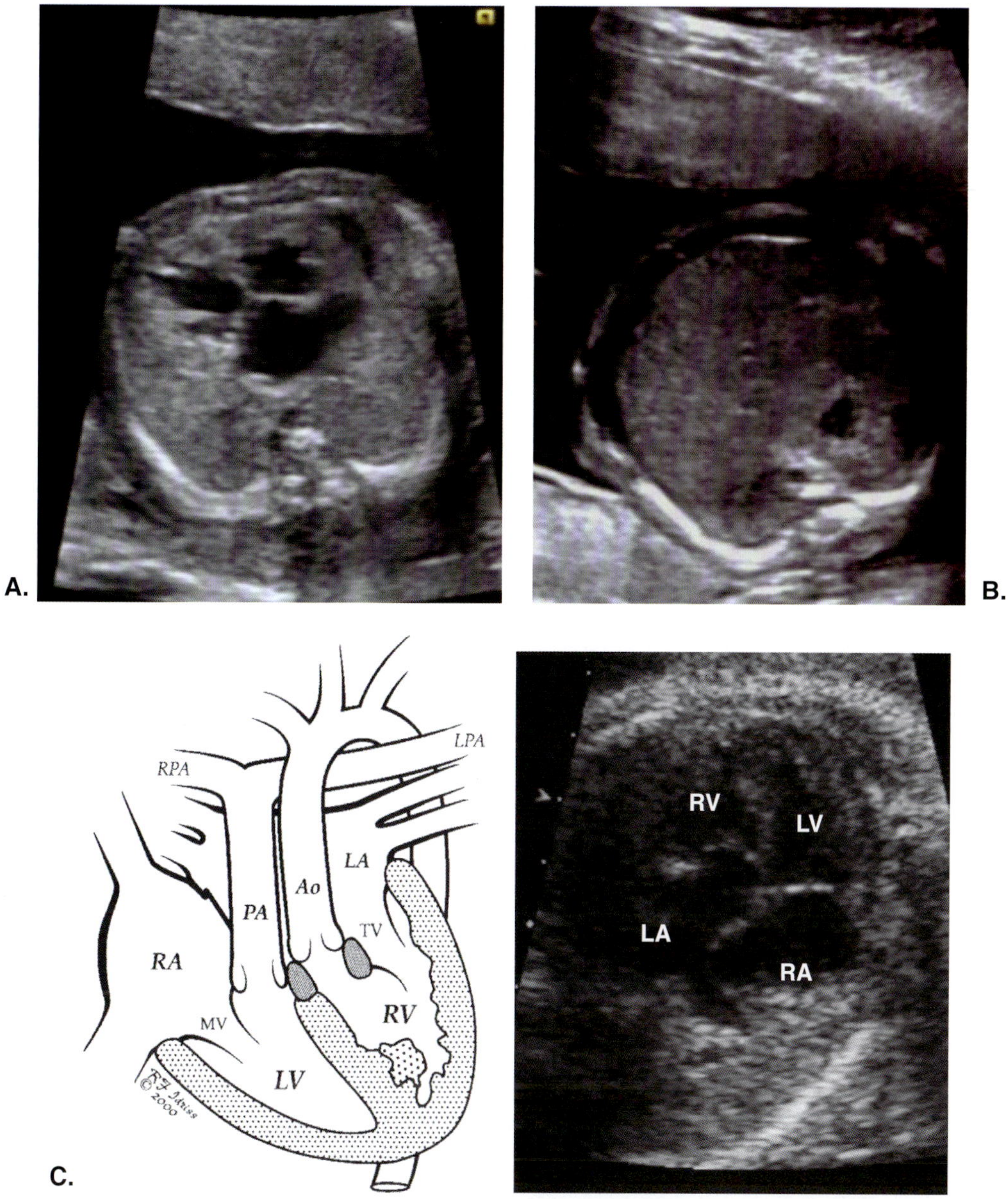

FIGURE 3.4.2 Congenital heart defects associated with AV block. **A:** Axial view of the fetal chest. The apex of the heart is pointing left, but even in this still frame, only one AV valve is seen. There is a small pericardial effusion (PE). To the left of the spine is the aorta and the azygous vein, suggesting an interrupted inferior vena cava. **B:** Caudal to figure **A**, the stomach is on the right. Ascites is seen. **C:** Congenitally corrected transposition of the great arteries (cc-TGA). Diagram and four-chamber view of cc-TGA showing atrioventricular and ventriculo-arterial discordance. (C, Reprinted from Maizels M, Cuneo BF, Sabbagha RE, eds. *Fetal Anomalies: Ultrasound Diagnosis and Postnatal Management*. New York, NY: Wiley-Liss; 2002.)

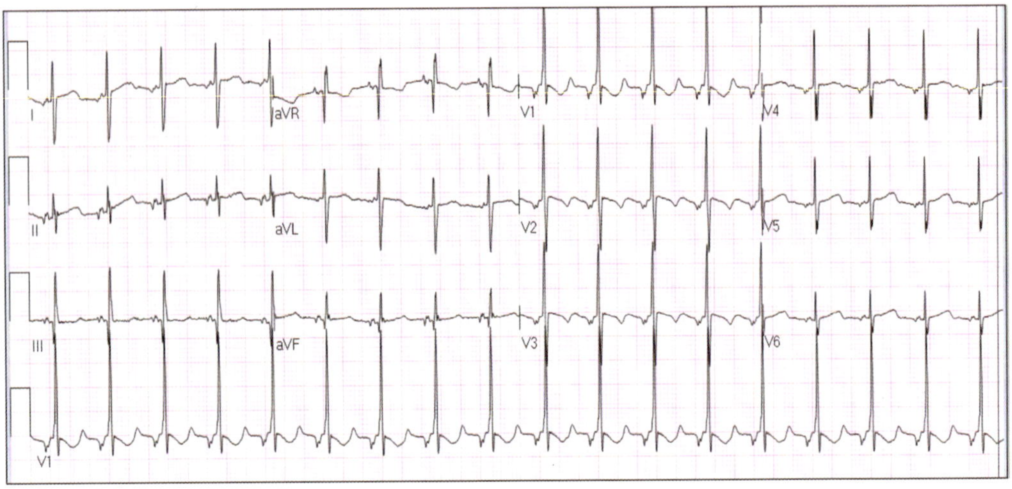

FIGURE 3.4.3 Twelve-lead ECG of an infant with right atrial isomerism (RAI). The P-wave is bifed but mostly inferior in lead 1, suggesting the pacemaker of the heart arises in the lower right atrium.

Other features of LAI include ipsilateral pulmonary venous return, an interrupted inferior vena cava with azygous continuation to the right or left superior vena cava, bilateral vena cava, and a spongy myocardium (ventricular noncompaction)[11-18] (FIGS. 3.4.5 and 3.4.6). Conduction system disease in LAI can present before 13 weeks and be progressive (FIGS. 3.4.7 and 3.4.8). In subjects with cc-TGA, the inversion of the ventricles often leads to disruption of the AV conduction axis and AV block, which usually appears in the third trimester. Familial recurrence of LAI has been documented in some case series,[14,15] raising the possibility of an underlying heritable pathogenic variant, while recurrence of cc-TGA has not been reported.

A.

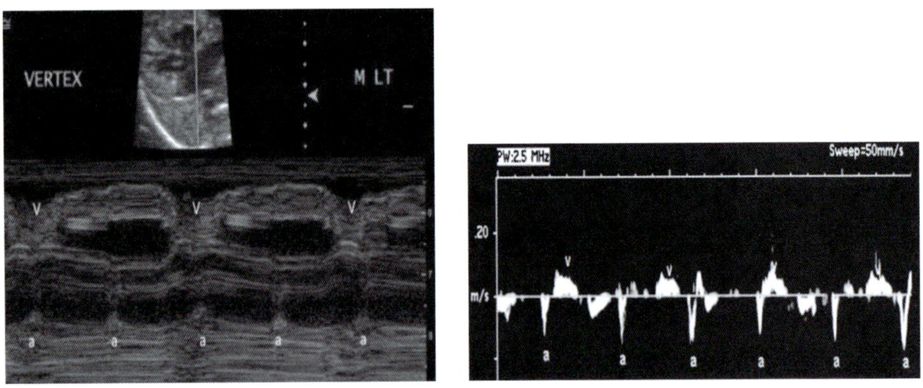

B.

FIGURE 3.4.4 Congenital heart disease (CHD) and 3° AV block. **A:** Simultaneous ventricular (v) and atrial (a) M-mode of a fetus with AV block and a slow (95 bpm) atrial rate. **B:** Mitral valve tissue Doppler of the same fetus.

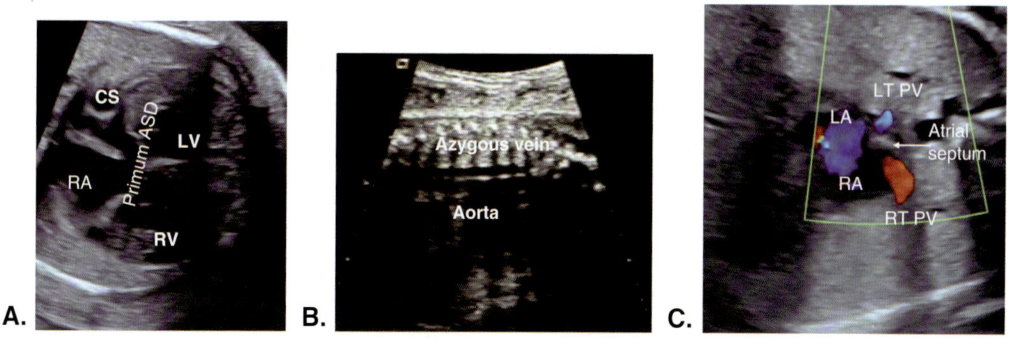

FIGURE 3.4.5 Echocardiographic features of left atrial isomerism (LAI). **A:** Four-chamber view showing a dilated coronary sinus (which received a left superior vena cava (not shown), a large primum atrial septal defect consistent with an AV sepal defect. **B:** Sagittal view of the azygous vein seen posterior to the aorta. This indicates an interrupted inferior vena cava with azygous connection to the right or left superior vena cava, seen in about 90% of fetuses with LAI. **C:** Ipsilateral pulmonary venous drainage: the right pulmonary veins (red) drain to the right-sided atrium and the left pulmonary veins drain to the left-sided atrium.CS, coronary sinus; LA, left atrium; Lt PV, left pulmonary vein; LV, left ventricle; RA, right atrium; Rt PV, right pulmonary vein; RV, right ventricle.

Outcome of Congenital Heart Disease Associated With AV Block and Bradycardia

Heterotaxy

The outcome of LAI with AV block is far worse than the outcome of LAI with sinus rhythm (FIG. 3.4.9). Therefore, fetuses with isomerism and either AV block or sinus bradycardia should receive increased surveillance after reaching a potentially viable gestational age, to look for new cardiac dysfunction and/or hydrops which if present would impact management options and counseling.

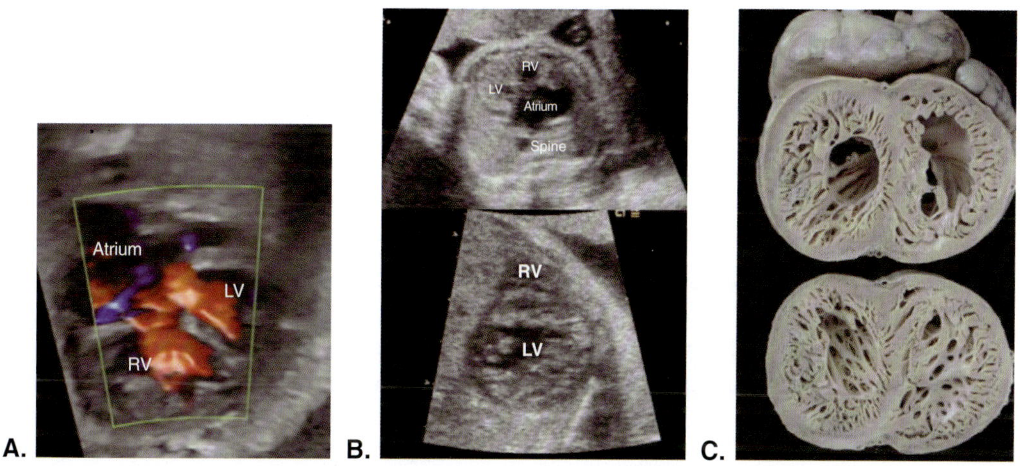

FIGURE 3.4.6 Ventricular noncompaction cardiomyopathy (also called "spongy myocardium") seen with left atrial isomerism (LAI) and AV block. **A** and **B:** Fetal echocardiogram and **C:** Pathologic specimen demonstrating spongiform appearance of the right and left ventricular myocardium. LV, left ventricle; RV, right ventricle. (C, This image is from the Web Portal of the Archiving Working Group of The International Society for Nomenclature of Paediatric and Congenital Heart Disease [ISNPCHD] [http://ipccc-awg.net] and courtesy of Diane E. Spicer BS, PA (ASCP) (The Congenital Heart Institute of Florida [CHIF]).)

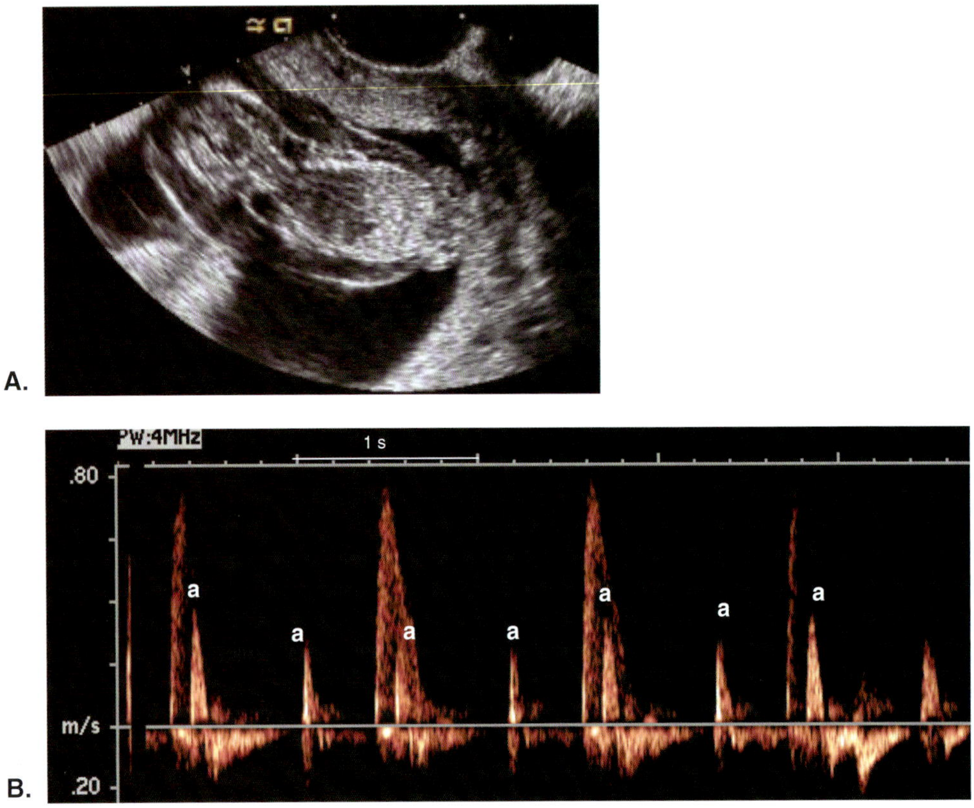

FIGURE 3.4.7 Transvaginal ultrasound of a 13-week fetus with bradycardia. **A:** Isolated levocardia and ventricular noncompaction were seen (not shown), and the fetus is severely hydropic. **B:** The rhythm is 3° AV block with a ventricular rate of 53 bpm. a, atrial contractions.

Three large studies have evaluated outcome of fetal heterotaxy. The first single center study from 1995 to 2011[18] reported 91 fetuses with LAI, 22 of whom had AV block or sinus bradycardia. Fifteen survived to birth. Predictors of mortality included hydrops and ventricular dysfunction. Surprisingly, fetuses with sinus bradycardia were at similar risk of mortality (50% of deaths) as those with AV block. A second retrospective study from 1980 to 2017 reported 177 fetuses with LAI, with 40% (n = 70) having AV block. Almost 50% of the LAI and AV block pregnancies were interrupted, and none of the remaining fetuses with LAI, outflow tract obstruction, and AV block survived.[19] The third study reported 40 fetal cases with AV block with no survivors by 3 months of age.[3]

A unique feature of some fetuses with LAI is a spongy or non-compacted myocardium (FIG. 3.4.6).[11-17] The combination of a spongy myocardium, CHD, and AV block is almost uniformly fatal, if not in utero, in the neonatal period.

A. C.

B. D.

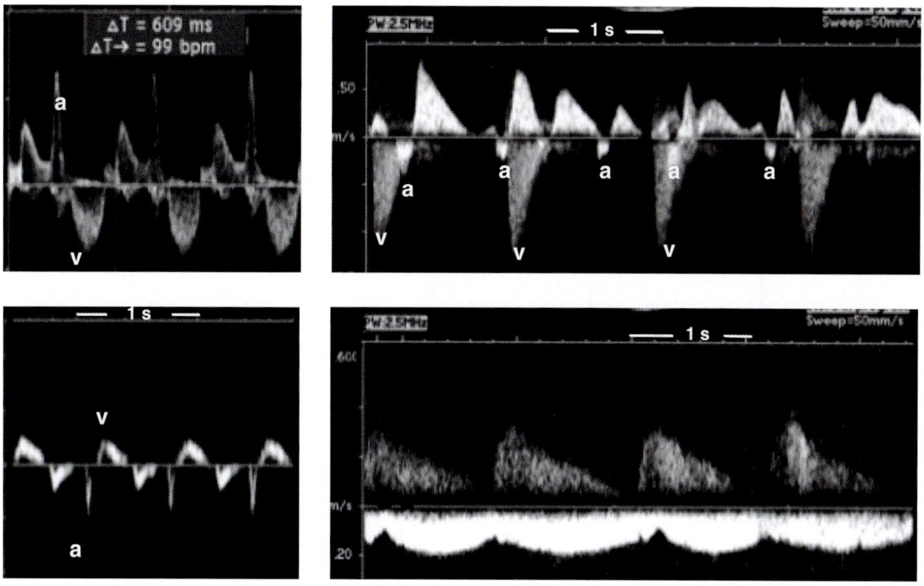

FIGURE 3.4.8 Evolution of AV block in left atrial isomerism (LAI). **A:** Pulsed Doppler of mitral (top tracings) and aortic valves and **(B)**, tissue Doppler at the lateral tricuspid annulus showing bradycardia with 1:1 AV conduction at 19 weeks (FHR 99 bpm). At 29 weeks, the rhythm evolved to 3° AV block with atrial bradycardia (90 bpm) and a low ventricular escape rate (50 bpm) as seen by superior vena cava (SVC)–aorta Doppler **(C)** and umbilical Doppler **(D)**. Note that in **(C** and **D)**, there is no relationship between the atrial (a) and the ventricular (v) contractions.

Congenitally Corrected Transposition of the Great Arteries

Hearts with cc-TGA are the second most frequently associated CHD with AV block, yet comprise fewer than 2% of reported fetal CHD cases. Cc-TGA should be considered in any case of intermittent or sustained 3° AV block, and fetuses with cc-TGA and apparently normal conduction should be followed for development of AV block **(FIG. 3.4.10)**. Subjects with cc-TGA have a normally located SA node and so are not prone to sinus bradycardia, but because of abnormal formation of the AV junction, the conduction tissue is abnormal and there is a lifetime risk of developing AV block. The outcome in cc-TGA is usually much better than the outcome for heterotaxy.[20-23] However, AV block is a risk factor for mortality in cc-TGA, which further increases with associated malformations, such as Ebstein malformation of the tricuspid valve[20-22] **(FIG. 3.4.11)**.

Eighty prenatal cases of cc-TGA have been described in three retrospective studies[20-23] **(TABLE 3.4.1)**. Of these cases, only seven developed AV block: three in the third trimester and four in the neonatal period. All seven cases received pacemakers as neonates. One patient died during infancy, and there were two intrauterine deaths.

Other Types of CHD Associated With AV Block

Other types of CHD associated with AV block are rare and sporadic and do not follow any pattern. In a large retrospective series,[3] >90% of AV block cases were associated with LAI or cc-TGA.

(text continued on page 150)

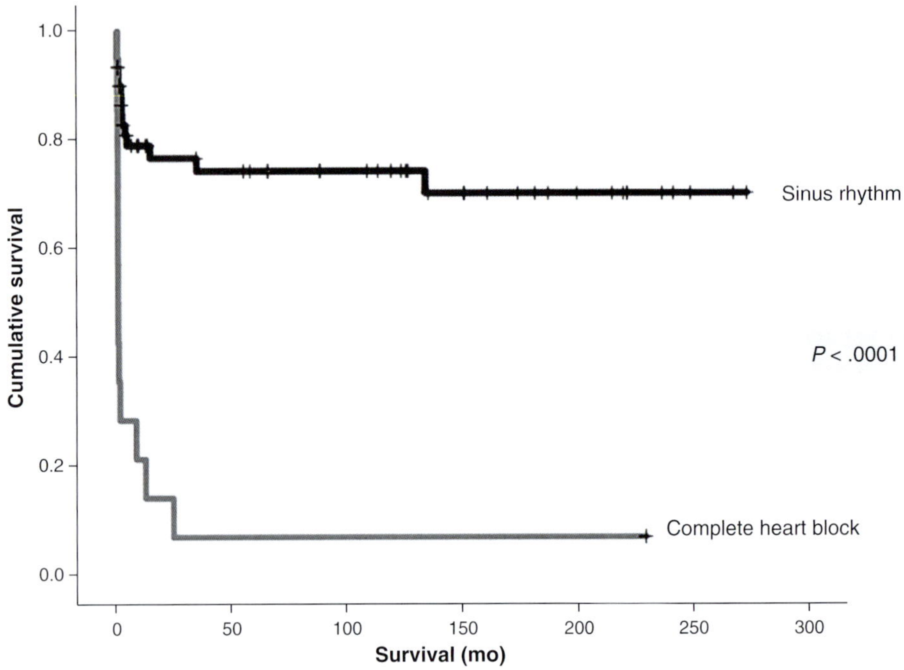

FIGURE 3.4.9 Kaplan-Meier survival curve of 70 infants with left atrial isomerism (LAI) and sinus rhythm (dark line) and those with complete heart block (gray line). (Reprinted from Vigneswaran TV, Jones CB, Zidere V, et al. Effect of prenatal laterality disturbance and its accompanying anomalies on survival. *Am J Cardiol*. 2018;122(4):663-671.)

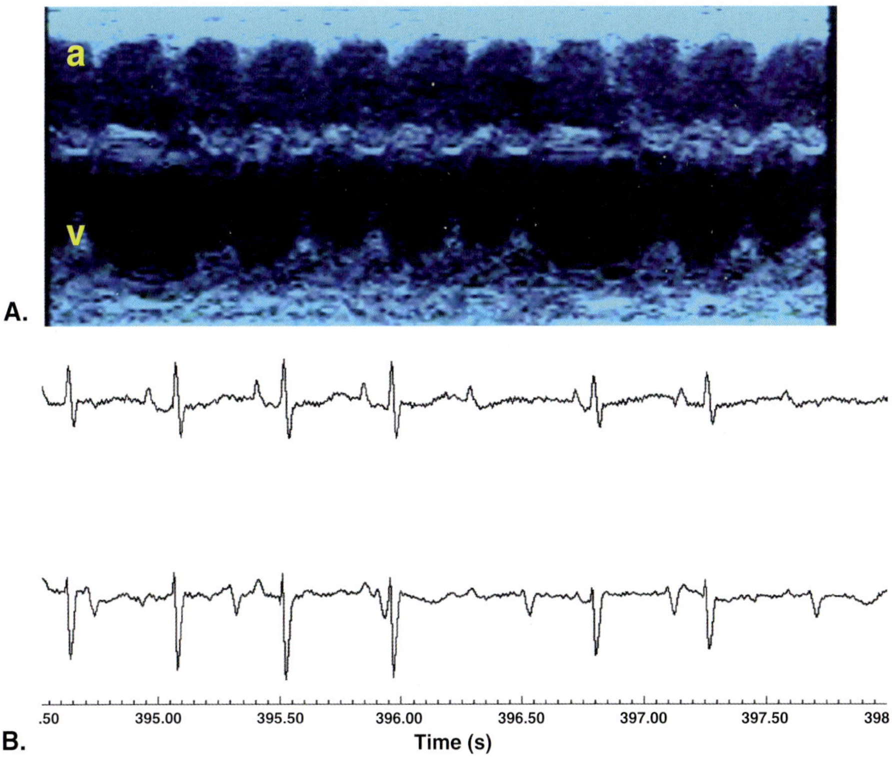

FIGURE 3.4.10 cc-TGA and AV block. **A:** Simultaneous atrial (a) and ventricular (v) M-mode of a 34-week fetus followed since early gestation with cc-TGA with intermittent AV block, seen as ventricular silence following an atrial contraction. **B:** Fetal magnetocardiogram of the same fetus shows intermittent type 2, 2° AV block (*).

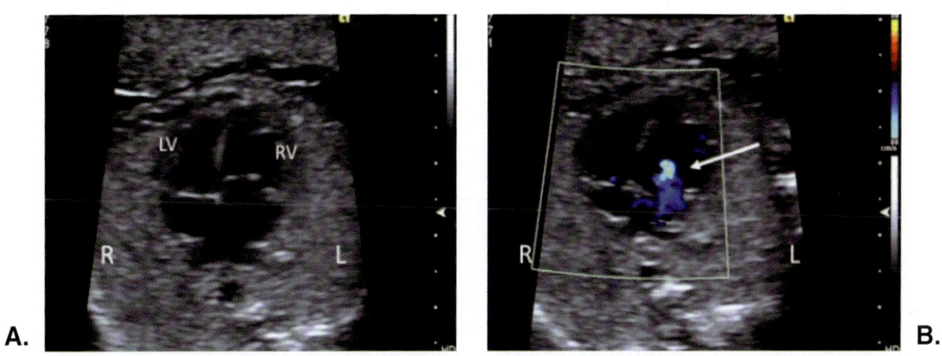

FIGURE 3.4.11 **A:** cc-TGA with Epstein anomaly of the posterior left-sided tricuspid valve. Since the AV valve always follows its ventricle, the right ventricle is posterior and to left and receives blood from the left atrium. **B:** The color Doppler demonstrates mild tricuspid insufficiency (arrow).

FETAL DIAGNOSIS AND EVALUATION

Early Diagnosis

Most of the cases described to date reported average gestational age at diagnosing CHD and AV block to be around 20 weeks, at time of routine second trimester obstetrical anomaly scan. As the main etiology of AV block associated with CHD lies in defective cardiac embryogenesis, the bradycardia of AV block can be detected at the time of nuchal translucency screening. However, <10% of reported cases of CHD and AV block are diagnosed at <15 weeks. Indications for early second trimester evaluation are sustained bradycardia (FIG. 3.4.7), an increased nuchal translucency at 10 to 12 weeks, or the history of a previously affected child.[3,24]

General Evaluation

If a fetal echocardiogram shows a regular ventricular rhythm and 1:1 AV relationship, then the fetus is considered to be in sinus rhythm. However, if the atrial rate is slower than ~110 beats bpm, the atrial focus may be nonsinus or ectopic, suggesting the possibility of displaced, duplicated, or even absent SA node. The AV interval should be measured and recorded, as progression of AV conduction disease during gestation is common and higher degrees of AV block may be preceded by 1° block.

In addition to assessing mechanisms of fetal bradyarrhythmia, cardiac anatomy, and overall fetal well-being, evidence of cardiac decompensation and other associated conditions that might worsen clinical outcome should also be evaluated. Traditional methods of assessing hemodynamic "well-being" are difficult in the fetus with 2° or 3° AV block as intermittent atrial contraction against a closed AV valve may produce a reflected A-wave in the ductus venosus, which in sinus rhythm, would imply decreased compliance. Furthermore, flow disturbance in the umbilical vein in the fetus with AV block should not be misinterpreted as the pulsations associated with imminent fetal death (FIG. 3.4.12). Fetal cardiomegaly, FHR < 50 bpm, and fetal hydrops portend a poor outcome. If fetal hydrops is present, an assessment of maternal health status including elevation in blood pressure and/or liver enzymes that may indicate development of "mirror" syndrome should be carried out.

The familial nature of heterotaxy has been noted raising and considerable progress made in defining the genetic underpinnings.[25] Consequently, a family history of heterotaxy warrants fetal echocardiographic screening in future pregnancies. Inheritance may be autosomal dominant, autosomal recessive, or X-linked. Interestingly, the pattern of inheritance favors lateral recurrence (siblings) rather than vertical recurrence (offspring).

Delivery

The biophysical profile may be helpful to assess the timing of delivery. For all fetuses with structural disease and bradycardia, avoidance of unnecessary iatrogenic premature delivery is key to improved survival; planning for administration of appropriate inotropic and chronotropic support after birth may stabilize the infant.[26] Fetuses with

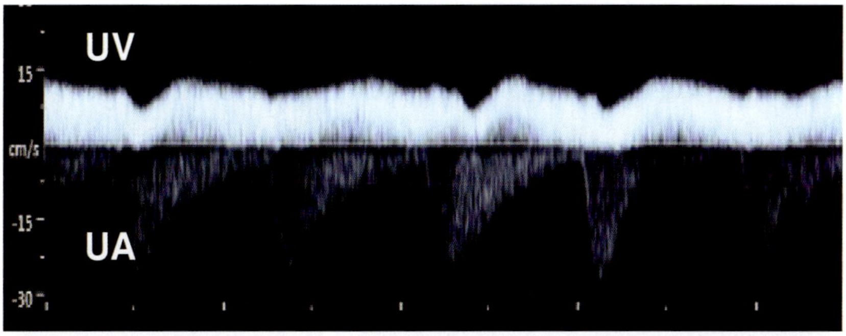

A.

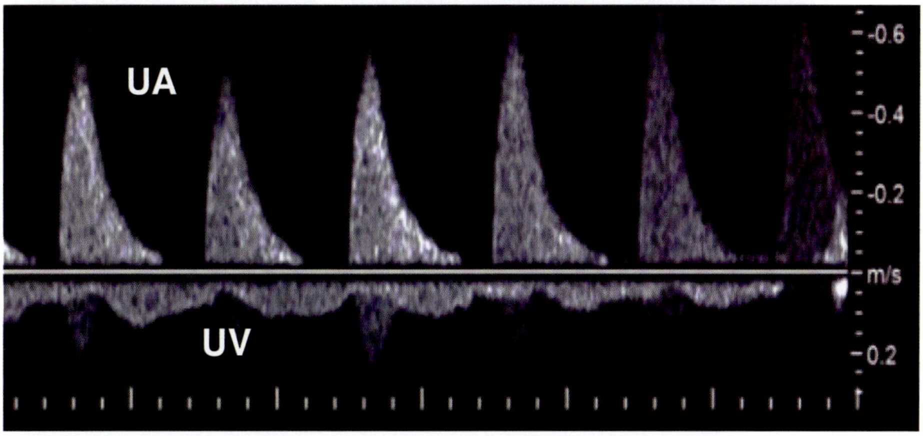

B.

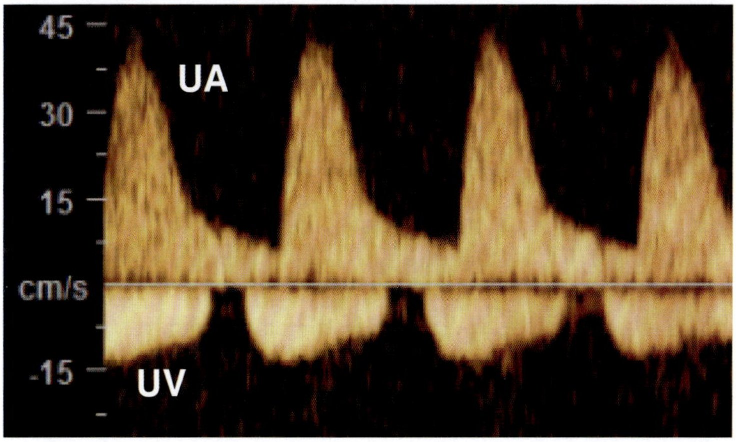

C.

FIGURE 3.4.12 Umbilical vein (UV) and ductus venosus (DV) Doppler flow patterns in the fetus with AV block compared to a fetus with normal rhythm and severe cardiac dysfunction. **A:** This 21-week fetus with occasional UV pulsations was in 3° AV block for <1 week had subjectively normal function and no AV valve insufficiency. **B:** UV pulsations are more consistent in this older fetus but do not reach the baseline. **C:** True UV "notching" in a severely compromised fetus. **D** and **E:** Intermittent A-wave flow reversal (above baseline) in the DV which occurs in AV block when the atrium contracts against a closed AV valve ("cannon waves"). **F** and **G:** The A-wave does not reverse but comes all the way to baseline. **H:** A-wave reversal with each atrial beat (arrow) consistent with a compromised fetus. a, atrial contraction; D, diastole; S, systole.

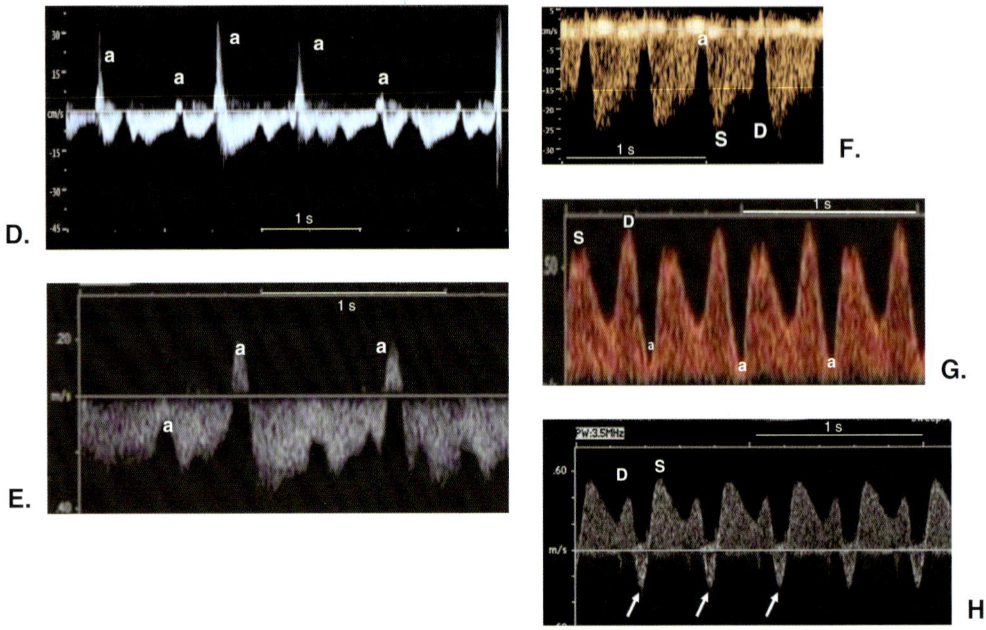

FIGURE 3.4.12 Cont'd

normal cardiac function and without hydrops can be delivered near term; however, decisions regarding the mode of delivery are ultimately the choice of the obstetrician. Delivery, regardless of mode and timing, should occur in a tertiary care center with the ability to institute ventricular pacing expeditiously or provide cardiac transplantation.

IN UTERO AND POSTNATAL TREATMENT

There is no effective in utero therapy for fetuses with fetal bradycardia or AV block in the presence of CHD. Transplacental beta-sympathomimetics administered to fetuses with LAI have increased the ventricular rate much as 12 to 16 bpm[26,27] but did not affect survival, as all treated fetuses died in the immediate neonatal period. In general, fetuses with cc-TGA and AV block in general have adequate ventricular rates, and most survive the neonatal period. Unfortunately, despite successful postnatal pacing, 1-year survival in LAI is at best 20%,[3,26,27] most likely because of CHD and diastolic dysfunction. Cardiac transplantation may thus be the best option especially when LAI is complicated by ventricular noncompaction.

SUMMARY

The prognosis of a fetus with 3° AV block in the setting of CHD depends on the associated lesion, but in nearly all circumstances, the neonatal outcome is poor. Treatment with sympathomimetic agents has been employed in hydropic fetuses with slow heart rates but with only variable short-term response and no long-term success. Experimental treatment with prenatal pacing is now available in humans in cases of anti-Ro–mediated 3° AV block and may prove to be the best transitional therapy for CHD disease and fetal 3° AV block in the future[28] (see Part 6, Chapter 3). The finding of sustained fetal bradycardia at any gestational age should prompt a thorough echocardiographic evaluation, given the high risk and poor prognosis of CHD and 3° AV block.

References

1. American College of Obstetricians and Gynecologists. Intrapartum fetal heart rate monitoring: nomenclature, interpretation and general management principals. *Obstet Gynecol.* 2009;114:192-202.
2. Mitchell JL, Cuneo BF, Etheridge SP, Horigome H, Weng HY, Benson DW. Fetal heart rate predictors of long QT syndrome. *Circulation.* 2012;126:2688-2695.
3. Lopes LM, Tavares GM, Damiano AP, et al. Perinatal outcome of fetal atrioventricular block: one-hundred-sixteen cases from a single institution. *Circulation.* 2008;118:1268-1275.
4. Jaeggi E, Ohman A. Fetal and neonatal arrhythmias. *Clin Perinatol.* 2016;43:99-112.
5. Jaeggi ET, Hamilton RM, Silverman ED, Zamora SA, Hornberger LK. Outcome of children with fetal, neonatal or childhood diagnosis of isolated congenital atrioventricular block. A single institution's experience of 30 years. *J Am Coll Cardiol.* 2002;39:130-137.
6. Schmidt KG, Ulmer HE, Silverman NH, Kleinman CS, Copel JA. Perinatal outcome of fetal complete atrioventricular block: a multicenter experience. *J Am Coll Cardiol.* 1991;17:1360-1366.
7. Cuneo B, Hughes S, Benson DW Jr. Heart rate perturbation in the stage 17-27 chick embryo: effect on stroke volume and aortic flow. *Am J Physiol.* 1993;264:H755-H759.
8. Zhu MY, Jaeggi E, Roy CW, Macgowan CK, Seed M. Reduced combined ventricular output and increased oxygen extraction fraction in a fetus with complete heart block demonstrated by MRI. *HeartRhythm Case Rep.* 2016;2:164-168.
9. Jacobs JP, Anderson RH, Weinberg PM, et al. The nomenclature, definition and classification of cardiac structures in the setting of heterotaxy. *Cardiol Young.* 2007;17(suppl 2):1-28.
10. Ho SY, Fagg N, Anderson RH, Cook A, Allan L. Disposition of the atrioventricular conduction tissues in the heart with isomerism of the atrial appendages: its relation to congenital complete heart block. *J Am Coll Cardiol.* 1992;20:904-910.
11. Arunamata A, Punn R, Cuneo B, Bharati S, Silverman NH. Echocardiographic diagnosis and prognosis of fetal left ventricular noncompaction. *J Am Soc Echocardiogr.* 2012;25:112-120.
12. Friedberg MK, Ursell PC, Silverman NH. Isomerism of the left atrial appendage associated with ventricular noncompaction. *Am J Cardiol.* 2005;96:985-990.
13. Punn R, Silverman NH. Cardiac segmental analysis in left ventricular noncompaction: experience in a pediatric population. *J Am Soc Echocardiogr.* 2010;23:46-53.
14. Stollberger C, Wegner C, Benatar A, et al. Postnatal outcome of fetal left ventricular hypertrabeculation/noncompaction. *Pediatr Cardiol.* 2016;37:919-924.
15. Guntheroth W, Komarniski C, Atkinson W, Fligner CL. Criterion for fetal primary spongiform cardiomyopathy: restrictive pathophysiology. *Obstet Gynecol.* 2002;99:882-885.
16. Digilio MC, Marino B, Bevilacqua M, Musolino AM, Giannotti A, Dallapiccola B. Genetic heterogeneity of isolated noncompaction of the left ventricular myocardium. *Am J Med Genet.* 1999;85:90-91.
17. Moura C, Hillion Y, Daikha-Dahmane F, et al. Isolated non-compaction of the myocardium diagnosed in the fetus: two sporadic and two familial cases. *Cardiol Young.* 2002;12:278-283.
18. Escobar-Diaz MC, Tworetzky W, Friedman K, et al. Perinatal outcome in fetuses with heterotaxy syndrome and atrioventricular block or bradycardia. *Pediatr Cardiol.* 2014;35:906-913.
19. Vigneswaran TV, Jones CB, Zidere V, et al. Effect of prenatal laterality disturbance and its accompanying anomalies on survival. *Am J Cardiol.* 2018;122:663-671.
20. Sharland G, Tingay R, Jones A, Simpson J. Atrioventricular and ventriculoarterial discordance (congenitally corrected transposition of the great arteries): echocardiographic features, associations, and outcome in 34 fetuses. *Heart.* 2005;91:1453-1458.
21. Paladini D, Volpe P, Marasini M, et al. Diagnosis, characterization and outcome of congenitally corrected transposition of the great arteries in the fetus: a multicenter series of 30 cases. *Ultrasound Obstet Gynecol.* 2006;27:281-285.
22. Wan AW, Jevremovic A, Selamet Tierney ES, et al. Comparison of impact of prenatal versus postnatal diagnosis of congenitally corrected transposition of the great arteries. *Am J Cardiol.* 2009;104:1276-1279.

23. Berg C, Geipel A, Kohl T, et al. Atrioventricular block detected in fetal life: associated anomalies and potential prognostic markers. *Ultrasound Obstet Gynecol.* 2005;26(1):4-15.
24. Baschat AA, Gembruch U, Knopfle G, Hansmann M. First-trimester fetal heart block: a marker for cardiac anomaly. *Ultrasound Obstet Gynecol.* 1999;14:311-314.
25. Li AH, Hanchard NA, Azamian M, et al. Genetic architecture of laterality defects revealed by whole exome sequencing. *Eur J Hum Genet.* 2019;27:563-573.
26. Jaeggi ET, Hornberger LK, Smallhorn JF, Fouron JC. Prenatal diagnosis of complete atrioventricular block associated with CHD: combined experience of two tertiary care centers and review of the literature. *Ultrasound Obstet Gynecol.* 2005;26:16-21.
27. Miyoshi T, Maeno Y, Sago H, et al. Fetal bradyarrhythmia associated with congenital heart defects - nationwide survey in Japan. *Circ J.* 2015;79:854-861.
28. Bar-Cohen Y, Loeb GE, Pruetz JD, et al. Preclinical testing and optimization of a novel fetal micropacemaker. *Heart Rhythm.* 2015;12:1683-1690.
29. Machado MV, Tynan MJ, Curry PV, Allan LD. Fetal complete heart block. *Br Heart J.* 1988;60(6):512-515.
30. Gembruch U, Hansmann M, Redel DA, Bald R, Knöpfle G. Fetal complete heart block: prentenatal diagnosis, significance and management. *Eur J Obstet Gynecol Reprod Biol.* 1989;31(1):9-22.
31. Lim JS, McCrindle BW, Smallhorn JF, et al. Clinical features, management and outcome of children with fetal and postnatal diangosis of isoermism syndromes. *Circulation.* 2005;112(16):2454-2461.

Immune-Mediated Atrioventricular Block

Helena M. Gardiner • Bettina F. Cuneo

INTRODUCTION

Complete atrioventricular (AV) block was first described 119 years ago as "impaired atrioventricular syndrome."[1] The association of a slow heart rate in two daughters of a mother with "Mikulicz disease" (Sjogren syndrome) was reported in 1928.[2] The description of the affected daughters from that report by Dr. RD Alyward is timeless, and the hypothesis of the underlying etiology posited by Dr. Janet Aiken 4 years later is remarkably prescient[3]:

> … The first child, a girl…had a pulse of 40 soon after birth; she was puny baby lacking energy and was cyanosed at times. She still survives and is a healthy girl, although quiet…. The fourth was another girl and in this case a slow foetal heart rate was noted…she suffered from occasional attacks of cyanosis; at 3 months old during one of these attacks, her pulse became irregular and she died.[2]

> The introduction of toxic bodies into the blood stream in utero would have a transient effect except…they might cause direct interference with development of the conducting system…in congenital heart-block there must have been prenatal direct interference with the conducting tract above its division….[3]

The association of maternal anti-Ro/SSA antibodies with fetal AV block was not reported until 1957.[4] The affected infant with "congenital acute lupus erythematosus" was born with a heart rate of 45 beats per minute and died 25 min later. Postmortem cardiac examination revealed extensive endocardial fibroelastosis (EFE); no AV node or His bundle was identifiable. In 1988, Lindsey Allan and colleagues at Guy's Hospital published the first series of 16 fetuses born to anti-Ro/SSA positive mothers with AV block.[5] Twelve were liveborn, and all with fetal hydrops died.

Since these first reports of maternal anti-Ro/SSA antibody–mediated fetal and neonatal AV block, it has been recognized that inflammation and fibrosis occur not only in the AV node but also in other parts of the conduction system. Manifestations of anti-Ro-SSA–mediated conduction system disease include AV block, sinus bradycardia, junctional ectopic tachycardia, and ventricular tachycardia. These arrhythmias can be independent of AV nodal disease, herald, or co-occur with it.

This chapter will concentrate primarily on the diagnosis and presentation of AV block associated with maternal anti-Ro/SSA antibodies. Treatment of fetal AV block will be discussed in Part 4, Chapter 3, and surveillance of anti-Ro antibody positive pregnancies will be discussed in Part 5, Chapter 2.

DEFINITION OF AV BLOCK

AV block is defined as a progressive disease of the AV node (AVN) culminating in the absence of the normal electrical communication between the atrium and ventricle. In the absence of an electrocardiogram, AV conduction can be evaluated by simultaneous interrogation of flow in a vein and an artery or by mitral inflow and aortic outflow measurements, as described in Part 2, Chapter 2 **(FIG. 3.5.1)**. 1° AV block is present when the atrial impulse is delayed, but there is still 1:1 AV conduction. 2° AV block occurs when some but not all the atrial beats are conducted to the ventricles, and 3° AV block is complete AV dissociation with no relationship between atrial and ventricular contractions **(FIGS. 3.5.2-3.5.5)**.

Just under half of the reported fetal cases of AV block have structurally normal hearts and the AV block is secondary to inflammation and fibrosis of a structurally normal AVN due to maternal anti-Ro/SSA antibodies.[6,7] The remainder of this chapter will be discussion of anti-Ro/SSA–mediated AV block. Other causes of fetal AV block were discussed in previous chapters. Lastly, a small proportion of pregnant women whose fetuses have 2° or 3° AV block and normally connected hearts are antibody negative. In such cases, disease may be due to a viral myocarditis, such as parvovirus,[8] long QT syndrome,[9] or heritable progressive cardiac conduction disorders.[10]

(text continued on page 163)

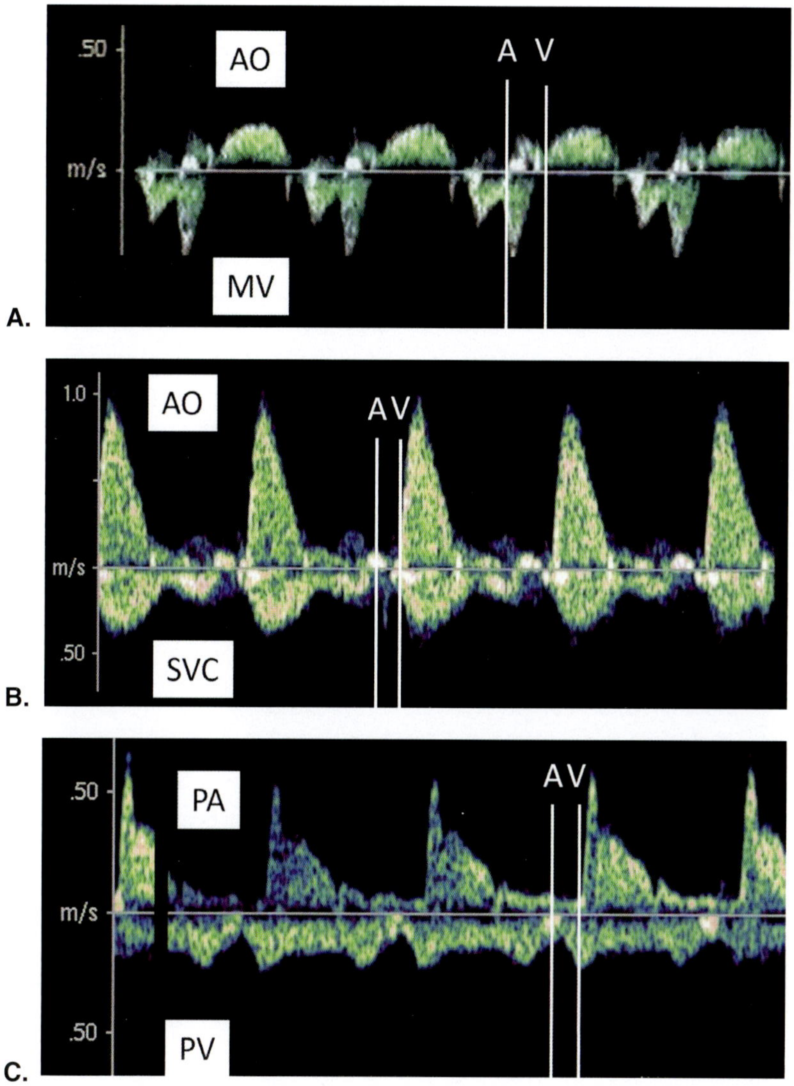

FIGURE 3.5.1 A-C: Doppler recordings of atrial and arterial waveform pairs recorded using a single gate. They demonstrate the atrioventricular (AV) time interval may be measured from a variety of sites: the mitral valve (MV) inflow and aortic valve (AV) outflow, the aorta (Ao) and superior vena cava (SVC), and a branch pulmonary artery (PA) and a pulmonary vein (PV).

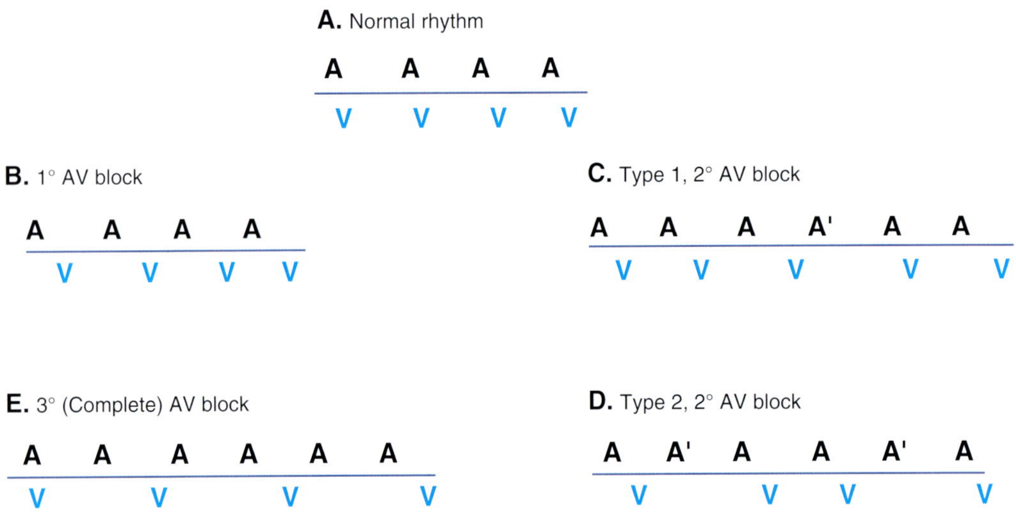

FIGURE 3.5.2 Cartoon showing various degrees of fetal atrioventricular (AV) block associated with anti-Ro/SSA antibody–mediated cardiac disease. Blue V, conducted ventricular beats. A, conducted atrial beats; A′, blocked atrial beats. **A:** Normal sinus rhythm with 1:1 conduction. **B:** 1° AV block. The AV interval is prolonged but each beat is conducted, **C:** Type 1, 2° AV block. The AV interval prolongs until a ventricular beat is dropped. **D:** Type 2, 2° AV block. A ventricular beat is dropped without a preceding prolonged AV interval. **E:** 3° AV block: no relationship between atrial and ventricular contractions.

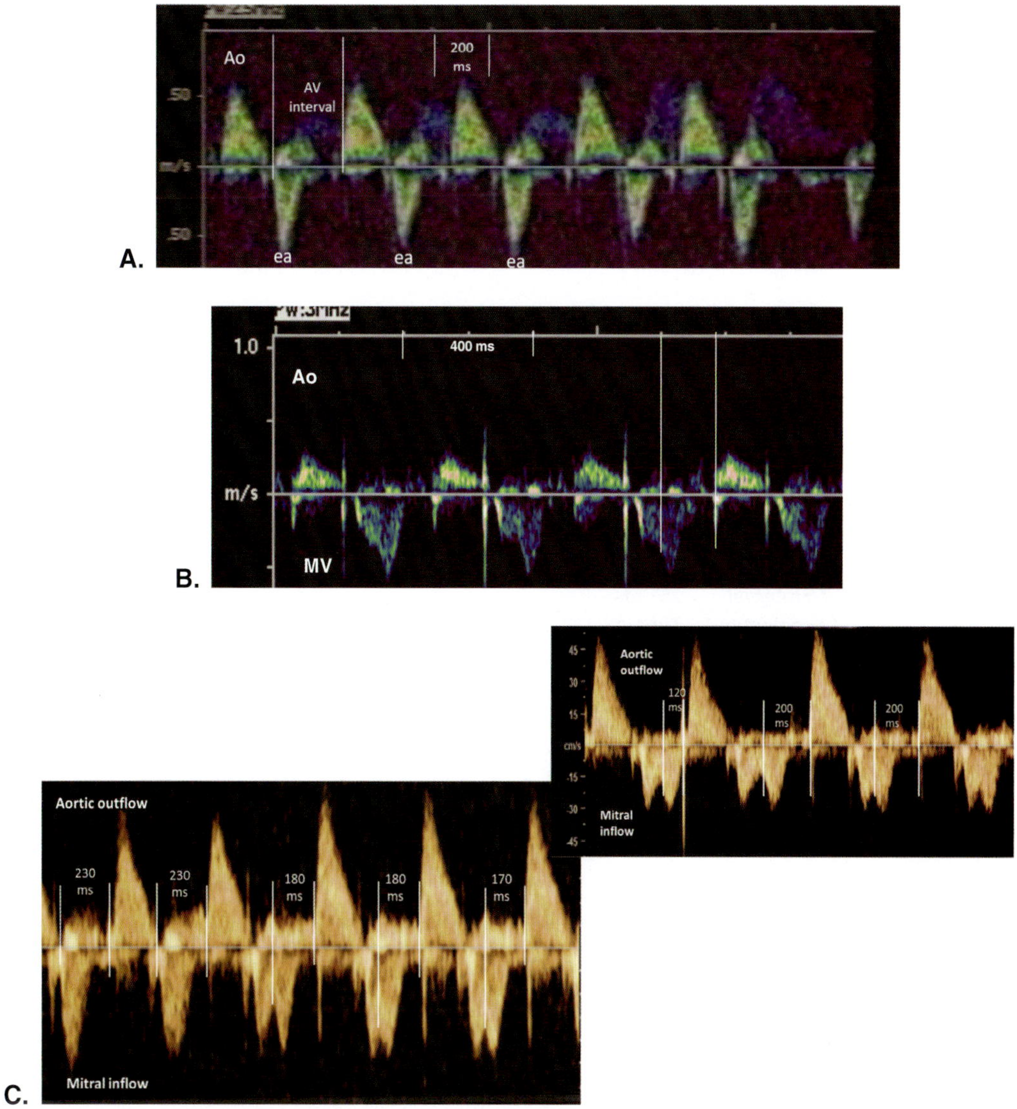

FIGURE 3.5.3 **1° Atrioventricular (AV) block.** Spectral Doppler of mitral inflow (below baseline) and aortic outflow (above baseline) in two fetuses. **A:** The mitral E- and A-waves are fused (ea), and the AV interval is >200 ms. This fetus was also having rare episodes of type 2, 2° AV block (not shown). **B:** The AV interval is prolonged to about 180 ms, but there are still distinct mitral E- and A-waves. **C:** Varying AV intervals in a fetus developing 1° AV block shown by spectral Doppler. **D:** Signal-averaged fetal electrocardiogram showing a prolonged PR interval consistent with 1° AV block.

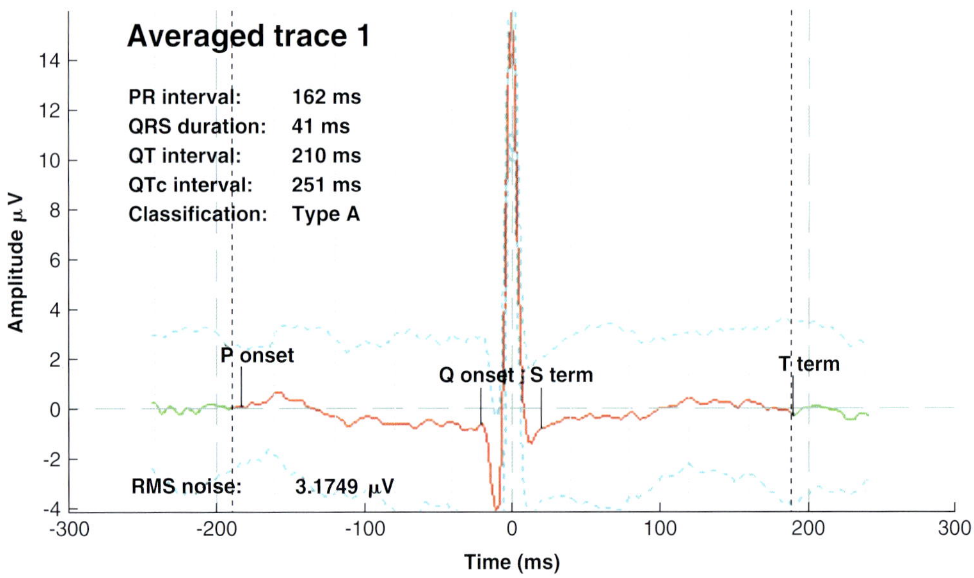

D.

FIGURE 3.5.3 Cont'd

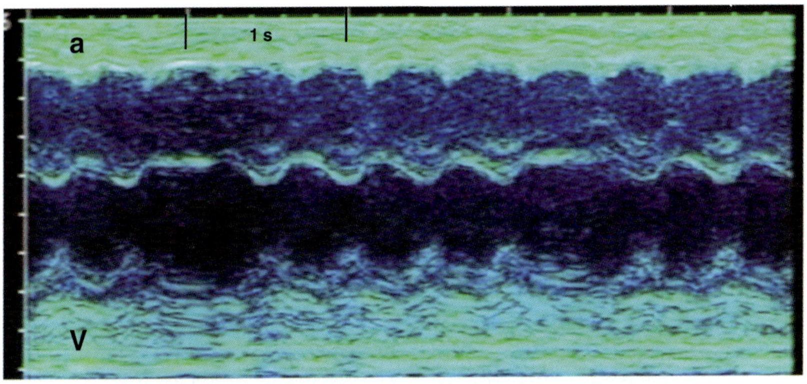

A.

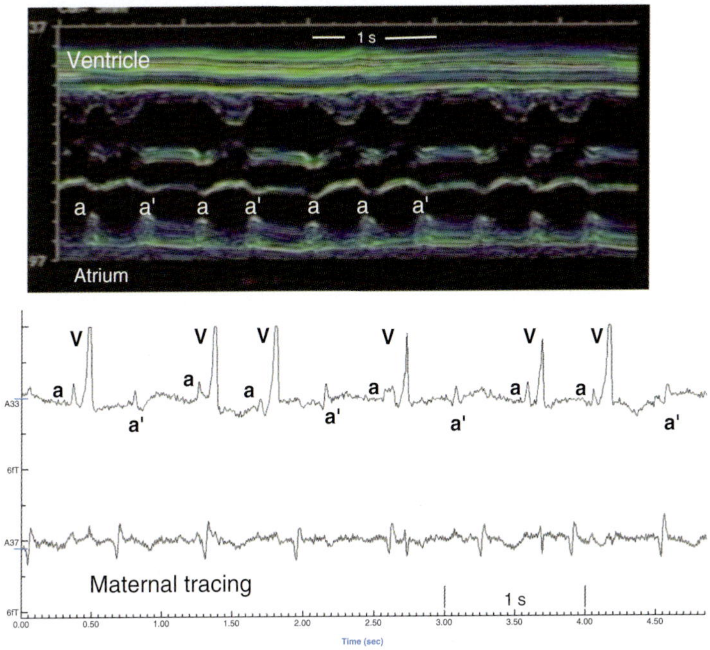

B.

FIGURE 3.5.4 **2° Atrioventricular (AV) block. A:** Simultaneous M-mode through the atrium (a) and the ventricle (V) showing a regular atrial rhythm. Occasionally the ventricle does not contract. Although this is 2° AV block, one cannot tell if it is type 1 or type 2. **B:** M-mode and fetal magnetocardiography (fMCG) of a fetus with intermittent type 2, 2° AV block. a, atrial contractions that are conducted; a′, atrial contractions that are blocked. Note that occasionally two atrial beats in a row are conducted. The maternal rhythm tracing is shown in the bottom tracing and the fetal tracing is shown on the top tracing of the fMCG. **C:** Spectral Doppler showing mitral inflow (above baseline) and aortic outflow (below baseline) of a fetus in type 1, 2° AV block. The a to Ao interval prolongs between the first and second beats, and the third atrial beat (*) is not conducted. **D:** Spectral Doppler of superior vena cava (SVC) and aorta (Ao). Reverse flow in the SVC corresponds to atrial contractions. **E:** Spectral Doppler of mitral inflow with fused ea waves and aortic outflow. Note the a-Ao interval (the a-v interval) is equal for each conducted ventricular beat. (B, Modified from Cuneo BF, Strasburger JF, Wakai RT, Ovadia M. Conduction System Disease in Fetuses Evaluated for Irregular Cardiac Rhythm. *Fetal Diagn Ther*. 2006;21:307-313.)

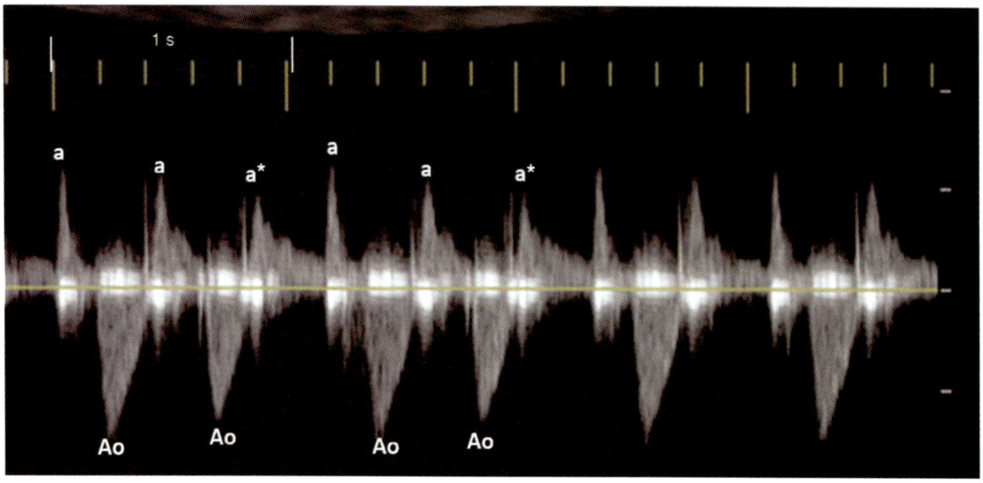

C.

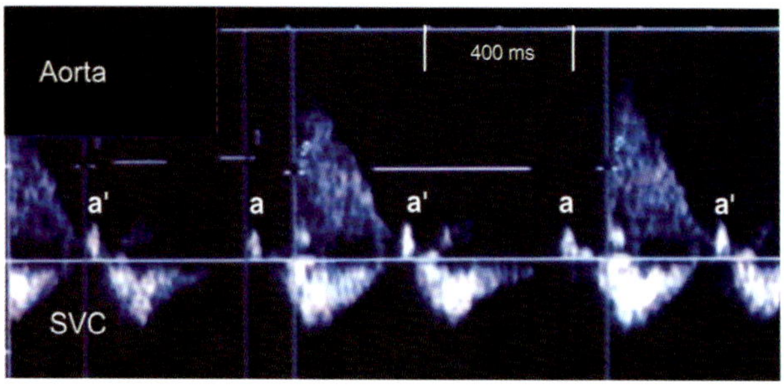

D.

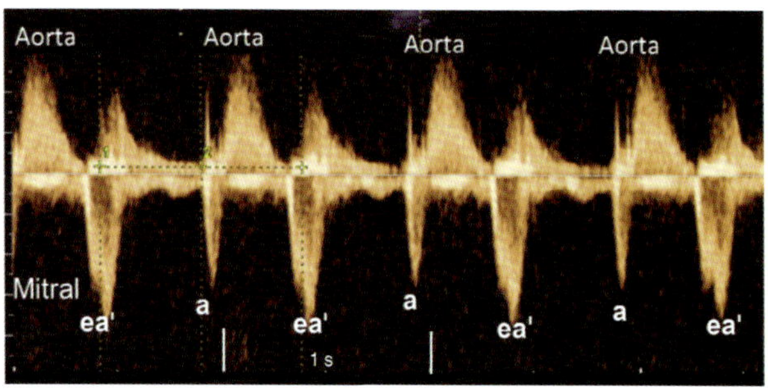

E.

FIGURE 3.5.4 Cont'd

A.

B.

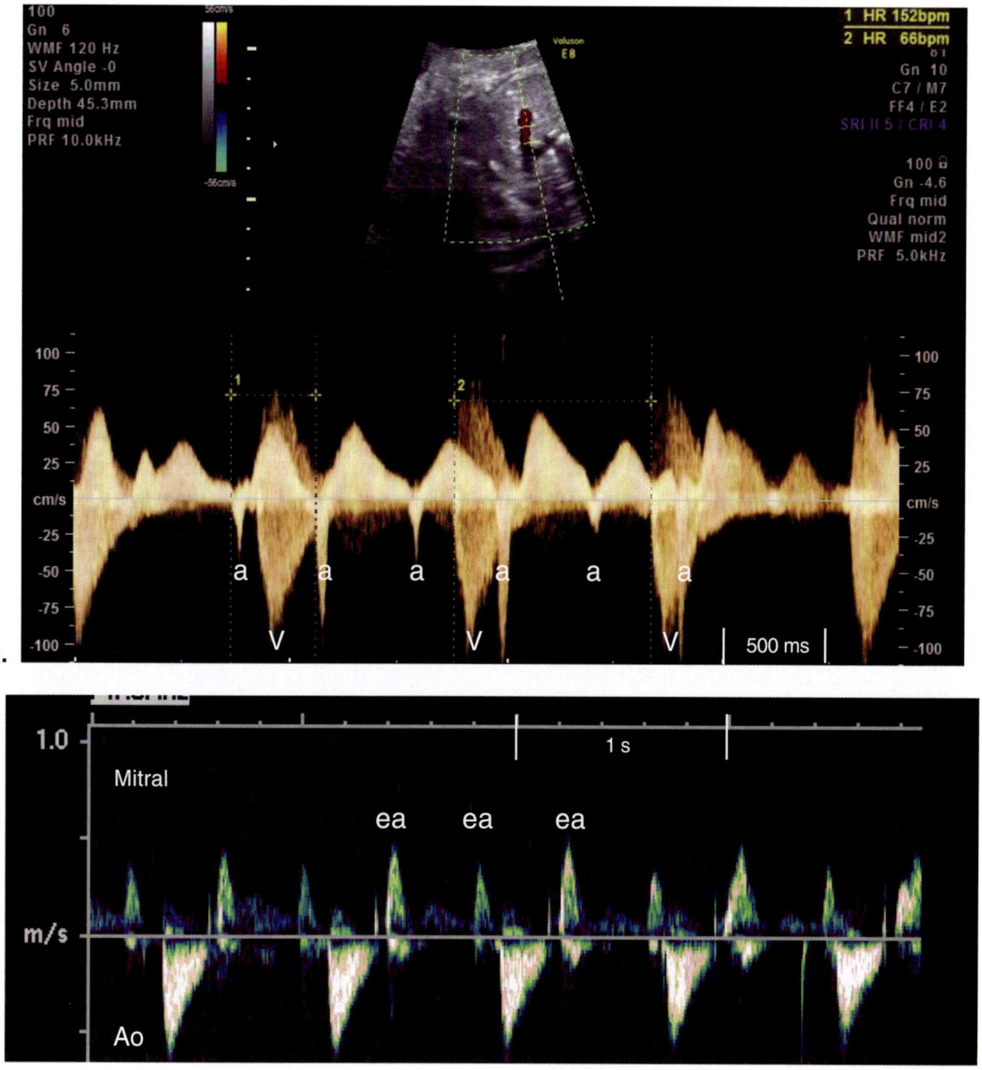

FIGURE 3.5.5 Complete atrioventricular (AV) block. A: Spectral Doppler of superior vena cava (above baseline) and aortic flow (below baseline). Atrial contractions (a) (below baseline) bear no relation to ventricular contractions (V). The atrial rate is 152 bpm and the ventricular rate is 66 bpm. **B:** Mitral inflow and aortic Doppler showing fused ea waves. Close appraisal of the AV interval shows it is not consistent, thus there is 3° AV block.

PREVALENCE OF ANTI-RO/SSA ANTIBODIES

Anti-Ro/SSA antibodies are detected in 1% to 2% of all women,[11] many of whom have no symptoms of connective tissue disease. Maternal anti-Ro/SSA antibodies cross the placenta from about 12 gestational weeks, and set up an inflammatory process, usually in the fetal AVN and myocardium that may result in fibrosis. Most fetuses with AV block are detected between 18 and 25 gestational weeks.[12,13] Women with thyroid disease have a higher risk of fetal AV block,[14] as do babies born in the spring or to non-white women.[15,16] Prenatal AV block is reported in only 2% to 3% of the population of pregnant women who have anti-Ro/SSA antibodies, but this risk increases to 15% to 20% for subsequent pregnancies, and recurrence of 3° AV block is more common in female fetuses.[17]

SPECTRUM OF ANTI-RO/SSA–MEDIATED CARDIAC DISEASE

The spectrum of fetal cardiac disease associated with maternal anti-Ro/SSA antibodies includes a more generalized inflammatory process in the fetus and neonate, including a classical skin rash (FIG. 3.5.6). The cardiac component is often referred to as cardiac neonatal lupus erythematosus (cardiac-NLE),[15,18] even though the infant does not have lupus erythematosus. Both the sinoatrial node and AVN may be involved, the former resulting in sinus bradycardia[19,20] (FIG. 3.5.7), atrial flutter,[20] or atrial standstill.[21] More commonly, maternal anti-Ro/SSA antibodies cause an early second trimester generalized myocarditis in the fetus characterized by AV valve regurgitation and, more rarely, rupture of the chordae.[22] Myocardial fibrosis, suggesting EFE may be seen on echocardiography, with or without signs of AV block (FIG. 3.5.8).[23,24]

The signature finding of anti-Ro/SSA antibody–mediated cardiac disease is AV block. In the most usual form of 3° AV block, there is inflammation predominantly of the AVN; thus, the atrial rate usually lies within the normal range and is regular, while the ventricular rate arises independently and is slow at less than or equal to 70 beats per minute. Clinically, gestational age at onset may be helpful in differentiating the likely cause of fetal bradycardia: anti-Ro/SSA antibody–mediated 3° AV block is usually established at 18 to 25 weeks of gestation. In contrast, blocked atrial bigeminy often presents later and resolves spontaneously either near term or after birth (see Part 1, Chapter 3). Long QT syndrome tends to present with 2°, not 3° AV block later in the third trimester (see Part 3, Chapter 7). However, age at presentation and age at arrhythmia onset are not the same. The gestational age at last documented normal heart rate is an important piece of information in the evaluation of the fetus with AV block, regardless of the etiology.

The development of 3° AV block is believed to be progressive, from 1° to 2° to 3°. Consequently, screening efforts have focused on ultrasound evaluation of anti-Ro/SSA antibody-positive pregnancies to detect a prolonged AV interval (1° AV block) or signs of myocardial inflammation.[25] The hypothesis was that treatment of 1° AV block would forestall progression to more advanced AV block. Surveillance of the anti-Ro/SSA positive pregnancy will be discussed in detail in Part 5, Chapter 2.

Older studies reported poor survival in fetuses and babies with cardiac-NLE, often with around 30% mortality.[15,26,27] In contrast, large single-center and national studies have reported outcomes of above 80% survival out to 10 years, in the absence of dilated cardiomyopathy (DCM). If the infant is born with 1° or 2° AV block, there may be progression after birth. In general, at least 70% of babies with 3° AV block are paced by 3 months of age.[15] Fetal cardiac dysfunction and myocardial damage may be recognized prenatally on ultrasound. DCM cardiomyopathy has been reported in between 7% and 23% of older children in larger multicenter or population registries and is associated with poor outcomes.[28-34]

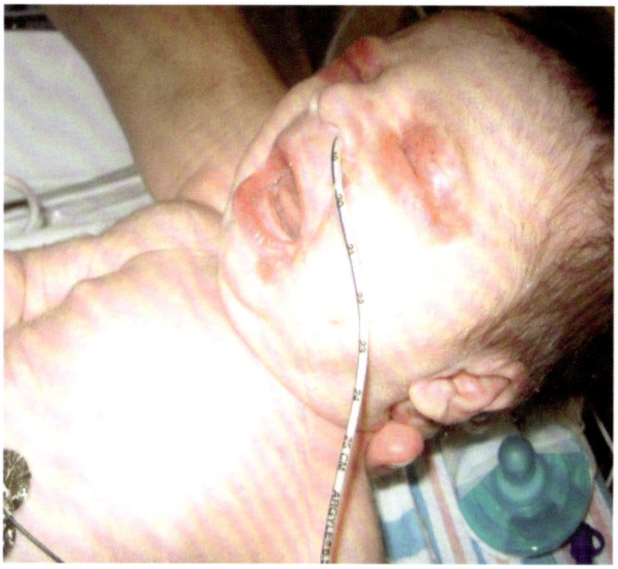

FIGURE 3.5.6 **Neonatal lupus rash.** This photo of a newborn with 1° atrioventricular block shows the typical erythematous rash around the eyes and mouth, which resolved in 2 to 3 months.

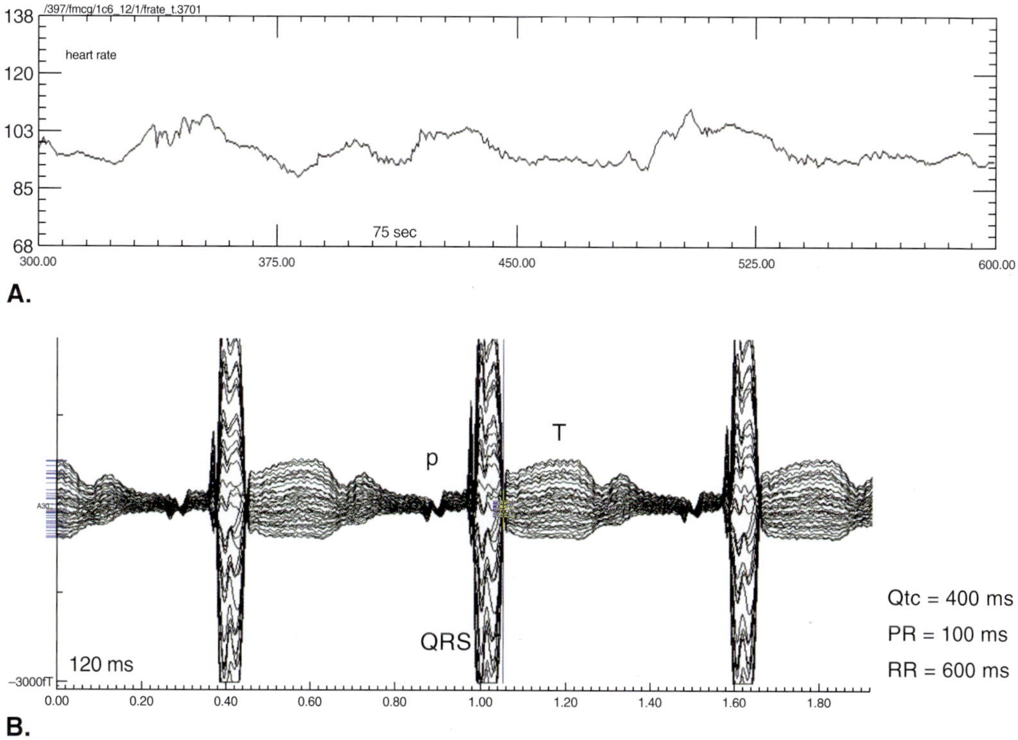

FIGURE 3.5.7 **Fetal magnetocardiography of anti-Ro/SSA antibody–mediated sinus bradycardia. A:** Fetal heart rate over time, varying from about 90 to 105 beats per minute. There is normal heart rate variability. **B:** Signal-averaged butterfly plot of the same fetus showing normal PR and QTc intervals (100 and 400 ms, respectively). The heart rate is about 100 bpm.

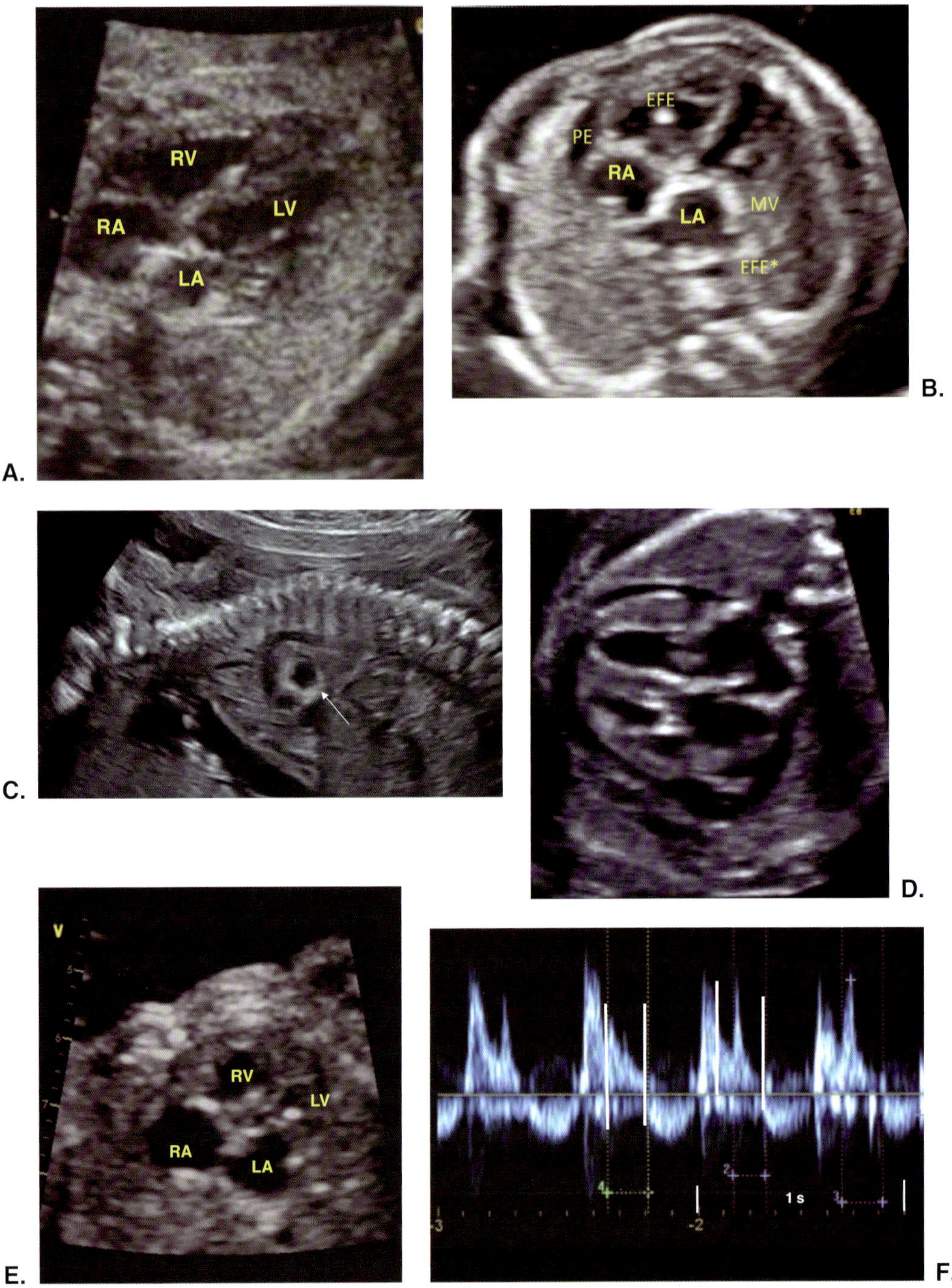

FIGURE 3.5.8 Two-dimensional images of endocardial fibroelastosis (EFE). A: Four-chamber view showing EFE in the septum but especially in the left atrium (LA). LV, left ventricle; RA, right atrium; RV, right ventricle. **B:** More extensive EFE is seen in this four-chamber view and includes both atrial walls, the both AV valves. There is also an echogenic spot on the tricuspid valve chordae. LA, left atrium; MV, mitral valve; PE, pericardial effusion; RA, right atrium. **C:** EFE limited to the left atrium. This is clearly seen in the sagittal view of the aortic arch (arrow). **D:** Patchy EFE in the septum, the right AV valve apparatus, and the left atrial wall. There is also a circumferential and prominent pericardial effusion. **E:** Another expression of EFE associated with 1° AV block. **F:** The AV interval is 165 ms.

The most devastating consequence of anti-Ro/SSA antibody–mediated disease is DCM (FIG. 3.5.9). DCM is reported in long-term national or multicenter studies to be between 7% and 18.8% and is associated with poor outcomes.[26-32,34,35] One recent national report from France found the probability of survival at 10 years was 23.1% for those diagnosed neonatally with DCM, 53.9% for those who developed late-onset DCM, and 98.6% for those without DCM.[33]

The causative factors of DCM have been elusive. One of the earliest reports of 16 children with DCM described normal cardiac function in utero, and before cardiac pacing (generally elective at 2 weeks). Twelve babies developed congestive heart failure before 2 years of age, with poor outcome (death or cardiac transplantation) in 75%, while four children recovered. Myocardial biopsy revealed hypertrophy in 11, interstitial fibrosis in 11, and myocyte degeneration in 2 children.[34] In light of the poor outcomes associated with DCM, antenatal steroid administration has been proposed to reduce the prevalence of DCM in hopes of improving outcomes. However, opinion remains divided, in part because supportive evidence is lacking. One study reported a reduced prevalence of DCM in childhood in a cohort treated with fluorinated steroids

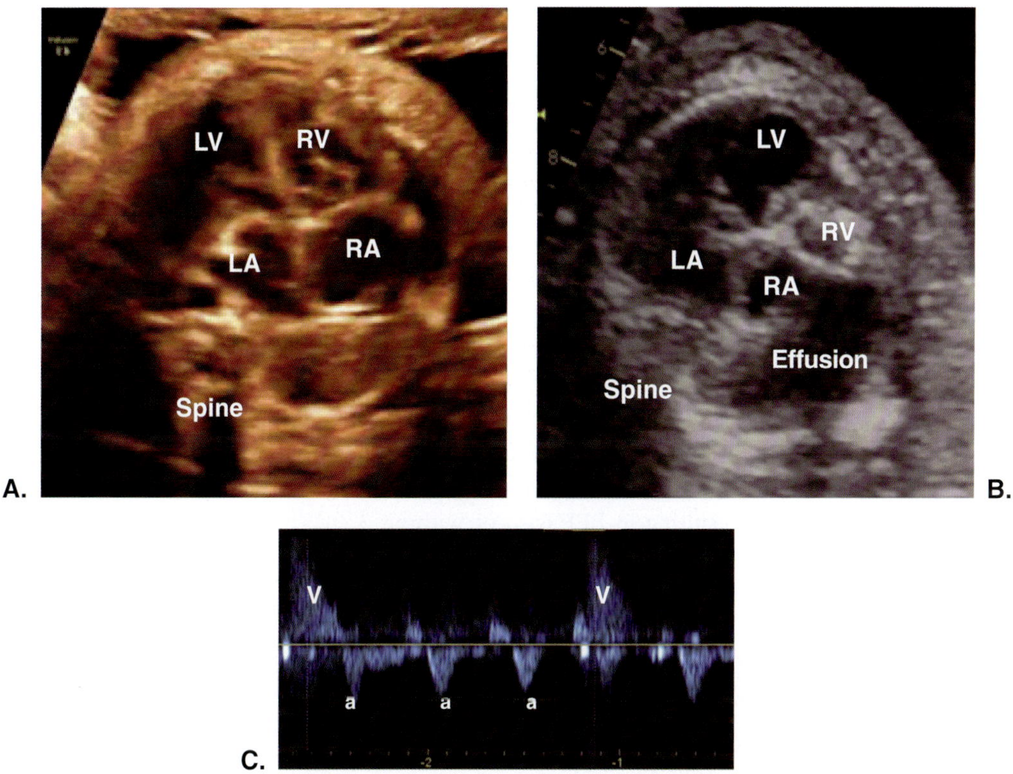

FIGURE 3.5.9 Dilated cardiomyopathy. A: Enlarged and poorly contractile heart with areas of patchy endocardial fibroelastosis (EFE). This infant was delivered at 32 weeks with a heart rate of 35 bpm and could not be resuscitated. **B:** Severe EFE of the right ventricle and a large pericardial effusion at 28 weeks of gestation. At this time the ventricular rate was 40 bpm **(C)**. The fetus died in utero a few days later. LA, left atrium; LV, left ventricle; RA, right atrium; RV, right ventricle.

during pregnancy compared with untreated historical controls. However, the historical controls were more severely affected than the treated cohort; and additionally as the majority of children with 3° AV block are paced from infancy, pacing-related cardiomyopathy is another plausible explanation for DCM, particularly when historical controls are used as they may have been exposed to less sophisticated pacing systems.[28] In the French national cohort study of 187 neonates, factors associated with DCM were characterized, and the authors proposed that neonatal and late-onset DCM were two different entities. Children presenting within the first week of life had fetal findings, including in utero DCM, hydrops, EFE, and pericardial effusion. However, those presenting later (at a median of 15.2 months, range 3.6 months-22.8 years) tended to be non-European in origin, had in utero mitral valve regurgitation, and had pacemaker implantation. Importantly, fluorinated steroids showed no protective effect against late-onset DCM ($P = .27$; HR = 1.65 [95% CI: 0.63-4.25]) and none of the known risk factors associated with neonatal DCM predicted late-onset DCM.[33] A recent Swedish study reported that subjects with antibody-mediated 3° AV block have an increased risk of DCM, myocardial and cerebral infarction, as well as a range of autoimmune diseases.[35]

PATHOGENESIS

Fetuses with cardiac-NLE usually have a normally structured heart with discontinuity between the atrial tissues and the ventricular conduction axis.[8] Recognition that only 2% of pregnancies with anti-Ro/SSA antibodies are affected by AV block has encouraged researchers to identify subgroups of women at higher risk of having an affected fetus.[11,12] The titer of antibodies is believed to be important: levels >100U/mL are associated with an 85% risk of disease developing in the fetus.[36] In addition, antibodies targeted at the 52-kd component of the Ro-antigen are purported by some investigators to be causative in 3° AV block[37,38] and also responsible for cardiomyopathy. The latter mechanism is thought to involve anti-Ro52 antibodies cross-reacting with a cardiomyocyte cell surface protein to induce dysregulation of intracellular calcium homeostasis.[38] Calcium is a main regulator of cardiomyocyte contraction, and thus myocardial contractility may be affected even in the absence of conduction system disease. The antibodies also have the potential to induce a diffuse immune response within the endomyocardial resulting in EFE with or without 3° AV block[23,24] and a high risk of end-stage heart failure and death.[26]

PRENATAL DETECTION OF ATRIOVENTRICULAR BLOCK

Doppler and M-Mode Modalities

Spectral Doppler and M-mode assessment of atrial and ventricular contraction and the AV interval have been discussed previously (Part 1, Chapter 1 and Part 2, Chapter 1).

The mechanical conduction time known as the AV interval is longer than concurrently measured electrical time intervals by 18 to 20 ms (comparing fetal magnetocardiography

PR interval with mitral inflow and aortic outflow AV interval 1) (FIG. 3.5.1).[39-41] There are several pitfalls associated with measurement and interpretation: the mechanical AV interval incorporates several time intervals, measurement of the intra-atrial conduction, conduction through the AVN, and the isovolumic conduction time, which represents the time between myocardial contraction and ventricular ejection. On the other hand, cardiac dysfunction may result in prolongation of the isovolumic conduction time which in turn prolongs the AV interval but does not necessarily indicate 1° AV block. This may be one explanation for the discrepancy between the relatively high prevalence of prolonged AV intervals described in pregnancies undergoing surveillance because of maternal anti-Ro/SSA antibodies and the reports of normal PR intervals on subsequent postnatal ECG.[41-43]

Fetal Magnetocardiography

More sophisticated methods of recording the fetal electrical cardiac conduction signals have been used in the research setting: fetal magnetocardiography (fMCG) and the fetal electrocardiogram (fECG). fMCG is noninvasive and can successfully record the magnetic fields of the fetal heart with high diagnostic quality from about 18 gestational weeks to term[44,45] (see Part 2, Chapter 3). The fMCG has revealed valuable new information, including that the development of 3° AV block may not always progress in a stepwise fashion from 1° to 2° to 3° and that a wide variety of electrical activity, including ventricular ectopy, junctional ectopic tachycardia, and ventricular tachycardia, may occur before 3° AV block develops.[46,47]

Fetal Electrocardiogram

fECG technologies have several potential advantages over fMCG including cost and portability. However, signal acquisition is not straightforward and clinical studies report periods of unsuccessful signal acquisition, likely due to the development of fetal vernix as well as signal loss associated with maternal muscle activity and fetal movement.[48-51] Systems vary and those using a higher number of electrodes and sophisticated signal separation techniques have reported good quality signal separation resulting in an ability to identify separate heart rate traces in multiple pregnancies. The more advanced systems can also separate the lower frequency "P" and "T" waves to produce the full fECG signature and its time intervals as well as record rhythm traces over several hours (in addition to averaged signals) and identify fetal arrhythmia.[48-52] fECG will be discussed in greater detail in Part 6, Chapter 1.

Pathophysiology of 3° AV Block

Ambulatory Doppler fetal heart rate (FHR) monitoring and fMCG and fECG of anti-Ro/SSA antibody positive pregnancies have shown that progression to 3° AV block is rapid, sometimes occurring even over a few hours. Furthermore, complex electrical patterns, such as ventricular ectopy or tachycardia and slow junctional ectopic tachycardia, may be identified soon before or concomitantly with 3° AV block[46,47] (FIG. 3.5.10).

In addition to these complex and changing patterns, the FHR patterns in 3° AV block can be identified as reactive or nonreactive. The pattern is more likely to be reactive if the ventricular rate is >56 bpm, and if the etiology is autoimmune, whereas lower heart rates and structural CHD are associated with nonreactive patterns.[46,47] Pharmacological use of betamimetics may increase the FHR by about 5 bpm but cannot reestablish reactivity.[47]

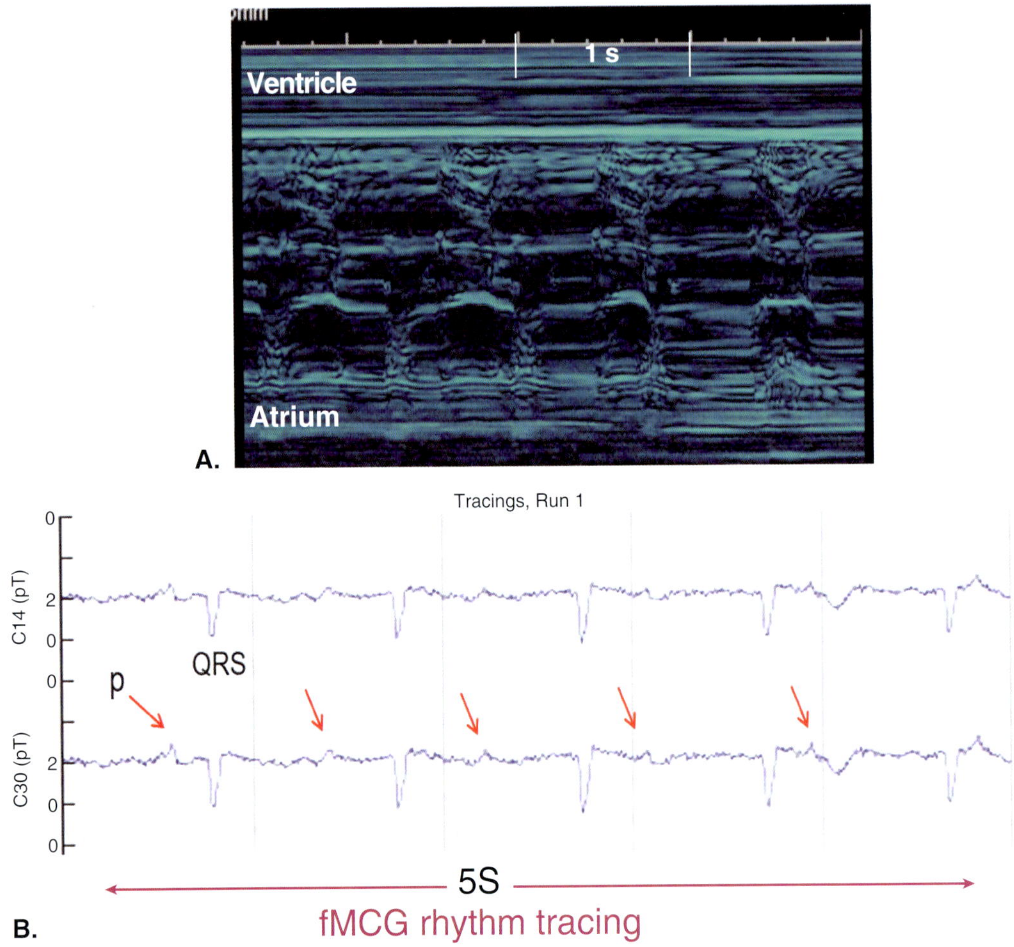

FIGURE 3.5.10 Anti-Ro/SSA antibody–mediated junctional ectopic tachycardia (JET) and AV block. A: M-mode showing atrial and ventricular rates are equal and about 65 bpm. **B:** The rhythm of junctional bradycardia and complete AV block was confirmed by fetal magnetocardiography. **C** and **D:** The ventricular rate (V) of 65 bpm is interrupted by a run of JET at a rate of about 150 bpm seen on the M-mode **(C)** and the spectral Doppler **(D)**. Aortic outflow is below baseline and mitral inflow is above baseline. V, ventricular. **E** and **F:** A second fetus that presented at 19 weeks with 1° AV block and normal fetal heart rate **(E)**. The episodes of the long RP tachycardia at 220 bpm were not recognized to be JET. The fetus was seen 2 days later and the rhythm was 3° AV block. No JET was seen at then or in subsequent examinations.

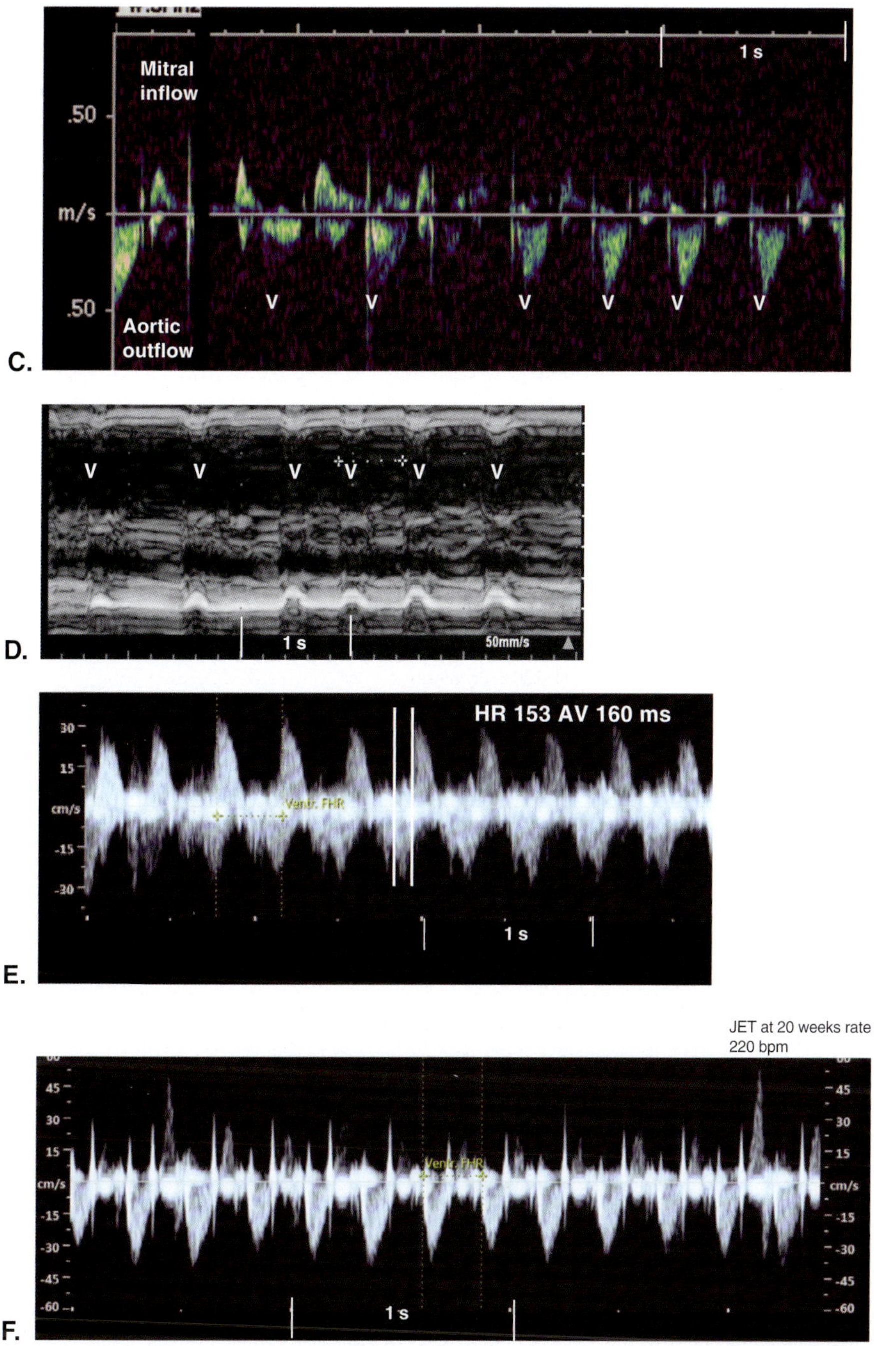

FIGURE 3.5.10 Cont'd

SUMMARY

Anti-Ro/SSA antibody–mediated AV block typically occurs at 18 to 25 weeks of gestation. It can occur in women with a known rheumatologic disorder, such as Sjogren syndrome, or it can be the first sign of anti-Ro/SSA antibody positivity in an asymptomatic mother. The spectrum of anti-Ro/SSA–mediated cardiac disease includes myocardial dysfunction, EFE, and AV valve insufficiency, but the signature finding is 1°, 2°, or 3° AV block. The risk of fetal AV block in anti-Ro/SSA antibody positive mothers is 1% to 2%, appears to be related to maternal antibody levels, and increases to 10% to 18% if the mother has a previously affected child with cardiac disease or a neonatal lupus rash. Surveillance of anti-Ro-positive pregnancies to management of fetal AV block are discussed in the following chapters.

References

1. Hogg GR. Congenital, acute lupus erythematosus associated with subendocardial fibroelastosis; report of a case. *Am J Clin Pathol.* 1957;28(6):648-654.
2. Aylward RD. Congenital heart block. *Br Med J.* 1928;(3517)1:943.
3. Aitken JK. Congenital heart-block. *Lancet.* 1932;220:1375-1379.
4. Hull D, Binns BA, Joyce D. Congenital heart block and widespread fibrosis due to maternal lupus erythematosus. *Arch Dis Child.* 1966;41(220):688-690.
5. Machado VL, Tynan MJ, Curry PVL, Allan LD. Fetal complete heart block. *Br Heart J.* 1988;60:512-515.
6. Scott JS, Maddison PJ, Taylor PV, Esscher E, Scott O, Skinner RP. Connective-tissue disease, antibodies to ribonucleoprotein, and congenital heart block. *N Engl J Med.* 1983;309:209-212.
7. Buyon JP, Winchester RJ, Slade SG, et al. Identification of mothers at risk for congenital heart block and other neonatal lupus syndromes in their children. Comparison of enzyme-linked immunosorbent assay and immunoblot for measurement of anti-SS-A/Ro and anti-SS-B/La antibodies. *Arthritis Rheum.* 1993;36(9):1263-1273.
8. Fishman SG, Pelaez LM, Baergen RN, Carroll SJ. Parvovirus-mediated fetal cardiomyopathy with atrioventricular nodal disease. *Pediatr Cardiol.* 2011;32(1):84-86.
9. Cuneo BF, Etheridge SP, Horigome H, et al. Arrhythmia phenotype during fetal life suggests long-QT syndrome genotype: risk stratification of perinatal long-QT syndrome. *Circ Arrhythm Electrophysiol.* 2013;6(5):946-951.
10. Baruteau AE, Pass RH, Thambo JB, et al. Congenital and childhood atrioventricular blocks: pathophysiology and contemporary management. *Eur J Pediatr.* 2016;175(9):1235-1248.
11. Hornberger LK, Al Rajaa N. Spectrum of cardiac involvement in neonatal lupus. *Scand J Immunol.* 2010;72(3):189-197.
12. Buyon JP. Neonatal lupus and autoantibodies reactive with SSA/Ro-SSB/La. *Scand J Rheumatol Suppl.* 1998;107:23-30.
13. Ambrosi A, Wahren-Herlenius M. Congenital heart block: evidence for a pathogenic role of maternal autoantibodies. *Arthritis Res Ther.* 2012;14(2):208.
14. Spence D, Hornberger L, Hamilton R, Silverman ED. Increased risk of complete congenital heart block in infants born to women with hypothyroidism and anti-Ro and/or anti-La antibodies. *J Rheumatol.* 2006;33(1):167-170.
15. Izmirly PM, Saxena A, Kim MY, et al. Maternal and fetal factors associated with mortality and morbidity in a multi-racial/ethnic registry of anti- SSA/Ro associated cardiac neonatal lupus. *Circulation.* 2011;124:1927-1935.
16. Ambrosi A, Salomonson S, Eliasson H, et al. Development of heart block in childrens of SSA/SSB autoantibody positive women is associated with maternal age and displays a season of birth pattern. *Ann Rheum Dis.* 2012;71(3):334-340.
17. Julkunen H, Eronen M. The rate of recurrence of isolated congenital heart block: a population based study. *Arthritis Rheum.* 2001;44:487-488.
18. Askanase AD, Friedman DM, Copel J, et al. Spectrum and progression of conduction abnormalities in infants born to mothers with anti-SSA/Ro-SSB/La antibodies. *Lupus.* 2002;11(3):145-151.

19. Chockalingam P, Jaeggi ET, Rammeloo LA, et al. Persistent fetal sinus bradycardia associated with maternal anti-SSA/Ro and anti-SSB/La antibodies. *J Rheumatol.* 2011;38(12):2682-2685.
20. Cuneo BF, Strasburger JF, Niksch A, Ovadia M, Wakai RT. An expanded phenotype of maternal SSA/SSB antibody-associated fetal cardiac disease. *J Matern Fetal Neonatal Med.* 2009;22(3):233-238.
21. Jaeggi ET, Chitayat D, Taylor G. Atrial standstill associated with loss of atrial myocytes: a rare cause of fetal bradyarrhythmia. *Heart Rhythm.* 2009;6(9):1370-1372.
22. Cuneo BF, Fruitman D, Benson DW, et al. Spontaneous rupture of atrioventricular valve tensor apparatus as late manifestation of anti-Ro/SSA antibody-mediated cardiac disease. *Am J Cardiol.* 2011;107(5):761-766.
23. Nield LE, Silverman ED, Smallhorn JF, et al. Endocardial fibroelastosis associated with maternal anti-Ro and anti-La antibodies in the absence of atrioventricular block. *J Am Coll Cardiol.* 2002;40:796-802.
24. Nield LE, Silverman ED, Taylor GP, et al. Maternal anti-Ro and anti- La antibody-associated endocardial fibroelastosis. *Circulation.* 2002;105:843-848.
25. Friedman DM, Kim MY, Copel JA, et al; PRIDE Investigators. Utility of cardiac monitoring in fetuses at risk for congenital heart block: the PR Interval and Dexamethasone Evaluation (PRIDE) prospective study. *Circulation.* 2008;117(4):485-493.
26. Jaeggi ET, Hamilton RM, Silverman ED, Zamora SA, Hornberger LK. Outcome of children with fetal, neonatal or childhood diagnosis of isolated congenital atrioventricular block. A single institution's experience of 30 years. *J Am Coll Cardiol.* 2002;39:130-137.
27. Eronen M, Sirèn MK, Ekblad H, Tikanoja T, Julkunen H, Paavilainen T. Short- and long-term outcome of children with congenital complete heart block diagnosed in utero or as a newborn. *Pediatrics.* 2000;106(1 pt 1):86-91.
28. Jaeggi ET, Fouron JC, Silverman ED, et al. Transplacental fetal treatment improves the outcome of prenatally diagnosed complete atrioventricular block without structural heart disease. *Circulation.* 2004;110:1542-1548.
29. Lopes LM, Tavares GM, Damiano AP, et al. Perinatal outcome of fetal atrioventricular block: one-hundred-sixteen cases from a single institution. *Circulation.* 2008;118:1268-1275.
30. Eliasson H, Sonesson SE, Sharland G, et al; Fetal Working Group of the European Association of Pediatric Cardiology. Isolated atrioventricular block in the fetus: a retrospective, multinational, multicenter study of 175 patients. *Circulation.* 2011;124:1919-1926.
31. Fredi M, Andreoli L, Bacco B, et al. First report of the Italian registry on immune-mediated congenital heart block (Lu.Ne registry). *Front Cardiovasc Med.* 2019;6:11.
32. Levesque K, Morel N, Maltret A, et al. "Lupus néonatal" group; Group of collaborators. Description of 214 cases of autoimmune congenital heart block: results of the French neonatal lupus syndrome. *Autoimmun Rev.* 2015;14(12):1154-1160.
33. Morel N. Incidence, risk factors, and mortality of neonatal and late onset dilated cardiomyopathy associated with cardiac neonatal lupus. *Int J Cardiol.* 2017;248:263-269.
34. Moak JP, Barron KS, Hougen TJ, et al. Congenital heart block: development of late-onset cardiomyopathy, a previously underappreciated sequela. *J Am Coll Cardiol.* 2001;37(1):238-242.
35. Mofors J, Eliasson H, Ambrosi A, et al. Comorbidity and long-term outcome in patients with congenital heart block and their siblings exposed to Ro/SSA autoantibodies in utero. *Ann Rheum Dis.* 2019;78(5):696-703.
36. Jaeggi E, Laskin C, Hamilton R, Kingdom J, Silverman E. The importance of the level of maternal anti-Ro/SSA antibodies as a prognostic marker of the development of cardiac neonatal lupus erythematosus a prospective study of 186 antibody-exposed fetuses and infants. *J Am Coll Cardiol.* 2010;55(24):2778-2784.
37. Salomonsson S, Dorner T, Theander E, Bremme K, Larsson P, Wahren-Herlenius M. A serologic marker for fetal risk of congenital heart block. *Arthritis Rheum.* 2002;46: 1233-1241.
38. Salomonsson S, Sonesson SE, Ottosson L, et al. Ro/SSA autoantibodies directly bind cardiomyocytes, disturb calcium homeostasis, and mediate congenital heart block. *J Exp Med.* 2005;201:11-17.
39. Kato Y, Takahashi-Igari M, Inaba T, Sumazaki R, Horigome H. Comparison of PR intervals determined by fetal magnetocardiography and pulsed Doppler echocardiography. *Fetal Diagn Ther.* 2012;32(1-2):109-115.
40. Cuneo BF, Bitant S, Strasburger JF, Kaizer A, Wakai RT. Assessment and outcome of AV conduction in normal and anti-Ro/SSA antibody positive pregnancies evaluated by echocardiography and magnetocardiography. *Ultrasound Obstet Gynecol.* 2019;54(5):625-633.
41. Sonesson SE, Salomonsson S, Jacobsson LA, Bremme K, Wahren-Herlenius M. Signs of first-degree heart block occur in one-third of fetuses of pregnant women with anti-SSA/Ro 52-kd antibodies. *Arthritis Rheum.* 2004;50:1253-1261.

42. Jaeggi ET, Silverman ED, Laskin C, Kingdom J, Golding F, Weber R. Prolongation of the atrioventricular conduction in fetuses exposed to maternal anti-Ro/SSA and anti-La/SSB antibodies did not predict progressive heart block. A prospective observational study on the effects of maternal antibodies on 165 fetuses. *J Am Coll Cardiol.* 2011;57:1487-1492.
43. Gardiner HM, Belmar C, Pasquini L, et al. Fetal ECG: a novel predictor of atrioventricular block in anti-Ro positive pregnancies. *Heart.* 2007;93:1454-1460.
44. Leuthold A, Wakai RT, Martin CB. Noninvasive in utero assessment of PR and QRS intervals from the fetal magnetocardiogram. *Early Hum Dev.* 1999;54(3):235-243.
45. Shah VK, Wakai RT. A compact, high performance atomic magnetometer for biomedical applications. *Phys Med Biol.* 2013;58(22):8153-8161.
46. Zhao H, Cuneo BF, Strasburger JF, Huhta JC, Gotteiner NL, Wakai RT Electrophysiological characteristics of fetal atrioventricular block. *J Am Coll Cardiol.* 2008;51(1):77-84.
47. Cuneo BF, Zhao H, Strasburger JF, Ovadia M, Huhta JC, Wakai RT. Atrial and ventricular rate response and patterns of heart rate acceleration during maternal-fetal terbutaline treatment of fetal complete heart block. *Am J Cardiol.* 2007;100(4):661-665.
48. Taylor MJ, Smith MJ, Thomas M, et al. Non-invasive fetal electrocardiography in singleton and multiple pregnancies. *BJOG.* 2003;110(7):668-678.
49. Taylor MJ, Thomas MJ, Smith MJ, et al. Non-invasive intrapartum fetal ECG: preliminary report. *BJOG.* 2005;112(8):1016-1021.
50. Graatsma EM, Miller J, Mulder EJ, Harman C, Baschat AA, Visser GH. Maternal body mass index does not affect performance of fetal electrocardiography. *Am J Perinatol.* 2010;27(7):573-577.
51. Arya B, Govindan R, Krishnan A, Duplessis A, Donofrio MT. Feasibility of noninvasive fetal electrocardiographic monitoring in a clinical setting. *Pediatr Cardiol.* 2015;36(5):1042-1049.
52. Gurve D, Pant JK, Krishnan S. Real-time fetal ECG extraction from multichannel abdominal ECG using compressive sensing and ICA. *Conf Proc IEEE Eng Med Biol Soc.* 2017;2017:2794-2797.

Channelopathies

Hitoshi Horigome

INTRODUCTION

Cardiac channelopathies are a group of inheritable disorders that predispose fetuses with primarily structurally normal hearts to arrhythmias through the alteration of ion channel currents of myocardial cells. Genetic variations in these channels affect their opening and closing functions, resulting in changes in the currents across the myocardial cell membranes that can lead to life-threatening arrhythmias.

The most common (~1/2000 individuals) cardiac channelopathy is congenital long QT syndrome (LQTS). There have been rare case reports of other cardiac channelopathies presenting in fetal life, including short QT syndrome and congenital sick sinus syndrome (SSS). Still other channelopathies including Brugada syndrome and catecholaminergic polymorphic ventricular tachycardia (CPVT) have not yet been reported during fetal life. This chapter will describe the current knowledge about the clinical presentation and diagnosis of the channelopathies. A discussion of genetic testing for the channelopathies can be found in Part 1, Chapter 3.

PRESENTATION OF LONG QT SYNDROME IN THE FETUS

The most common presentation of LQTS during fetal life is sinus bradycardia.[1-6] This bradycardia is frequently unrecognized and underappreciated because very few LQTS positive fetuses meet the obstetrical criteria for bradycardia, which is ≤110 bpm at any time during pregnancy.[3] In a large study, only 17% of fetuses with genetically confirmed LQTS met the obstetrical criteria, while 70% had a fetal heart rate (FHR) < third percentile for gestational age[2] **(FIG. 3.6.1)**. The degree of bradycardia seems to vary with pathogenic variant burden. For example, fetuses with homozygous *KCNQ1* variants have lower FHR than those with heterozygous *KCNQ1* variants[4]. In addition to sinus bradycardia, torsades de pointes (TdP), the signature rhythm of LQTS, often occurs with a 2° AV block **(FIG. 3.6.2)** and the two are easily recognized as abnormal.[7] However, TdP and/or 2° AV block occur in <25% of reported fetal LQTS cases.

There are three groups of fetuses at risk for LQTS. The first group are those with a parent carrier of a known pathogenic LQTS variant ("inherited LQTS"). In general,

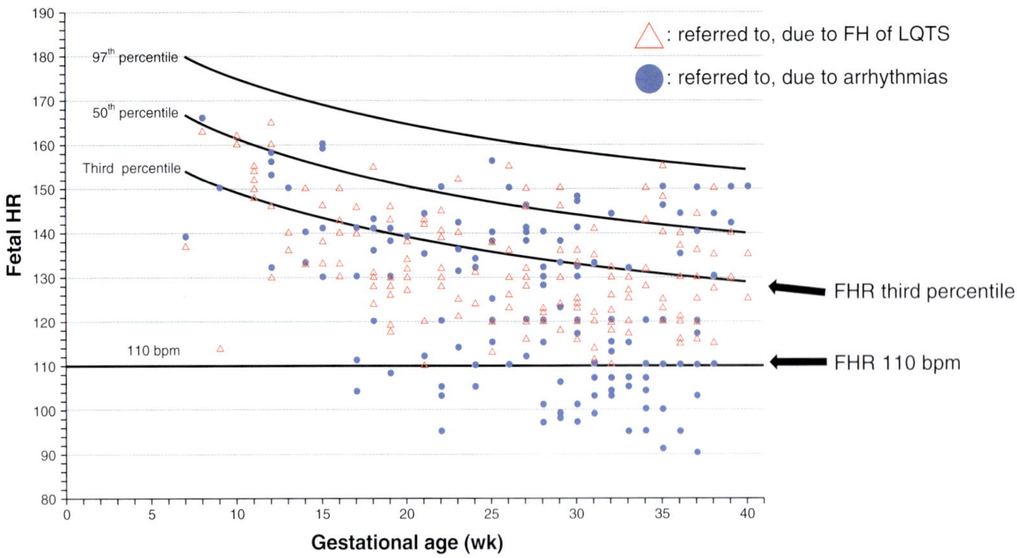

FIGURE 3.6.1 Screening of long QT syndrome (LQTS) based on fetal heart rate (FHR). If FHR 110 bpm is used for screening of LQTS, only 19% of LQTS cases are included below the screening line. However, if the third percentile line is adopted, 66% of LQTS cases are picked up. △, family history of LQTS; •, arrhythmia. (Reprinted from Mitchell JL, Cuneo BF, Etheridge SP, Horigome H, Weng HY, Benson DW. Fetal heart rate predictors of long QT syndrome. *Circulation*. 2012;126:2688-2695.)

the fetal presentation of inherited LQTS is mild and the arrhythmia burden is less compared with de novo LQTS. Exceptions are some familial *KCNH2* variants,[1,8-11] fetuses with homozygous or compound heterozygous variants, those with Jervell and Lange-Nielsen syndrome (homozygous variant of *KCNQ1* or *KCNE1*), and fetuses with maternal mosaicism for *SCN5A* R1623Q.[12-14] Recurrent stillbirth is another presentation of familial LQTS; compared to the general population stillbirths are 10 times higher in familial LQTS, and not all losses carry the family variant or have a history of TdP.[15] In familial LQTS, there are some genotype-phenotype–specific features. For example, fetal bradycardia is more pronounced in LQT1 (*KCNQ1*) and LQT2 (*KCNH2*) than in LQT3 (*SCN5A*).

The second group of fetuses at risk for LQTS are those presenting unexpected TdP, with or without 2° AV block (FIG. 3.6.3). These fetuses most frequently have de novo variants and can be identified as early as 19 weeks of gestation. Among these cases of early-onset LQTS with high arrhythmia burden, the two most prevalent genotypes are some *KCNH2* variants in the pore regions and *SCN5A* R1623Q or L409P variants.[1,3,16-19] The other rare but severe forms of early-onset LQTS include Timothy syndrome (*CACNA1C* variant)[20-22] and calmodulinopathy (*CALM1 or CALM2* variants).[23] Pathogenic variants are not identified or are uncharacterized in about 30% of these severe and early onset cases.

The third group are pregnant women with a history of stillbirths or unexplained neonatal or infant deaths. Approximately 12% of sudden infant death victims carry LQTS variants.[24] For example, using molecular autopsy, Crotti et al[25] found LQTS-associated gene variants in 8.8% of fetal demise. The role of LQTS-variants in stillbirths has yet to

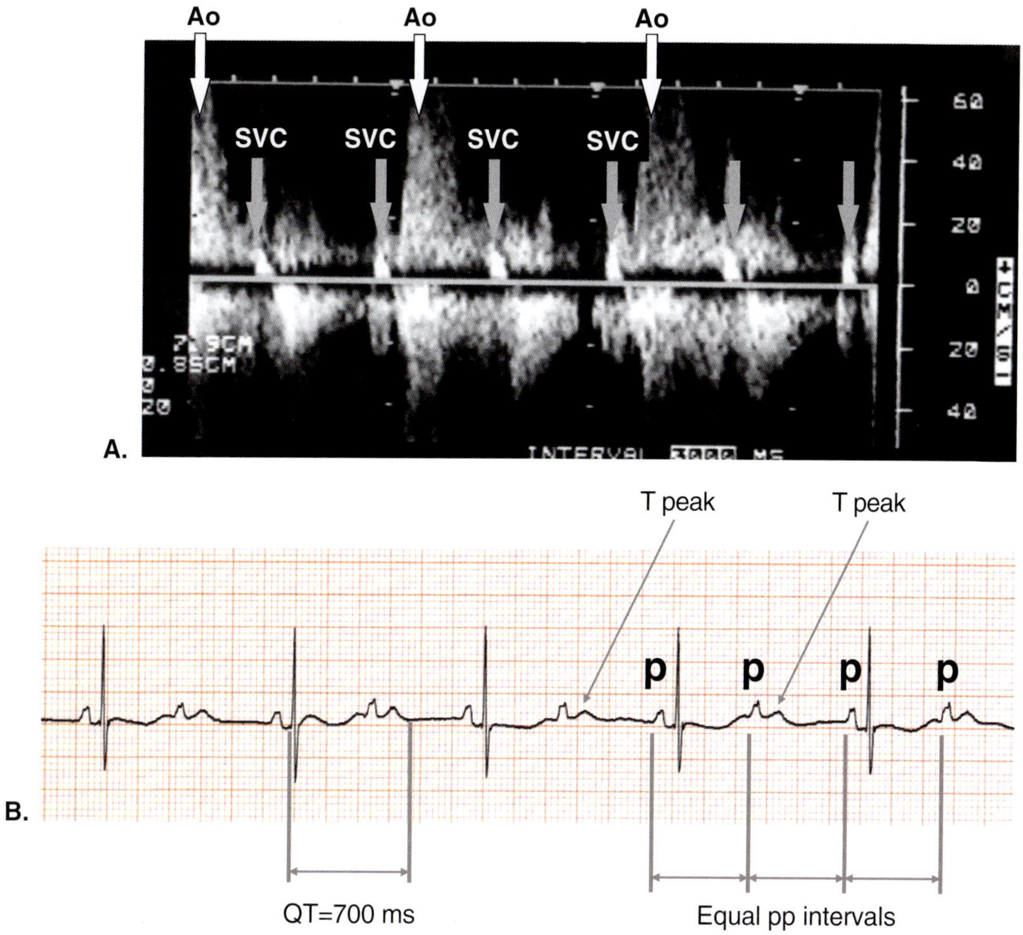

FIGURE 3.6.2 2° atrioventricular block observed in a fetus with long QT syndrome. **A:** Pulsed Doppler waveforms of ejection flow in the fetal aorta, showing fixed A-A (p-p) intervals with alternate atrioventricular (AV) conduction (2:1 AV block) due to extremely prolonged refractory period of the ventricle. The A rate is 106 bpm, and V rate is 53 bpm. SVC, inverse flow due to atrial contraction in the superior vena cava; Ao, ejection flow due to ventricular contraction in the aorta. **B:** Electrocardiogram recorded after birth in the same patient as **A**. Findings show that half of the P-waves are located on the T-waves without AV conduction due to extremely prolonged QT intervals (700 ms). PP (0.62 s) and VV (1.25 s) intervals are both regular.

be determined, but obstetricians, perinatal health providers, and cardiologists should be aware of these early-onset life-threatening types of LQTS and consider molecular autopsy when confronted with an unexplained stillbirth.

Literature Summary of Fetal LQTS Presentation (Table 3.6.1)

A search of English-language journals for case reports or series of LQTS diagnosed in utero revealed 55 cases, including 10 cases with LQT1, 23 with LQT2, 15 with LQT3, 3 with calmodulinopathy, 3 unknown, and 1 with multiple pathogenic variants. Investigation of the genotype-phenotype correlations revealed that all LQT1 fetuses showed only sinus bradycardia, whereas the frequencies of 2:1 AV block and TdP reached

(text continued on page 182)

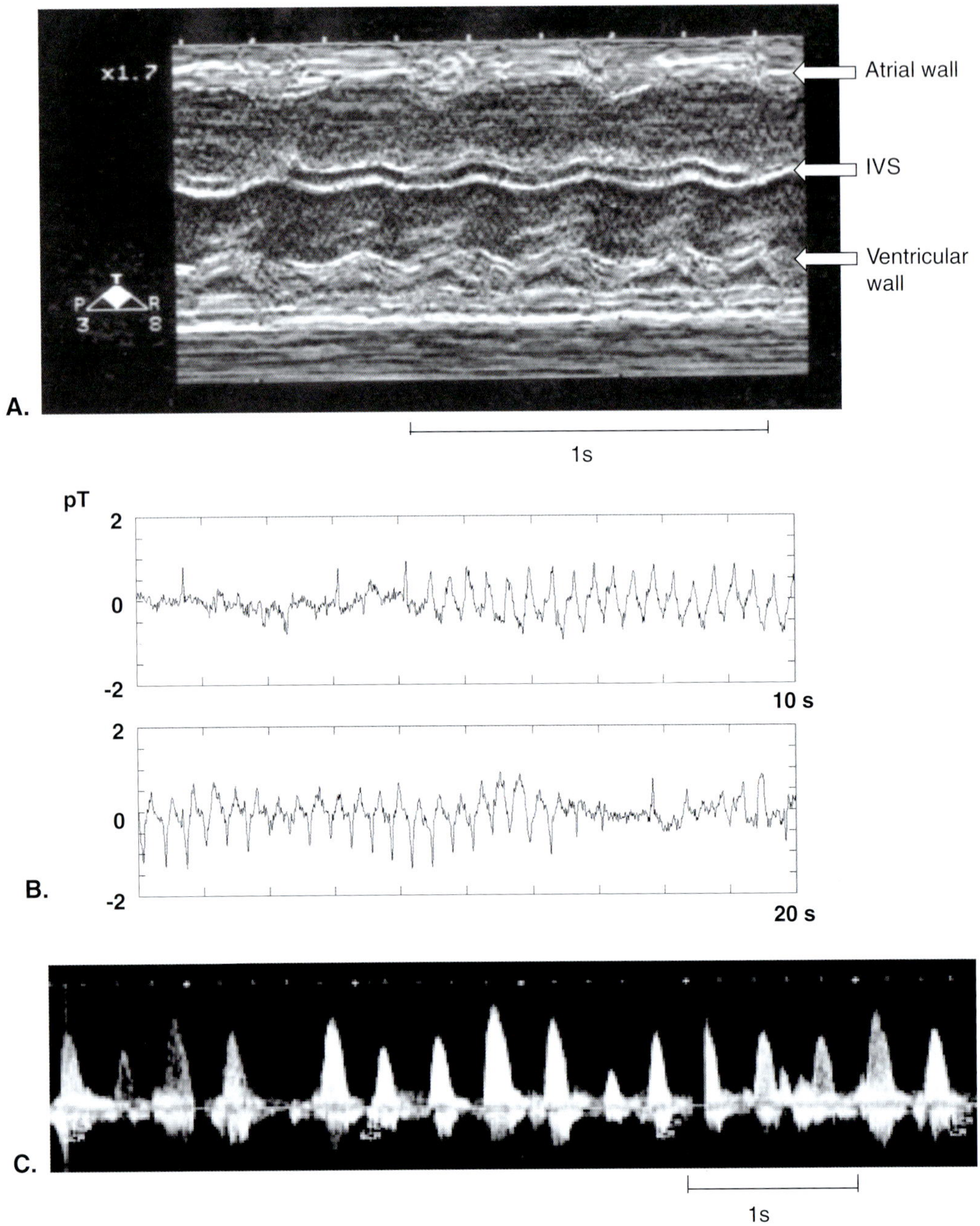

FIGURE 3.6.3 Torsade de pointes (TdP) observed in a fetus with long QT syndrome. **A:** M-mode fetal echocardiogram. The atrial wall movement is faster than that of the ventricular wall without any correlations, indicating ventricular tachycardia. Ventricular wall motion is a little irregular with a rate of 210 bpm. IVS, interventricular septum. **B:** Typical waveforms of TdP recorded with fetal magnetocardiography, showing polymorphic ventricular tachycardia (VT) with an irregular rhythm and QRS morphology. **C:** Pulsed Doppler waveforms of ejection flow in the fetal aorta, showing irregular intervals and amplitudes, which suggest polymorphic VT (TdP).

TABLE 3.6.1 LITERATURE SUMMARY OF FETAL LONG QT SYNDROME

Author (y)	Origin of LQTS	Hx of Fetal Loss	GA (wk)	Rhythm	Delivery (wk)	Variant
1. Vigliani (1995)	Mother	ND	38	Brady	VD (40)	ND
2. Donofrio (1999)		ND	32	Brady		ND
3. Hamada (1999)	Mother	No	37	Brady	VD (38)	*KCNQ1* A341V
4. Cuneo (2003)	De novo	No	30	VT, 2:1 AV block, SB (110 bpm)	CS (34)	*SCN5A* R1623Q
5. Johnson (2003)	Mother	ND	38	VT, SB (120 bpm)	ND (38)	*KCNH2* R725Q
6. Miller (2004)	Maternal mosaicism	SB × 2	28	VT^2, SB, 2:1 AV block	ECS (32)	*SCN5A* R1623Q
7. Chang (2004)	De novo	ND	ND	Tachy-brady	ND (38)	*SCN5A* V1763M
8. Lupoglazoff (2004)	Mother	ND	~30	2:1 AV block	ND	*KCNH2* T613M
9.	Mother	ND	~30	VT, 2:1 AV block	ND	*KCNH2* D501N
10.	M + F	ND	~30	VT, 2:1 AV block	ND	Multiple
11.	De novo	ND	~30	VT, 2:1 AV block	ND	*KCNH2* G628S
12.	De novo	ND	~30	VT, 2:1 AV block	ND	*KCNH2* Y93C
13.	Mother	ND	~30	SB	ND	*KCNQ1* R231C
14.	Mother	ND	~30	SB	ND	*KCNQ1* G325R
15.	Mother	ND	~30	SB	ND	*KCNQ1* R231C
16.	Mother	ND	~30	SB	ND	*KCNQ1* R231C
17.	Mother	ND	~30	SB	ND	*KCNQ1* G1258 insA
18. Schultz-Bahr (2004)	De novo	Primip	ND	Tachy-brady	CS (35)	*SCN5A* P1332L
19. Schneider (2005)	Mother	ND	32	SB	VD (38)	*KCNQ1* CTG to CCG
20. Ten Harkel (2005)	De novo	ND	29	Irregular	CS (33)	*SCN5A* R1623Q
21. Tomek (2008)	Father	Primip	22	2° AV block, SB		
			26	VT	CS (31)	*SCN5A* ND
22. Bhuiyan (2008)	M + F Consanguineous	MC × 2 SB × 2 homoz	22	2:1 AV block		

(Continued)

TABLE 3.6.1 LITERATURE SUMMARY OF FETAL LONG QT SYNDROME (CONTINUED)

Author (y)	Origin of LQTS	Hx of Fetal Loss	GA (wk)	Rhythm	Delivery (wk)	Variant
			29	PVC, VT	CS (32)	Homoz *KCNH2* Q1070X
23. Wang (2008)	Novel de novo		32	Arrhythmia	ECS (32)	
	Novel de novo		34	VT	ND	*SCN5A* G1631D
24. Simpson (2009)	De novo	No	30	VT[1,2,3]	ND (32)	*KCNH2* T613M
25. Horigome (2010)	+ FH	ND	ND	SB	ND	*KCNQ1* Thr587Met
26.	? de novo	ND	ND	SB	ND	*KCNQ1* Ala341Val
27.	? de novo	ND	ND	VT, 2:1 AV block	ND	*KCNH2* Gly628Ser
28.	? de novo	ND	ND	VT	ND	*KCNH2* Del(7)(q32qter)
29.	+ FH	ND	ND	ND	ND	*KCNH2* Ser243 + 112x
30.	? de novo	ND	ND	VT, 2:1 AV block	ND	*KCNH2* GM628Ala
31.	? de novo	ND	ND	VT, 2:1 AV block	ND	*KCNH2* Thr613met
32.	? de novo	ND	28	2:1 AV block	ND	*SCN5A* Ala1186Thr
33.	? de novo	ND	ND	VT, 2:1 AV block	ND	*SCN5A* Asn1774Asp
34. Murphy (2011)	De novo	No	19	VT[1,2,3]	FD(25)	*SCN5A* L409B
35. Donofrio (2012)	De novo	No	19	Irregular		
			26	2:1 AV block		
			30	VT[1,2], 2:1 AV block	ECS (30)	*SCN5A* R1623Q
36. Chabaneix (2012)	ND (but no FH)	No	36	PVCs, VT, SB (120 bpm)		
			37	VT[1], 2:1 AV block	ND (37)	*KCHN2* Gly628Ser
37. Kormarlu (2012)	Father	Primip		Tachy[1,2,3]	ECS	*KCNH2* ND
38. Theeuws (2013)	De novo	No	32	VT[1,2,3]	ECS (32)	UK
39. Crotti (2013)	De novo	No	21	SB (110 bpm)		
			27	SB (90 bpm)	CS (37)	*CALM2* D96V
40. Cuneo (2013)	De novo	ND	28	VT, 2:1 AV block	CS (33)	*KCNH2* G628S

TABLE 3.6.1 LITERATURE SUMMARY OF FETAL LONG QT SYNDROME (CONTINUED)

Author (y)	Origin of LQTS	Hx of Fetal Loss	GA (wk)	Rhythm	Delivery (wk)	Variant
41.	Mother novel	1 SB	34	VT, 2:1 AV block	NSVD (38)	*KCNH2* Thr613Lys Lys897Thr
42.	De novo	ND	30	VT, 2:1 AV block	CS (35)	*SCN5A* R1623Q
43.	De novo twins	ND	30	VT[1,3], 2:1 AV block	ECS (31)	*SCN5A* R1623Q
44. Flock (2014)	Mother	Prim	29	SB	CS (39)	*KCNQ1* G350V
45.	De novo	No	27	VT[1,2,3], SB, 2:1 AV block	ECS (27)	*KCNH2* G682S
46.	Mother	Prim	27	SB, 2:1 AV block	CS (38)	*KCNH2* T613M
47. Priest (2014)	Father	No	ND	Brady	CS (38)	*KCNH2* T613M
48. Reed (2015)	De novo	No		Brady	VD (38)	*CALM3* D130G
49. Chaix (2016)	De novo	30		SB (109 bpm)		
		36		2:1 AV block		
		37		SB (85 bpm)	CS (37)	*CALM3*
50. Magnusson (2017)	Mother	MC × 1 SB × 1	ND	ND	VD	*SCN5A* C1231G>A
51. Blais (2017)	De novo	No	26	VT, 2:1 AV block	CS (37)	*SCN5A* R1623Q
52. Miyake (2017)	De novo	MC × 1	28	2:1 AV block		
			30	VT[3], SB	CS (35)	*KCNH2* S624R
53.	Father	ND	24	VT, SB		
			26	VT[3], SB	CS (37)	*KCNH2* T613M
54. Tuveng (2018)	Mother, novel variant	Fetal loss × 1	ND	SB	ND	*KCNH2* R62Q
55. Crimmins (2018)	De novo	None	27	VT, 2:1 AV block	CS (30)	*KCNH2* G628S

Brady, bradycardia; CS, cesarean section; ECS, emergency cesarean section; FD, fetal demise; +FH, positive family history; homoz, homozygous for the LQTS variant; M + F, mother and father; MC, miscarriage; ND, no data; prim, primiparous mother; SB, sinus bradycardia; Tachy-brady, tachycardia and bradycardia; UK, tested for common variants but negative; VD, vaginal delivery; VT, ventricular tachycardia; 1, cardiac dysfunction; 2, biventricular hypertrophy; 3, hydrops.

approximately 60% and 80%, respectively, in both LQT2 and LQT3 fetuses. Babies with LQT2 and LQT3 were delivered at a gestational age of 27 to 38 (median 35) weeks, via cesarean delivery in ~75% of the pregnancies of which one-third were emergency cesarean deliveries.

A family history of LQTS or sudden cardiac death was a common clue to the diagnosis of LQT1, but it was infrequent in LQT2 (36%) and LQT3 (13%), meaning that prenatal screening for these LQTS genotypes based on family history results in incomplete ascertainment. Furthermore, clinical experience has revealed that some of the more severe cases of fetal LQTS are due to de novo variants which have a negative family history. As for the genotypes identified, it is worth noting that locations of LQT2 variants are almost exclusively at the pore region of the *KCNH2* gene.[1] These variants at the pore region are also known to be associated with life-threatening clinical course in later life. Among them, T613M (6 cases) and G628S (5 cases) should be recognized as hot spots. On the other hand, the LQT3 variant sites are distributed throughout the *SCN5A* gene, with R1623Q being the most frequent missense variant (7/15 cases). Although R1623Q variants were mostly reported as de novo cases, 10% to 20% of them were possibly inherited by germ-line mosaicism, which was demonstrated in one case.[14] Also, it is worth noting that no fetal cases with *SCN5A*-E1784K, the most prevalent *SCN5A* variant in childhood/adulthood with rather favorable outcome,[26] have been reported.

DIAGNOSIS OF FETAL LQTS

Prenatal diagnosis of LQTS is challenging because direct recording of electrocardiogram (ECG) is not possible and availability of fetal magnetocardiography is limited. Therefore, the diagnosis rests on a positive family history as described in Part 1, Chapter 3, or suspicion based on the FHR and rhythm, regardless of family history.

Doppler Echo Diagnosis of LQTS

The Doppler echo diagnosis of LQTS relies on recognition of the LQTS rhythms. Sinus bradycardia may be subtle as it frequently does not even meet obstetrical criteria for bradycardia; nonetheless, findings of a prolonged isovolumic relaxation time should raise suspicion for LQTS[27]. The LQTS rhythms can be assessed by M-mode and simultaneous spectral Doppler interrogation of the superior vena cava and the aorta.[28,29] In fetal LQTS, 2° AV block may be mistaken for blocked atrial bigeminy, but the a-a′ and a′-a interval will be regular in 2° AV block. Lastly, even though the ventricular rates may be similar TdP should not be mistaken for supraventricular tachycardia. In TdP, the atrial rate is slower as AV dissociation is present. There will also be an intermittent irregular pattern of ejection flow of the aorta or a "wax and wane" pattern (FIG. 3.6.3) in fetuses with TdP. These Doppler patterns have been proven to reflect TdP by simultaneous MCG recording.[30] More details on the diagnosis of TdP can be found in Part 3, Chapter 3.

Magnetocardiographic Diagnosis of LQTS

Measurement of QTc can establish the diagnosis of fetal LQTS. Using a threshold of QTc > 490 ms, LQTS can be diagnosed correctly, and QTc > 620 ms predicts development of TdP.[11] Appearance of intermittent 2:1 AV block is also a risk factor for development of TdP. If repeated nonsustained ventricular tachycardia (VT) is recorded, the possibility of TdP is high and transplacental pharmacotherapy should be considered.

IN UTERO MANAGEMENT OF THE FETUS WITH LQTS (FIG. 3.6.4)

If possible, the first step in the management of the fetus suspected of LQTS by a parent with LQTS, a family history of sudden infant death or stillbirth, or an LQTS rhythm, is a fetal magnetocardiography (fMCG). As noted above, sensitivity and specificity of fMCG for LQTS is high. However, regardless if fMCG is available to confirm the diagnosis, the management of the fetus is still based on the rhythm phenotype. Note, however, that because of the increased risk for stillbirth in familial LQTS, obstetrical monitoring should be more frequent and detailed in all cases of suspected or confirmed LQTS.

Although sinus bradycardia is an important marker for LQTS, fetuses are usually asymptomatic and require only obstetrical monitoring with a baseline fetal echocardiogram. More vigilant follow-up is suggested after 28 weeks, as this is often when TdP will first present.

2° AV block can be isolated, herald the onset of TdP, or co-occur with TdP. Treatment is generally unnecessary but monitoring for TdP should be intensified. If fMCG is available, it should be repeated, as if intermittent, it is not always detected by echocardiography.

VT (TdP) is a serious and life-threatening arrhythmia for the fetus, and treatment should be strongly considered to avert a preterm delivery, development of hydrops, or intrauterine demise. Fetal treatment of LQTS is discussed in Part 4, Chapter 3.

If the fetus is suspected of LQTS or there is a family history of LQTS, the mother's vitamin D (25,OH) and magnesium levels should be optimized. Many pregnant women have low <2 ng/dL magnesium levels. Anecdotal reports show prolonged QT-intervals in normal fetuses whose mothers are severely vitamin D deficient. The QT intervals normalized after maternal vitamin D treatment (J. Strasburger, MD, personal communication).

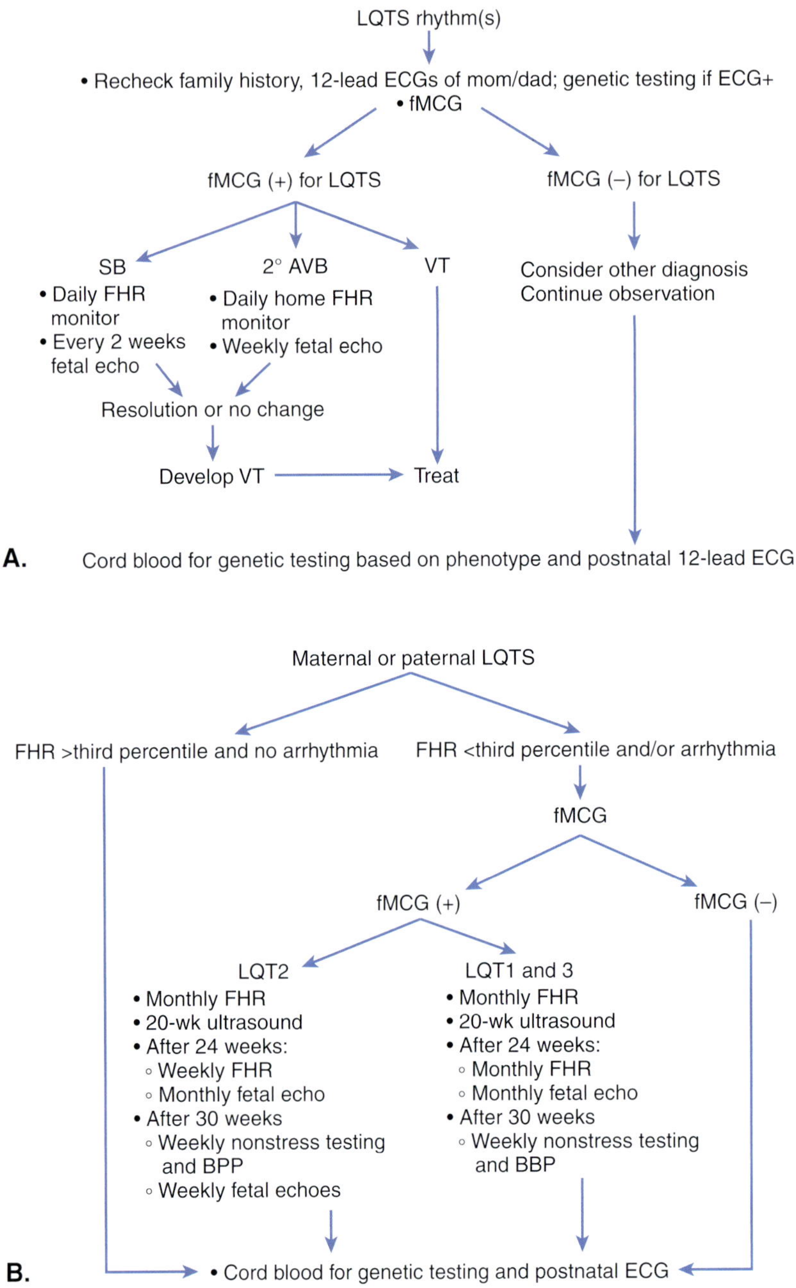

FIGURE 3.6.4 Decision tree for suspected fetal long QT syndrome (LQTS). **A:** The fetus without a family history of LQTS. **B:** The fetus with a family history of LQTS.

FETAL PRESENTATION AND DIAGNOSIS OF OTHER CHANNELOPATHIES

As previously stated, data are sparse or nonexistent regarding the fetal presentation channelopathies other than LQTS. There is one report on a fetus with short QT syndrome[31] (*KCNQ1* gain-of-function variant) who presented with atrial fibrillation in utero. Congenital SSS has also been reported in association with sinus bradycardia in fetal/neonatal life due to *SCN5A* or *HCN4* variant, which are involved in sinus node dysfunction,[32,33] or more interestingly, in association with noncompaction cardiomyopathy, which develops concurrently with changes in *HCN4* expression in conduction system.[33] The etiology of bradycardia in the fetus may in the future be expanded to CPVT, as bradycardia was recently found to be a marker for CPVT in children younger than 10 years.[34] While CPVT has not yet been described in the fetus, it was found in an infant dying suddenly.[35]

SUMMARY

The fetal channelopathies constitute a growing pool of patients who require careful diagnosis and diligent management. Although not every fetus is at risk of in utero demise, primary prevention of life-threatening arrhythmias in LQTS and CPVT are highly successful. Clinical experience has indicated that the earlier these channelopathies can be identified, the better the protection from adverse cardiac events. Greater suspicion for the channelopathies and referrals to fetal arrhythmia centers by obstetrical care providers, as well as moving fECG and fMCG from the research to the clinical arena, will improve the detection of these sometimes subtle but high-risk group of arrhythmias.

References

1. Horigome H, Nagashima M, Sumitomo N, et al. Clinical characteristics and genetic background of congenital long-QT syndrome diagnosed in fetal, neonatal, and infantile life: a nationwide questionnaire survey in Japan. *Circ Arrhythm Electrophysiol.* 2010;3:10-17.
2. Mitchell JL, Cuneo BF, Etheridge SP, Horigome H, Weng HY, Benson DW. Fetal heart rate predictors of long QT syndrome. *Circulation.* 2012;126:2688-2695.
3. ACOG Committee on Practice Bulletins. Intrapartum fetal heart rate monitoring: nomenclature, interpretation and general management principals. *Obstet Gynecol.* 2009;114:192-202.
4. Winbo A, Fosdal I, Lindh M, et al. Third trimester fetal heart rate predicts phenotype and mutation burden in the type 1 long QT syndrome. *Circ Arrhythm Electrophysiol.* 2015;8(4):806-814.
5. Vigliani M. Romano-Ward syndrome diagnosed as moderate fetal bradycardia. A case report. *J Reprod Med.* 1995;40(10):725-728.
6. Beinder E, Grancay T, Menéndez T, Singer H, Hofbeck M. Fetal sinus bradycardia and the long QT syndrome. *Am J Obstet Gynecol.* 2001;185(3):743-747.
7. Donofrio MT, Gullquist SD, O'Connell NG, Redwine FO. Fetal presentation of congenital long QT syndrome. *Pediatr Cardiol.* 1999;20(6):441-444.
8. Cuneo BF, Etheridge SP, Horigome H, et al. Arrhythmia phenotype during fetal life suggests long-QT syndrome genotype: risk stratification of perinatal long-QT syndrome. *Circ Arrhythm Electrophysiol.* 2013;6:946-951.
9. Lupoglazoff JM, Denjoy I, Villain E, et al. Long QT syndrome in neonates: conduction disorders associated with HERG mutations and sinus bradycardia with KCNQ1 mutations. *J Am Coll Cardiol.* 2004;43:826-830.
10. Miyake A, Sakaguchi H, Miyazaki A, Miyoshi T, Aiba T, Shiraishi I. Successful prenatal management of ventricular tachycardia and second-degree atrioventricular block in fetal long QT syndrome. *HeartRhythm Case Rep.* 2016;3:53-57.

11. Cuneo BF, Strasburger JF, Yu S, et al. In utero diagnosis of long QT syndrome by magnetocardiography. *Circulation*. 2013;128:2183-2191.
12. Bhuiyan ZA, Momenah TS, Gong Q, et al. Recurrent intrauterine fetal loss due to near absence of HERG: clinical and functional characterization of a homozygous nonsense HERG Q1070X mutation. *Heart Rhythm*. 2008;5:553-561.
13. Uysal F, Turkgenc B, Toksoy G, et al. Homozygous, and compound heterozygous mutation in 3 Turkish family with Jervell and Lange-Nielsen syndrome: case reports. *BMC Med Genet*. 2017;18:114.
14. Miller TE, Estrella E, Myerburg RJ, et al. Recurrent third-trimester fetal loss and maternal mosaicism for long- QT syndrome. *Circulation*. 2004;109:3029-3034.
15. Cuneo BF, Kaizer AM, Clur SA, et al. Mothers with long QT syndrome are at increased risk for fetal death: findings from a multicenter international study. *Am J Obstet Gynecol*. 2020;222(3):263.e1-263.e11.
16. Simpson JM, Maxwell D, Rosenthal E, Gill H. Fetal ventricular tachycardia secondary to long QT syndrome treated with maternal intravenous magnesium: case report and review of the literature. *Ultrasound Obstet Gynecol*. 2009;34:475-480.
17. Greene EA, Berul CI, Donofrio MT. Prenatal diagnosis of long QT syndrome: implications for delivery room and neonatal management. *Cardiol Young*. 2013;23(1):141-145.
18. Cuneo BF, Ovadia M, Strasburger JF, et al. Prenatal diagnosis and in utero treatment of torsades de pointes associated with congenital long QT syndrome. *Am J Cardiol*. 2003;91(11):1395-1398.
19. Murphy LL, Moon-Grady AJ, Cuneo BF, et al. Developmentally regulated SCN5A splice variant potentiates dysfunction of a novel mutation associated with severe fetal arrhythmia. *Heart Rhythm*. 2012;9:590-597.
20. Splawski I, Timothy KW, Sharpe LM, et al. Ca(V)1.2 calcium channel dysfunction causes a multisystem disorder including arrhythmia and autism. *Cell*. 2004;119(1):19-31.
21. Corona-Rivera JR, Barrios-Prieto E, Nieto-García R, et al. Unusual retrospective prenatal findings in a male newborn with Timothy syndrome type 1. *Eur J Med Genet*. 2015;58(6-7):332-335.
22. Dufendach KA, Timothy K, Ackerman MJ, et al. Clinical outcomes and modes of death in Timothy syndrome: a multicenter international study of a rare disorder. *JACC Clin Electrophysiol*. 2018;4(4):459-466.
23. Crotti L, Spazzolini C, Tester DJ, et al. Calmodulin mutations and life-threatening cardiac arrhythmias: insights from the International Calmodulinopathy Registry. *Eur Heart J*. 2019;40(35):2964-2975. doi:10.1093/eurheartj/ehz311.
24. Ioakeimidis NS, Papamitsou T, Meditskou S, Iakovidou-Kritsi Z. Sudden infant death syndrome due to long QT syndrome: a brief review of the genetic substrate and prevalence. *J Biol Res (Thessalon)*. 2017;24:6. doi:10.1186/s40709-017-0063-1.
25. Crotti L, Tester DJ, White WM, et al. Long QT syndrome-associated mutations in intrauterine fetal death. *J Am Med Assoc*. 2013;309:1473-1482.
26. Wilde AA, Moss AJ, Kaufman ES, et al. Clinical aspects of type 3 long-QT syndrome: an international multicenter study. *Circulation*. 2016;134:872-882.
27. Clur SB, Vink AS, Etheridge SP, et al. Left ventricular isovolumetric relaxation time is prolonged in fetal long-QT syndrome. *Circ Arrhythm Electrophysiol*. 2018;11(4):e005797. doi:10.1161/CIRCEP.117.005797.
28. Chabaneix J, Andelfinger G, Fournier A, Fouron JC, Raboisson MJ. Prenatal diagnosis of long QT syndrome with the superior vena cava–aorta Doppler approach. *Am J Obstet Gynecol*. 2012;207:e3-e7.
29. Miyoshi T, Sakaguchi H, Shiraishi I, Yoshimatsu J, Ikeda T. Potential utility of pulsed-wave Doppler for prenatal diagnosis of fetal ventricular tachycardia secondary to long QT syndrome. *Ultrasound Obstet Gynecol*. 2018;51:697-699.
30. Horigome H, Iwashita H, Yoshinaga M, Shimizu W. Magnetocardiographic demonstration of torsade de pointes in a fetus with congenital long QT syndrome. *J Cardiovasc Electrophysiol*. 2008;19:334-335.
31. Hong K, Piper DR, Diaz-Valdecantos A, et al. De novo KCNQ1 mutation responsible for atrial fibrillation and short QT syndrome in utero. *Cardiovasc Res*. 2005;68:433-440.
32. Benson DW, Wang DW, Dyment M, et al. Congenital sick sinus syndrome caused by recessive mutations in the cardiac sodium channel gene (SCN5A). *J Clin Invest*. 2003;112:1019-1028.
33. Ishikawa T, Ohno S, Murakami T, et al. Sick sinus syndrome with HCN4 mutations shows early onset and frequent association with atrial fibrillation and left ventricular noncompaction. *Heart Rhythm*. 2017;14:717-724.
34. Miyata K, Ohno S, Itoh H, Horie M. Bradycardia is a specific phenotype of catecholaminergic polymorphic ventricular tachycardia induced by RYR2 mutations. *Intern Med*. 2018;57(13):1813-1817.
35. Tester DJ, Dura M, Carturan E, et al. A mechanism for sudden infant death syndrome (SIDS): stress-induced leak via ryanodine receptors. *Heart Rhythm*. 2007;4:733-739.

PART

4

Treatment of Fetal Arrhythmias

Treatment of Supraventricular Tachyarrhythmias

Stacy Ann Stratemann Killen • Frank A. Fish

INTRODUCTION

The goal of fetal arrhythmia treatment is the vaginal delivery of a full-term, nonhydropic infant in sinus rhythm. Fetuses with supraventricular tachyarrhythmias (SVT) are at risk for preterm cesarean delivery with its associated morbidities and mortalities for baby and mother.[1,2] In the modern era, successful in utero treatment of SVT is the rule rather than the exception; nonetheless, management of fetal SVT can be challenging for several reasons. First, the provider is caring for two (and with twins, three) patients, only one of whom can be monitored directly for "well-being" and antiarrhythmic medication side effects. Second, successful management depends on a team of obstetricians, nurses, and fetal cardiologists who may view the management of the pregnancy differently (delivery vs treatment). Third, conversion to sinus rhythm can take many days, require several medications and necessitate different routes of medication delivery. However, understanding the tachycardia mechanisms, the pharmacology of the antiarrhythmic medications, and facilitating effective communication between family and care team can lead to excellent outcomes.

This chapter will describe the management, including treatment, of fetal SVT, which includes atrial flutter, atrioventricular reentrant tachycardia (AVRT), permanent junctional reciprocating tachycardia (PJRT), and atrial ectopic tachycardia as defined in Part 3, Chapter 2. The general approach to the fetus with tachycardia has been described in Part 1, Chapter 1.

WHEN TO TREAT FETAL SVT

The decision to treat fetal SVT depends on several factors, including tachycardia duration, the fetal hemodynamics and well-being, and, to some extent, the gestational age. Treatment is recommended if tachycardia is sustained or incessant, defined as ≥12 hours of uninterrupted tachycardia or tachycardia present ≥50% of the echocardiographic monitoring time (typically ~30 minutes).[1,3,4] Intermittent tachycardia is diagnosed if present <50% of the echocardiographic monitoring time or in <12 hours of a 24-hour fetal monitoring period.[1,3] If there is uncertainty regarding the duration of tachycardia, the mother can undergo continuous electronic fetal heart rate monitoring for several hours or overnight, with the caveat that in tachycardia, electronic fetal heart rate monitors often halve the true heart rate. Thus, a monitor rate of 130 beats per minute (bpm) without variability may represent a true fetal heart rate of 260 bpm (see Part 2, Chapter 1, for more discussion of fetal monitoring). Intermittent tachycardia without hydrops or other signs of hemodynamic compromise may not require treatment but close fetal monitoring is essential.[1] Home monitoring by mothers using a handheld Doppler device can successfully detect tachycardia recurrence.[4]

Regardless of tachycardia rate or duration, any fetus with evidence of hemodynamic compromise (cardiomegaly plus cardiac dysfunction, more than mild atrioventricular [AV] valve insufficiency, or hydrops) should be treated, because in these settings mortality can be 30% to 50%.[5,6] Forty percent of fetuses with SVT, especially AVRT, are hydropic at presentation.

The cardiovascular profile, a 10-point score assessing the degree of cardiac compromise based on Doppler flow patterns in the ductus venosus, umbilical vein and artery, AV valve function, hydrops, and shortening fraction,[7] is not accurate in the presence of sustained SVT. This is because flow in the ductus venosus will be abnormal (to-and-fro flow) based on heart rate alone.

The decision to treat is also influenced by the gestational age at presentation. In the presence of a fetal arrhythmia, many obstetricians will perform a cesarean delivery since fetal well-being, as determined by fetal heart rate variability and absence of decelerations, cannot be assessed unless the rhythm is normal. With agreement of the parents, obstetricians, and fetal cardiologists, pharmacological conversion can be successful after 37 weeks with the goal of a spontaneous vaginal delivery shortly thereafter. One may set a time limit for successful conversion such as "if the fetus has not converted in 3, 5, or 7 days, he will be delivered." On the other hand, if a >37-week fetus is severely hydropic and has a nonreassuring biophysical profile score, Cesarean delivery and tachycardia conversion in the operating room with ECMO on standby may be the best option.

A current approach to fetal SVT therapy based on tachycardia duration, associated fetal compromise, and gestational age is presented in TABLE 4.1.1. In addition to these parameters, tachycardia mechanism and duration, the biophysical profile score, and maternal risk factors for tolerating therapy are important to consider when choosing whether to initiate fetal antiarrhythmic therapy, selecting the type of therapy or electing to proceed with premature, Cesarean delivery.[1]

TABLE 4.1.1 CURRENT APPROACH TO FETAL SUPRAVENTRICULAR TACHYARRHYTHMIAS (SVT)

Tachycardia Duration	Treatment Strategy
Intermittent SVT without hydrops	• Ambulatory monitoring or twice-weekly fetal heart rate auscultation and frequent fetal echoes
Sustained SVT with/without hydrops OR Intermittent SVT with hemodynamic compromise	• <37 wk of gestation → drug therapy • >37 wk of gestation → delivery or drug therapy

PHARMACOLOGY OF ANTIARRHYTHMIC THERAPIES (TABLE 4.1.2)

Most types of fetal SVT respond to treatment with survival rates of 80% to 100%,[5,8] but it is important to remember that both mother and fetus are affected by the therapy. Current pharmaceutical agents are administered "off-label" via the maternal circulation ("transplacental therapy") or directly into the fetus (intracordal or intramuscular injection) to treat fetal SVT. The primary antiarrhythmic agents used for treating fetal SVT include digoxin, sotalol, and flecainide.[5] Amiodarone is typically reserved for refractory tachycardia with hydrops given its significant side effect profile.[5,8] Standard doses of the antiarrhythmics and side effects are shown in TABLE 4.1.2.

Digoxin inhibits the Na^+/K^+ ATPase to prolong refractoriness of the AV node and slow the sinus node. Digoxin is usually well absorbed in the absence of hydrops and reaches steady state in 3 to 5 days after loading. Fetal levels are 20% to 40% lower than maternal levels.[9] Because flecainide and amiodarone can increase digoxin levels, digoxin doses should be decreased when used in combination with these drugs. Digoxin is generally safe for mothers and fetuses but is commonly associated with significant the following side effects: maternal nausea, vomiting, anorexia, and extreme fatigue.[10] Other possible side effects include blurred vision, headache, dizziness, and nocturnal Wenckebach (Mobitz type 1°, 2° AV block).[5,10-12] Signs of digoxin effect must be separated from signs of toxicity, the former including PR interval prolongation, sinus bradycardia and ST-T wave changes. Signs of digoxin toxicity include symptomatic bradycardia or AV block, ventricular tachycardia or fibrillation, hypotension, altered mental status, weakness, abdominal pain, and visual changes. No serious adverse events related to digoxin have occurred in healthy women, but digoxin is contraindicated in mothers with hypertrophic cardiomyopathy, AV block, and Wolff-Parkinson-White syndrome. A recent study demonstrated that transplacental digoxin given orally to the mother was just as effective as IV digoxin at reaching therapeutic serum concentrations.[13,14]

Sotalol is a K+ channel blocker and β-adrenergic receptor-blocker with the combined effect of prolonging action potential duration and cardiac tissue refractoriness, slowing AV node conduction, and decreasing heart rate. It is well transferred across the placenta, even with hydrops. Fetal levels are similar to maternal levels within 2 to 4 hours after oral administration.[15] After prolonged treatment, fetal levels can be even higher than maternal levels. Common maternal side effects of sotalol include nausea, dizziness, fatigue, hypotension, depression, insomnia, worsening asthma, bradycardia, QTc prolongation, and 1° AV block/PR prolongation.[1] Acquired long QT syndrome with torsades de pointes is the most important risk of sotalol administration. Therefore, serial ECG monitoring or telemetry; withholding other QT prolonging medications; maximizing vitamin D, potassium, and magnesium levels; and keeping QTc duration <500 ms are essential if sotalol treatment is given. In the setting of prolonged treatment, fetal magnetocardiography (fMCG) can be considered to assess the fetal QTc interval.

Flecainide inhibits Na+ channels and has weak β-adrenergic receptor-blocker properties, thus prolonging conduction and refractoriness of all cardiac tissues, including accessory pathways and, to a lesser extent, the AV node. This drug usually reaches therapeutic concentrations within 3 days.[16] Common maternal side effects of flecainide include headache, dizziness, visual disturbances/blurred vision, nausea, con-

TABLE 4.1.2 PHARMACOLOGIC TREATMENT OF FETAL SUPRAVENTRICULAR TACHYARRHYTHMIAS

Drug	Standard Transplacental Dosages	Common Side Effects	ECG Effects
Digoxin	Load: 375-500 micrograms (μg) every 8 h × 3 doses or 500 μg every 12 h × 4 doses Maintenance: 250-500 μg every 12 h (goal drug levels 1.5-2.5 ng/mL) Intramuscular digoxin = 88 μg/kg estimated fetal weight	Nausea, vomiting, fatigue, blurred vision, sinus bradycardia	1° and 2° AV block, including nocturnal Wenckebach (Mobitz type 1 2° AV block)
Flecainide	300 mg daily (100 mg every 8 h or 150 mg every 12 h) Goal drug levels 0.2-1 μg/mL If using a combination of digoxin and flecainide, decrease digoxin dose by 50%	Headache, dizziness, visual disturbances	QRS widening (intraventricular conduction delay/ bundle branch block), QTc prolongation, 1° AV block
Sotalol	240-480 mg daily (120-160 mg every 12 or 8 h); 160 mg every 12 h (starting dose with hydrops)	Nausea, dizziness, fatigue, hypotension, bradycardia	QRS widening (QTc prolongation, 1° AV block
Amiodarone	Load: 600 mg every 6-8 h (1800-2400 mg/d) × 2-5 d Maintenance: 200-600 mg/d Goal drug levels 0.7-2.8 μg/mL Must decrease doses of digoxin (by 50%) and flecainide if these are being used in combination with amiodarone Intraperitoneal amiodarone	Nausea, thrombocytopenia, photosensitivity, rash, maternal/fetal thyroid dysfunction, liver dysfunction, visual disturbance, gait/ coordination/movement problems, peripheral neuropathy/paresthesia	QRS widening (intraventricular conduction delay), QTc prolongation; wide P-waves, QTc ~0.48, bradycardia, 1° AV block

Adapted from Donofrio MT, Moon-Grady AJ, Hornberger LK, et al. Diagnosis and treatment of fetal cardiac disease: a scientific statement from the American Heart Association. *Circulation*. 2014;129(21): 2183-2242.

stipation, QRS widening (intraventricular conduction delay or bundle branch block), QTc prolongation, and 1° AV block/PR prolongation.[1] Proarrhythmia risk can be minimized by keeping maternal serum concentrations <1 μg/mL and by avoiding excessive QRS prolongation (>50% change from baseline or >100 ms). Mothers with coronary artery disease, ventricular arrhythmias, Brugada syndrome, and congestive heart failure should not be treated with flecainide.[17]

Amiodarone inhibits K+ channels, Na+ channels, Ca++ channels, and β-adrenergic receptors and thus prolongs cardiac tissue refractoriness and slows conduction throughout atrial and ventricular myocardia. High doses are needed to treat fetal tachycardia, because amiodarone and its active metabolite incompletely cross the placenta.[18] This drug is a pregnancy class D therapy, because it is associated with known fetal risk. Common maternal side effects of amiodarone include nausea, thrombocytopenia, photosensitivity, rash, thyroid dysfunction, liver dysfunction, visual disturbance, gait/coordination/ movement problems, peripheral neuropathy/paresthesia, intraventricular conduction delay or bundle branch block, QTc prolongation (rarely, torsades de pointes), and bradycardia. Pulmonary toxicity and hepatotoxicity are rare but serious complications usually associated with chronic use. Fetal thyroid dysfunction, growth restriction, and neurodevelopmental abnormalities can also occur.[9,12,19-21] Because amiodarone elimination is slow (via shedding of epithelial cells of the skin and gastrointestinal tract), drug effects may persist for weeks after amiodarone is discontinued.

Verapamil, procainamide, and quinidine are no longer recommended for treatment of fetal tachycardia, and there are no significant data to suggest that *propranolol* (pure β-adrenergic receptor-blockers) can achieve rhythm control at currently recommended maternal doses.[1]

EFFICACY OF CURRENT THERAPIES

Correct and timely identification of fetal tachycardia type and assessment of fetal well-being are important when determining pharmacological therapy and mode of drug delivery. Absence of movement and breathing, with or without poor tone, indicates a sick fetus needing conversion to sinus rhythm quickly. In this situation, simultaneous direct and transplacental treatment should be considered. Alternatively, even with hydrops, if the fetus is moving and breathing and has normal tone, transplacental therapy (typically with two agents) can be initiated; the mother should be hospitalized, and frequent modified biophysical profile testing and continuous electronic fetal heart rate monitoring should be utilized.

Treatment of a hydropic fetus usually requires combination transplacental therapy or direct fetal treatment plus transplacental therapy. Digoxin has poor transplacental transfer in fetal hydrops[22] while flecainide and sotalol can cross the placenta effectively.[5,16,23] The combination of digoxin and sotalol is thought to be more effective for treatment of atrial flutter in the setting of fetal hydrops, while digoxin and flecainide are thought to be the best transplacental combination for AVRT.[5] Risk factors for developing hydrops include sustained/incessant SVT, AVRT as the tachycardia mechanism, onset of tachycardia before 32 weeks gestation, and co-occurrence of structural heart disease.[5,7] Faster ventricular rates have been found to be a risk factor for fetal hemodynamic compromise in some, but not all studies. As previously noted, flow in the ductus venosus will be abnormal in all fetuses with heart rates >190 bpm and should not be used to assess severity of fetal compromise.

In a retrospective multicenter study comparing nonrandomized treatment with digoxin, flecainide, and sotalol, tachycardia mechanism, tachycardia duration, and presence of associated hydrops/fetal hemodynamic compromise significantly influenced fetal response to therapy.[5] Digoxin or flecainide is currently considered first-line therapy for AVRT in many institutions,[5,24] while sotalol or digoxin is considered best first-line therapy for atrial flutter.[5,15,25,26] Flecainide as a single agent is not recommended for atrial flutter, as it can slow the atrial rate without corresponding delay in the AV node, leading to an increase in the ventricular response, including rapid 1:1 conduction. Ectopic atrial tachycardia often responds best to flecainide or digoxin,[1,24] while PJRT is often best treated with flecainide or sotalol.[1,27]

Retrospective studies report variable success rates for all antiarrhythmic agents used to treat fetal SVT. In utero conversion of SVT to sinus rhythm with oral digoxin monotherapy has occurred in 50% to 100% of patients without hydrops but in <40% of patients with hydrops.[5,6,12,24,28-35] Flecainide has converted 58% to 100% without hydrops and 43% to 86% with hydrops,[12,23,24,31,33,36-38] while sotalol monotherapy has converted 40% to 100% without hydrops and 50% to 67% with hydrops.[15,25,26,39,40]

Two recent meta-analyses evaluating transplacental therapies found that flecainide was more effective than digoxin at converting fetal AVRT to sinus rhythm, especially in the setting of fetal hydrops.[41,42] Strizek et al reported a 3-day (range 1-7 days) median time to conversion of AVRT with flecainide in both hydropic and nonhydropic fetuses,[37] which was substantially shorter than conversion to sinus rhythm with digoxin.[5]

Amiodarone is another important therapeutic option but is often reserved for refractory tachycardia with hydrops given its significant side effect profile.[9] It is effective for conversion of AVRT, ventricular tachycardia and junctional ectopic tachycardia, but was much less effective for atrial flutter. Discontinuing amiodarone treatment after resolution of hydrops is recommended to minimize the maternal and fetal side effects.[9] Thyroid function tests are recommended for mother and baby at birth, at 2 weeks of age, and then monthly for the first 3 months of life because of the risk of neonatal hypothyroidism.

Direct fetal treatment is typically reserved for fetuses who require a more rapid conversion to sinus rhythm because of a poor biophysical profile score or because of severe hydrops recalcitrant to transplacental therapy alone. Different antiarrhythmic agents have been given through specific routes. For example, intracordal injections of flecainide, adenosine, digoxin, and amiodarone have been reported, with some fetal deaths due to cardiac standstill, severe bradycardia, or cord accidents. Intracordal adenosine is not recommended in the treatment of fetal tachycardia because the risks of tachycardia recurrence and cord accidents outweigh the benefits. Antiarrhythmic injections into ascites (intraperitoneal route) have been reported without side effects in some series.[17] However, bowel fibrosis and strictures were seen in one fetus (B. Cuneo, personal communication). An efficacious direct fetal treatment is digoxin, 88 μg/kg of estimated fetal weight (based on head circumference) or the 50th percentile of weight for gestational age injected into the fetal thigh or buttock.[9,22,43] Repeat injections every 12 hours for 36 hours can be given if the first injection is not successful. Concurrent transplacental treatment is necessary to maintain fetal serum digoxin levels.

A prospective, multicenter study (Fetal Atrial Flutter & Supraventricular Tachycardia [FAST] therapy trial; https://www.fasttherapytrial.com/; https://clinicaltrials.gov/ct2/show/NCT02624765) to assess safety and efficacy of these agents is currently underway. This study includes three randomized clinical substudies comparing first-line treatment for atrial flutter without hydrops (RCT A), supraventricular tachycardia without hydrops (RCT B), and supraventricular tachycardia with hydrops (RCT C). There is also a prospective registry of nonrandomized study participants. Hopefully, the results of this study will clarify the optimal choice of therapy for fetal supraventricular tachyarrhythmias.

MATERNAL AND FETAL MONITORING

During Initiation of Therapy

The approach to the tachycardic fetus is shown in FIGURE 4.1.1. Prior to initiating fetal therapy, maternal assessment with ECG, +/−echocardiography, serum electrolytes (including calcium and magnesium), complete blood count, TSH/freeT4, 25(OH) vitamin D level, renal function, and liver function is recommended.[8] Evaluation for SS-A antibodies is recommended for junctional ectopic tachycardia (described in Part 3, Chapter 3) and fetal atrial flutter due to their association with immune-mediated carditis.[44-47] Correction of underlying maternal electrolyte abnormalities (calcium, potassium, and magnesium) and treatment of vitamin D deficiency can decrease risk of maternal proarrhythmia and may also facilitate pharmaco-conversion of fetal and maintenance of sinus rhythm once conversion occurs.[48]

Vigilant monitoring for fetal and maternal adverse events, including proarrhythmia, is important, especially during the initiation of antiarrhythmic treatment. Many protocols include inpatient monitoring for at least 48 to 72 hours (5-6 doses of therapy).[5] At some institutions maternal telemetry is performed; at others, daily ECG or ECGs prior to each medication dose have sufficed. Drug levels of digoxin and flecainide have been found to be helpful in SVT management only if very high doses of either medication are needed to convert SVT or maintain sinus rhythm or if the ECG does not reflect the clinical findings. An example would be if a mother treated with digoxin experiences severe nausea and vomiting without ECG findings of digoxin effect. Unfortunately, results of flecainide levels are usually not available for several days and thus are not helpful in acute management decisions.

Monitoring the fetus for antiarrhythmic drug effect is more difficult. fMCG and some fetal ECG can accurately detect ST-T-wave changes, and PR, QRS, and QT durations, but these technologies are not generally available.[49] Echocardiography can be helpful in monitoring the AV interval, which is generally 10 to 30 ms longer than the fMCG PR interval.[50]

After Conversion to Sinus Rhythm

Once tachycardia conversion or heart rate control is achieved, transplacental therapy is usually continued until delivery. However, the same dose and even the same antiarrhythmic medication used for conversion may not be necessary to maintain sinus rhythm. Once hydrops has resolved or SVT has been controlled for 2 to 3 weeks, one approach is to maintain sinus rhythm at the lowest dose of the medication that has the least proarrhythmic risk. This can be accomplished by slowly lowering the medication dose until SVT recurs, until the dose is low enough to substantially reduce the risk of proarrhythmia, or until the medication is discontinued. Close monitoring is essential during this titration and can be accomplished by frequent visits to the obstetrician for fetal heart rate auscultation and/or ultrasounds or by ambulatory fetal heart rate monitoring by the mother with occasional ultrasounds or echocardiograms.[4] If the

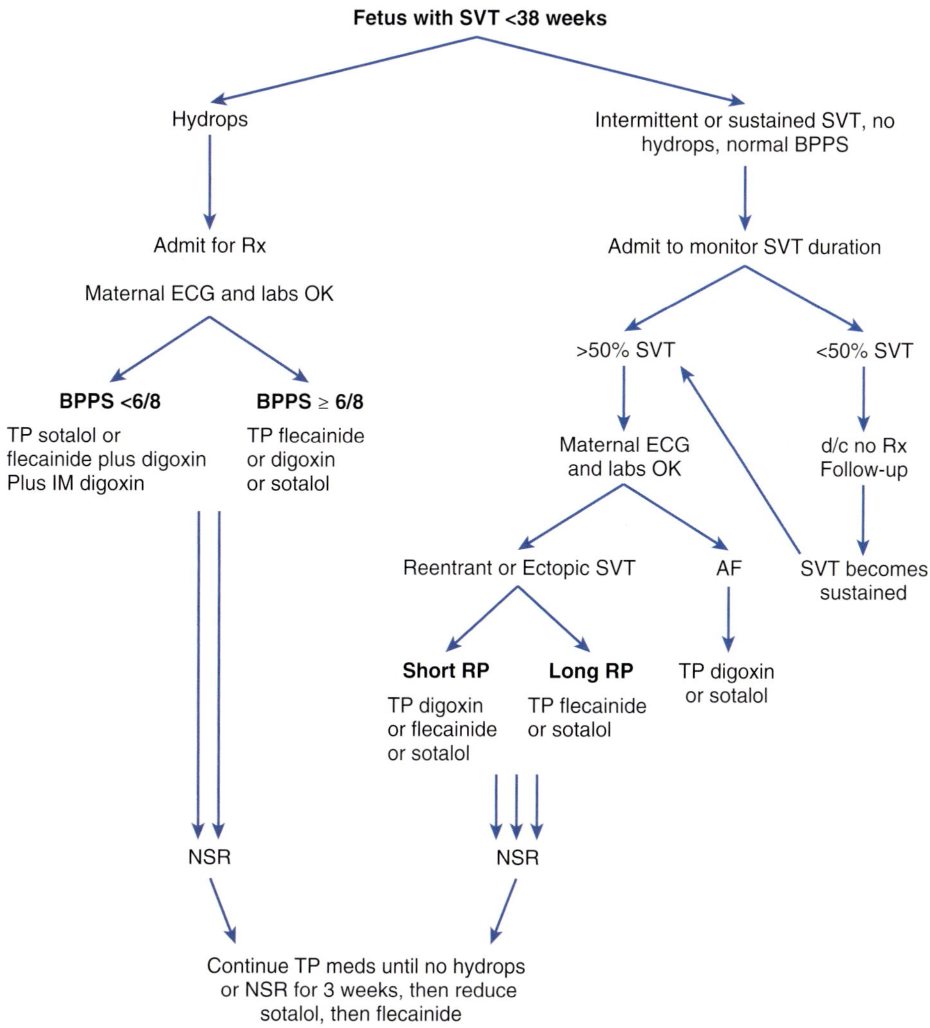

FIGURE 4.1.1 Approach to the fetus at gestational age <37 weeks presenting with tachycardia. AF, atrial flutter; BPPS, biophysical profile score (modified to exclude heart rate); ECG, electrocardiogram; IM, intramuscular (to fetus); NSR, normal sinus rhythm; Rx, treatment; SVT, supraventricular tachyarrhythmia; TP, transplacental.

mother suspects SVT recurrence, she can send an audiotext to the physician managing her care. The total medication dose or frequency can then be re-increased as an outpatient since the mother has been monitored at the higher dose during acute SVT treatment. Another approach is to wean the antiarrhythmic with the highest likelihood of proarrhythmia.[4]

Another important reason to monitor mother and fetus after SVT conversion is that in the hydropic fetus, diuresis after conversion can cause rapid, progressive polyhydramnios and preterm labor in up to 40% of fetuses.[48]

ADVERSE EVENTS ASSOCIATED WITH SVT THERAPIES

In a recent, prospective, multicenter study by Miyoshi and colleagues on behalf of the Japan Fetal Arrhythmia Group evaluating protocol-based treatment of fetal SVT, adverse events were observed in 78% (39/50) of mothers, with only one serious event (Mobitz type 2° AV block) that resolved with discontinuation of therapy.[13] Nausea and vomiting were the most common maternal side effects.[13] Fetal adverse events occurred in 24% (12/49) of fetuses, 4 of whom required discontinuation of therapy; two fetal deaths occurred during combination therapy with digoxin and sotalol.[13]

Despite vigilant fetal and maternal monitoring, fetal deaths, even in nonhydropic fetuses, have been reported in virtually every published series of fetal SVT treatment. These deaths have been reported with escalation of a drug dose but have also been observed after weeks of control with a stable dose. This raises concern about the potential of various antiarrhythmic agents to cause a new arrhythmia or worsen the existing arrhythmia.[14] Because sotalol and flecainide reach concentrations many times higher in amniotic fluid compared to in maternal serum, fetal toxicity can occur (through fetal swallowing of amniotic fluid) without maternal evidence of toxicity. This gives credence to reducing the maintenance dose of antiarrhythmics as low as possible, giving only one medication rather than two, substituting digoxin for sotalol or flecainide, if possible, and normalizing low levels of maternal vitamin D or magnesium.

SUMMARY

While fetal tachycardia with hydrops has a mortality rate as high as 30%, even a hydropic fetus has a >80% chance of a successful outcome with current approaches to transplacental antiarrhythmic therapy. The goal of fetal tachycardia treatment is conversion to sinus rhythm or heart rate reduction to increase cardiac output, thereby decreasing the risk of hydrops and enhancing hydrops resolution. Treatment is primarily transplacental (oral or intravenous maternal administration), while direct fetal treatment (cordocentesis, intramuscular, or intraperitoneal injections) is typically reserved for refractory tachycardia in severely hydropic fetuses or for fetuses with an abnormal biophysical profile score who are in urgent need of conversion.

Multiple studies reporting the safety and efficacy of digoxin, flecainide, and sotalol as monotherapy for SVT without hydrops and as combination therapy for SVT with hydrops support efforts for in utero treatment to avoid premature, cesarean deliveries when possible. At this time, data suggest that digoxin and flecainide are first-line for AVRT, flecainide or sotalol are first-line for long RP tachycardias (like atrial ectopic tachycardia), and sotalol is first-line for atrial flutter.

Irrespective of the choice of antiarrhythmic therapy, transplacental drug effects are not immediate and modifications in first-line therapy may be required to achieve tachycardia conversion or rate control. Also, monitoring for fetal and maternal adverse events, including proarrhythmia, remains paramount. For the medical teams caring for pregnancies complicated by fetal SVT, patience and vigilance are key to successful therapy.

References

1. Donofrio MT, Moon-Grady AJ, Hornberger LK, et al. Diagnosis and treatment of fetal cardiac disease: a scientific statement from the American Heart Association. *Circulation.* 2014;129(21):2183-2242.
2. Zoeller BB. Treatment of fetal supraventricular tachycardia. *Curr Treat Options Cardiovasc Med.* 2017;19(1):7.
3. Strasburger JF, Cheulkar B, Wichman HJ. Perinatal arrhythmias: diagnosis and management. *Clin Perinatol.* 2007;34(4):627-652.
4. MacIntosh A, Benson DW, Collins K, Von Alvensleben J, Cuneo BF. HRS abstract 2020.
5. Jaeggi ET, Carvalho JS, De Groot E, et al. Comparison of transplacental treatment of fetal supraventricular tachyarrhythmias with digoxin, flecainide and sotalol: results of a nonrandomized multicenter study. *Circulation.* 2011;124(16):1747-1754.
6. Simpson JM, Sharland GK. Fetal tachycardias: management and outcome of 127 consecutive cases. *Heart.* 1998;79(6):576-581.
7. Hofstaetter C, Hansmann M, Eik-Nes SH, Huhta JC, Luther SL. A cardiovascular profile score in the surveillance of fetal hydrops. *J Matern Fetal Neonatal Med.* 2006;19(7):407-413.
8. Strasburger JF, Cuneo BF, Michon MM, et al. Amiodarone therapy for drug-refractory fetal tachycardia. *Circulation.* 2004;109(3):375-379.
9. Syme MR, Paxton JW, Keelan JA. Drug transfer and metabolism by the human placenta. *Clin Pharmacokinet.* 2004;43(8):487-514.
10. Moatassim S, Touleimat S, Hazelzet T, et al. Maternal complications induced by digoxin treatment of fetal tachycardia: a retrospective series of 18 cases. *J Gynecol Obstet Hum Reprod.* 2018;47(2):35-38.
11. Miyoshi T, Maeno Y, Hamasaki T, Inamura N, et al; Japan Fetal Arrhythmia Group. Antenatal therapy for fetal supraventricular tachyarrhythmias: multicenter trial. *J Am Coll Cardiol.* 2019;74(7):874-885.
12. Bartalena L, Bogazzi F, Braverman LE, Martino E. Effects of amiodarone administration during pregnancy on neonatal thyroid function and subsequent neurodevelopment. *J Endocrinol Invest.* 2001;24(2):116-130.
13. Strasburger JF. Predictability in fetal supraventricular tachycardia management. *J Am Coll Cardiol.* 2019;74(7):886-888.
14. Oudijk MA, Michon MM, Kleinman CS, et al. Sotalol in the treatment of fetal dysrhythmias. *Circulation.* 2000;101:2721-2726.
15. Bourget P, Pons JC, Delouis C, Fermont L, Frydman R. Flecainide distribution, transplacental passage, and accumulation in the amniotic fluid during the third trimester of pregnancy. *Ann Pharmacother.* 1994;28(9):1031-1034.
16. Hopson JR, Buxton AE, Rinkenberger RL, Nademanee K, Heilman JM, Kienzle MG. Safety and utility of flecainide acetate in the routine care of patients with supraventricular tachyarrhythmias: results of a multicenter trial. The Flecainide Supraventricular Tachycardia Study Group. *Am J Cardiol.* 1996;77(3):72A-82A.
17. Gembruch U, Hansmann M, Redel DA, Bald R. Intrauterine therapy of fetal tachyarrhythmias: intraperitoneal administration of antiarrhythmic drugs to the fetus in fetal tachyarrhythmias with severe hydrops fetalis. *J Perinat Med.* 1988;16:39-42.
18. Jouannic JM, Delahaye S, Fermont L, et al. Fetal supraventricular tachycardia: a role for amiodarone as second-line therapy? *Prenat Diagn.* 2003;23(2):152-156.
19. Magee LA, Nulman I, Rovet JF, Koren G. Neurodevelopment after in utero amiodarone exposure. *Neurotoxicol Teratol.* 1999;21(3):261-265.
20. Vanbesien J, Casteels A, Bougatef A, et al. Transient fetal hypothyroidism due to direct fetal administration of amiodarone for drug resistant fetal tachycardia. *Am J Perinatol.* 2001;18(2):113-116.
21. Younis JS, Granat M. Insufficient transplacental digoxin transfer in severe hydrops fetalis. *Am J Obstet Gynecol.* 1987;157:1268-1269.
22. Alsaied T, Baskar S, Fares M, et al. First-line antiarrhythmic transplacental treatment for fetal tachyarrhythmia: a systematic review and meta-analysis. *J Am Heart Assoc.* 2017;6(12):e007164.
23. Ekman-Joelsson BM, Mellander M, Lagnefeldt L, Sonesson SE. Foetal tachyarrhythmia treatment remains challenging even if the vast majority of cases have a favourable outcome. *Acta Paediatr.* 2015;104(11):1090-1097.
24. Barjot P, Hamel P, Calmelet P, Maragnes P, Herlicoviez M. Flecainide against fetal supraventricular tachycardia complicated by hydrops fetalis. *Acta Obstet Gynecol Scand.* 1998;77(3):353-358.
25. Naheed ZJ, Strasburger JF, Deal BJ, Benson DW Jr, Gidding SS. Fetal tachycardia: mechanisms and predictors of hydrops fetalis. *J Am Coll Cardiol.* 1996;27(7):1736-1740.
26. Sridharan S, Sullivan I, Tomek V, et al. Flecainide versus digoxin for fetal supraventricular tachycardia: comparison of two drug treatment protocols. *Heart Rhythm.* 2016;13(9):1913-1919.

27. Shah A, Moon-Grady A, Bhogal N, et al. Effectiveness of sotalol as first-line therapy for fetal supraventricular tachyarrhythmias. *Am J Cardiol.* 2012;109(11):1614-1618.
28. Van der Heijden LB, Oudijk MA, Manten GT, ter Heide H, Pistorius L, Freund MW. Sotalol as first-line treatment for fetal tachycardia and neonatal follow-up. *Ultrasound Obstet Gynecol.* 2013;42(3):285-293.
29. Oudijk MA, Stoutenbeek P, Sreeram N, Visser GH, Meijboom EJ. Persistent junctional reciprocating tachycardia in the fetus. *J Matern Fetal Neonatal Med.* 2003;13(3):191-196.
30. Jaeggi E, Fouron JC, Drblik SP. Fetal atrial flutter: diagnosis, clinical features, treatment, and outcome. *J Pediatr.* 1998;132:335-339.
31. Fouron JC, Fournier A, Proulx F, et al. Management of fetal tachyarrhythmia based on superior vena cava/aorta Doppler flow recordings. *Heart.* 2003;89:1211-1216.
32. Jaeggi E, Fouron JC, Fournier A, et al. Ventriculo-atrial time interval emsrued on M-Mode echocardiography: a determining element in diagnosis treatment and prognosis of fetal supraventricular tachycardia. *Heart.* 1998;79:582-587.
33. Van Engelen AD, Weijtens O, Brenner JI, et al. Management, outcome and follow-up of fetal tachycardia. *J Am Coll Cardiol.* 1994;24:1371-1375.
34. Kleinman CS, Copel JA, Weinstein EM, Santulli TV Jr, Hobbins JC. Treatment of fetal supraventricular tachyarrhythmias. *J Clin Ultrasound.* 1985;13(4):265-273.
35. Frohn-Mulder IM, Stewart PA, Witsenburg M, Den Hollander NS, Wladimiroff JW, Hess J. The efficacy of flecainide versus digoxin in the management of fetal supraventricular tachycardia. *Prenat Diagn.* 1995;15(13):1297-1302.
36. Ebenroth ES, Cordes TM, Darragh RK. Second-line treatment of fetal supraventricular tachycardia using flecainide acetate. *Pediatr Cardiol.* 2001;22(6):483-487.
37. Allan LD, Chita SK, Sharland GK, Maxwell D, Priestley K. Flecainide in the treatment of fetal tachycardias. *Br Heart J.* 1991;65(1):46-48.
38. Strizek B, Berg C, Gottschalk I, Herberg U, Geipel A, Gembruch U. High-dose flecainide is the most effective treatment of fetal supraventricular tachycardia. *Heart Rhythm.* 2016;13(6):1283-1288.
39. Ekiz A, Kaya B, Bornaun H, et al. Flecainide as first-line treatment for fetal supraventricular tachycardia. *J Matern Fetal Neonatal Med.* 2017;31(4):407-412.
40. Sonesson SE, Fouron JC, Wesslen-Eriksson E, Jaeggi E, Winberg P. Foetal supraventricular tachycardia treated with sotalol. *Acta Paediatr.* 1998;87(5):584-587.
41. Oudijk MA, Ruskamp JM, Ververs FF, et al. Treatment of fetal tachycardia with sotalol: transplacental pharmacokinetics and pharmacodynamics. *J Am Coll Cardiol.* 2003;42(4):765-770.
42. Hill GD, Kovach JR, Saudek DE, Singh AK, Wehrheim K, Frommelt MA. Transplacental treatment of fetal tachycardia: a systematic review and meta-analysis. *Prenat Diagn.* 2017;37(11):1076-1083.
43. Parilla BV, Strasburger JF, Socol ML. Fetal supraventricular tachycardia complicated by hydrops fetalis: a role for direct fetal intramuscular therapy. *Am J Perinatol.* 1996;13(8):483-486.
44. Cuneo B, Strasburger JF, Niksch A, Ovadia M, Wakai RT. An expanded phenotype of maternal SSA/SSB antibody-associated fetal cardiac disease. *J Matern Fetal Neonatal Med.* 2009;22(3):233-238.
45. Sacks JH, Samai C, Gomez K, Kanaan U. Maternal antibody-associated fetal second-degree heart block and atrial flutter: case report and review. *Pediatr Cardiol.* 2013;34(8):2040-2043.
46. Zaidi SJ, Siddiqui S, Cuneo BF, Strasburger JF, McDuffie R, Wakai RT. Prenatal diagnosis and management of junctional ectopic tachycardia. *HeartRhythm Case Rep.* 2017;3(11):503-508.
47. Dubin AM, Cuneo BF, Strasburger JF, Wakai RT, Van Hare GF, Rosenthal DN. Congenital junctional ectopic tachycardia and congenital complete atrioventricular block: a shared etiology? *Heart Rhythm.* 2005;2(3):313-315.
48. Wacker-Gussmann A, Strasburger JF, Cueno BF, Wakai RT. Diagnosis and treatment of fetal arrhythmia. *Am J Perinatol.* 2014;31(7):617-628.
49. Campbell JQ, Best TH, Eswaran H, Lowery CL. Fetal and maternal magnetocardiography during flecainide therapy for supraventricular tachycardia. *Obstet Gynecol.* 2006;108(3 pt 2):767-771.
50. Cuneo BF, Bitant S, Strasburger JF, Kaizer AM, Wakai RT. Assessment of atrioventricular conduction by echocardiography and magnetocardiography in normal and anti-Ro/SSA-antibody positive pregnancies. *Ultrasound Obstet Gynecol.* 2019;54(5):625-633.

Treatment of Ventricular Tachycardias

Sally-Ann Barker Clur • Arja Suzanne Vink • Nico A. Blom • Hitoshi Horigome

INTRODUCTION

After establishing a diagnosis of ventricular tachycardia (VT), a major decision is to determine if the VT is torsades de pointes, the polymorphic VT of long QT syndrome (LQTS) or the VT is unrelated to LQTS. This is important because many antiarrhythmic medications used in treating VT prolong the QT interval and may exacerbate TdP leading to fetal demise. The decision to treat VT depends on numerous factors including etiology, gestational age, cardiac function, the presence of hydrops fetalis, duration and frequency of VT, and ventricular rate.

In general, a diagnosis of fetal VT requires hospital admission for continuous fetal heart rate monitoring and at least daily biophysical profile score testing and fetal echocardiograms regardless of the etiology. There is little consensus regarding the best treatment of fetal VT due to its rarity. Restoring sinus rhythm is often difficult, drug efficacy is variable, and multiple antiarrhythmic medications are frequently necessary.[1] Treatment should aim at maintaining the fetus in a stable condition with adequate cardiac output to allow for fetal maturation, restoration of sinus rhythm if possible, regression of hydrops, and the achievement of a normal vaginal delivery at term.

OVERVIEW OF VT ANTIARRHYTHMIC MEDICATIONS

Antiarrhythmic drugs are classified into five main classes depending on their mechanism of action (FIG. 4.2.1).[2] *Class I* agents interfere with the sodium channel. They depress the maximum rise of the cardiac action potential and slow conduction through the His-Purkinje system and myocardium. They are divided into three groups depending on their onset of depression, effect on the action potential duration, and effective recovery period. *Class Ia* drugs have an intermediate onset of depression and include quinidine, procainamide, and disopyramide. They also have potassium channel blocking effects. *Class Ib* agents have a fast onset of depression

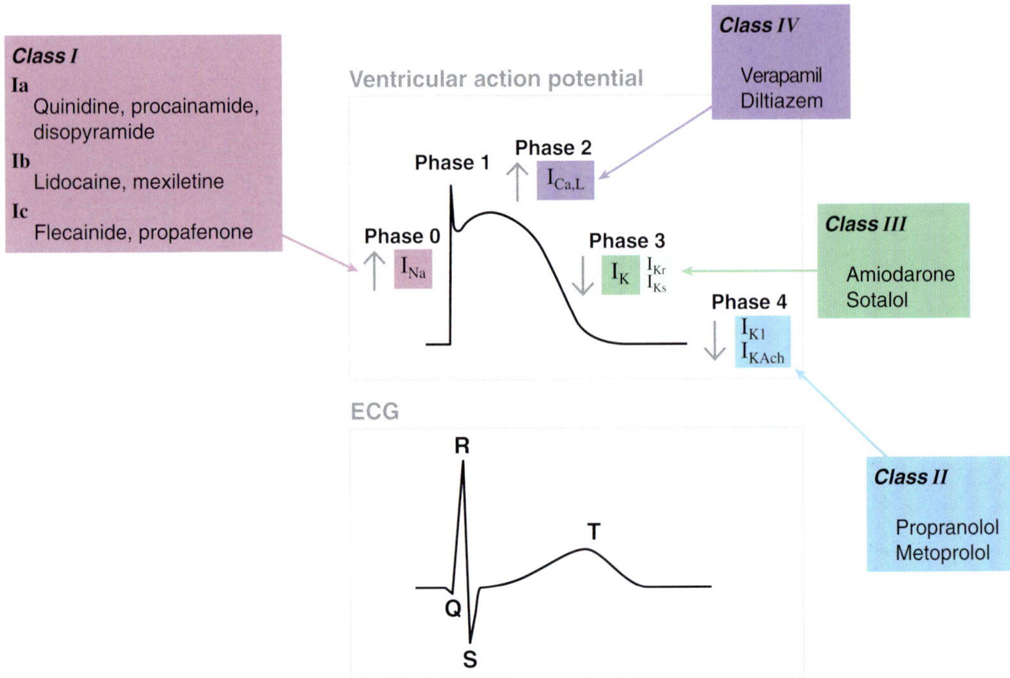

FIGURE 4.2.1 The cardiac action potential showing the four phases and the places where the different antiarrhythmic medications have their effects. A simultaneous ECG registration shows the relationship between the phases of the action potential and the ECG waves. Ca, calcium; K, potassium; Na, sodium.

and include lidocaine and mexiletine. Flecainide and propafenone are *Class Ic* drugs and have a slow onset of depression. *Class II* agents are antisympathetic nervous system agents and are predominantly beta-blockers, that is, propranolol and metoprolol. Propranolol also shows some class I effects. *Class III* agents affect potassium efflux and lengthen the action potential duration. Examples are amiodarone and sotalol. Sotalol has additional class II effects and amiodarone also has class I, II, and IV activity. *Class IV* agents such as verapamil and diltiazem affect calcium channels and the AV node. Usage of verapamil for fetal VT has not been described and it has been associated with sudden death when used in infants with supraventricular arrhythmias.[3] *Class V* agents, including digoxin and magnesium, work by other or unknown mechanisms.

GENERAL TREATMENT OF VT

All *class I* drugs have a negative inotropic effect and should be avoided during cardiac failure.[3] Quinidine[4] and procainamide[5] have been used for an intermittent fetal VT without a positive effect. Monomorphic VT unrelated to LQTS associated with a mild pericardial effusion responded to flecainide (SAB Clur, personal communication).

The first report describing successful intrapartum treatment of persistent fetal ventricular ectopy associated with fetal hemodynamic compromise was described in 1975. The fetus was treated with transplacental intravenous propranolol (5 mg × 2). Postnatally a short run of VT was recorded. Since then the positive effect of propranolol usage has been described in idiopathic VT and accelerated ventricular rhythm.[1,6] A potential problem associated with its use is the transplacental passage of only 25% to 35%.[7]

Improvement in fetal VT with sotalol has been described in one case.[8] Sotalol, alone or in combination with digoxin or propranolol, given in the treatment of VT in five fetuses that subsequently were diagnosed with LQTS resulted in either no improvement or worsening of the hydrops.[9,10] This is not surprising as sotalol prolongs the QTc interval and is thus contraindicated in LQTS.

Digoxin is contraindicated in treatment of VT. Digoxin use has been reported in two patients with LQTS, both with deleterious effects. In a patient with 2:1 AV block, VT, digoxin treatment exacerbated the hydrops and resulted in an emergency cesarean delivery at 28 weeks gestation.[11] In another case with VT and hydrops associated with ungenotyped LQTS, no improvement was seen with digoxin treatment, and a cesarean delivery followed at 36 weeks gestation.[12]

From 1999 onward, reports of transplacental therapy of fetal VT with amiodarone appeared.[13-15] In the absence of LQTS, the effect of amiodarone was favorable with a reduction of hydrops and the restoration of sinus rhythm.[13,14] The use of amiodarone in cases that subsequently were diagnosed with LQTS led to worsening hydrops.[10,14,16] Amiodarone has a very long half-life (6 weeks),[3,13] and a transient elevation of the thyroid-stimulating hormone in the fetus and mother postnatally, suggesting thyroid suppression, has been reported in some cases.[13,15]

PRENATAL TREATMENT OF TDP

Although the optimal prenatal therapy for the fetus with LQTS presenting with TdP has not yet been established, there are 16 such cases reported in the literature that were treated with maternal administrations of various antiarrhythmic drugs (TABLE 4.2.1). The findings in TABLE 4.2.1 underscore the importance of differentiating TdP from other fetal VT. Fetuses with TdP treated with amiodarone and/or sotalol had exacerbation of tachycardia (case #2) resulting in premature emergency delivery (cases #3 and 11) or stillbirth (case #4). TABLE 4.2.1 also suggests that the prenatal rhythms predict postnatal rhythm; thus, if a fetus has TdP, the postnatal care team should be prepared to treat TdP. However, if only 2° AV block is seen in utero, TdP may still occur after birth, as seen in case #5.

First-line treatment with IV magnesium sulfate (class V antiarrhythmic) is extremely successful in terminating or reducing salvos of TdP. Infusion of magnesium in tocolytic doses has a rapid onset of action, and most obstetricians are familiar with its usage in the management of maternal preeclampsia.[7,14] The mechanism of action of magnesium sulfate is only partially known. It is a cofactor of the sodium-potassium pump. By stimulating the efflux of sodium and influx of

TABLE 4.2.1 IN UTERO TREATMENT OF TDP IN FETAL LONG QT SYNDROME

Case	Author (y)	GA (wk) at Diagnosis	In Utero Rhythm	Hydrops	In Utero Therapy	Outcome	Gene Variant
1	Hamada (1999)	37	SB	No	BB[a]	Alive	KCNQ1-A341V
2	Cuneo (2003)[a]	30	2:1 AV block, SB, TdP	Yes	Amio, Mg, lido	Alive	SCN5A-R1623Q
3	Miller (2004)	28	2:1 AV block, SB, TdP	Yes	BB, amio	Alive	SCN5A-R1623Q
4	Bhuiyan (2008)	22	2:1 AV block, PVC, SB, TdP	Yes	Flec, sotalol, amio	Still birth	Homoz KCNH2-Q1070X
5		22	2:1 AV block, SB	Yes	Dex	Alive	Homoz KCNH2-Q1070X
6	Horigome (2008)[a]	28	2:1 AV block, SB, TdP	No	Lido, BB, mex, Mg	Alive	KCNH2-G628S
7	Simpson (2009)[a]	30	TdP	Yes	Flec, BB, Mg	Neurol, died	KCNH2-T613M
8	Cuneo (2013)	28[a]	2:1 AV block, TdP	No	BB, lido, Mex, Mg	Alive	KCNH2-G628S
9		34	2:1 AV block, TdP	ND	BB, Mg	Alive	KCNH2-T613K, K897T
10		30[a]	2:1 AV block, TdP	ND	BB, mex, Mg	CA	SCN5A-R1623Q
11		30[a]	2:1 AV block, TdP	ND	Sotalol	CA	SCN5A-R1623Q
12	Miyake (2017)[a]	28	2:1 AV block, SB, TdP	Yes	Mg, mex	Alive	KCNH2-S624R
13		24	2:1 AV block, SB, TdP	Yes	BB, Mg	Alive	KCNH2-T613M
14	Blais (2017)[a]	26	2:1 AV block, SB TdP	Yes	Mg, BB, mex	Alive	SCN5A-R1623Q
15	Crimmins (2017)[a]	27	2:1 AV block, TdP	Yes	Mg, lido	Alive	KCNH2-G628S
16	Miyoshi (2018)[a]	28	2:1 AV block, TdP	Yes	Mg	Alive	KCNH2-S624A

Amio, amiodarone; AV, atrioventricular; BB, beta-adrenergic blocking agent; CA, cardiac arrest; flec, flecainide; lido, lidocaine; mex, mexiletine; Mg, magnesium; SB, sinus bradycardia; TdP, torsades de pointes.
[a]de novo pathogenic variant.

TABLE 4.2.2 ANTIARRHYTHMIC MEDICATIONS IN FETAL VT

Medication	Dose	VT No LQTS	VT Suspected LQTS
Magnesium sulfate	LD 2-6 g IV; MD 1-2 g/h; Level <6 mEq/L	OK	OK
Lidocaine	LD 1-5 mg/kg IV MD 1-4 mg/min; Level 1.5-5 μg/mL	OK	OK
Propranolol	10-320 mg/d divided q 6 po	OK	OK
Mexiletine	600-900 mg/d divided q 8 po		
Flecainide	100-300 mg/d divided q 8 or q 12 po	OK	Do not use
Sotalol	160-480 mg/d divided q 8 or q 12 po	OK	Do not use
Amiodarone	LD 1200-1800 mg/d divided q 6 for 48 h; MD 200-600 po q day	OK	Do not use

IV, intravenous; g, grams; h, hours; L, liters; LD, loading dose; LQTS, long QT syndrome; mEq, milli-equivalents; mg, milligrams; mL, milliliters; MD, maintenance dose; po, given by mouth; q, every; VT, ventricular tachycardia.

potassium, it has effects opposite to digoxin and results in a decrease in intracellular calcium. It has been used with complete or partial success in the management of VT runs and TdP in fetal LQTS, either alone or in combination with intravenous lidocaine[16-19] or propranolol or mexiletine.[7,17,18,20-23] Propranolol decreases the transmural dispersion of repolarization and the induction of TdP and has been a successful adjunct therapy for TdP. However, because the transplacental transfer of propranolol is extremely low (25%-30%), higher doses may be necessary. See TABLE 4.2.2 for recommended doses of antiarrhythmic drugs used in the treatment of TdP.

Knowledge of the specific mutation and phenotype can assist with tailoring prenatal therapy; for TdP; however, most fetal cases have been de novo pathogenic variants (TABLE 4.2.1): in only 4/15 cases of LQTS with TdP was the variant familial. However, if the variant is known, Na+ channel–blocking agents such as lidocaine and mexiletine (class Ib) may be the best choice for LQTS caused by gain-of-function *SCN5A* variants. LQT2 patients have a loss of function in their potassium channels and a Na+ channel blocker will prolong their QT interval further. However, differential responses to Na+ channel blockade have been reported. For example, lidocaine (class Ib) successfully treated two cases of LQT2, both with the p.Gly628Ser mutation.[18,19] Flecainide has exacerbated VT in a fetus homozygous for LQT2[10] and in a fetus with 2:1 AV block, VT, and hydrops.[24] Based on this experience and the success of IV magnesium, lidocaine, or mexiletine and beta-blocker, flecainide is not a first- or second-line agent for treatment of TdP.[25,26]

SUMMARY

When VT is associated with 2° AV block and/or sinus bradycardia in a structurally normal heart, LQTS with TdP should be suspected (**FIG. 4.2.2**). For acute treatment of suspected TdP or with hemodynamic compromise, intravenous magnesium or magnesium and lidocaine with the possible addition of mexiletine and/or propranolol are recommended given the descriptions of successful therapy.[2,17,21,25,27] Given the proarrhythmic effects, previous association with sudden fetal death, and failure to improve outcome, flecainide is less attractive as treatment of TdP. As amiodarone and sotalol prolong the QT interval and have been associated with worsening of TdP, they should be avoided in LQTS cases. However, if LQTS is not suspected in cases of fetal VT, sotalol and amiodarone can successfully restore sinus rhythm. Digoxin should never be used in this setting.

Treatment strategies for isolated VT and VT with suspected or known LQTS are shown in **FIG. 4.2.3**.

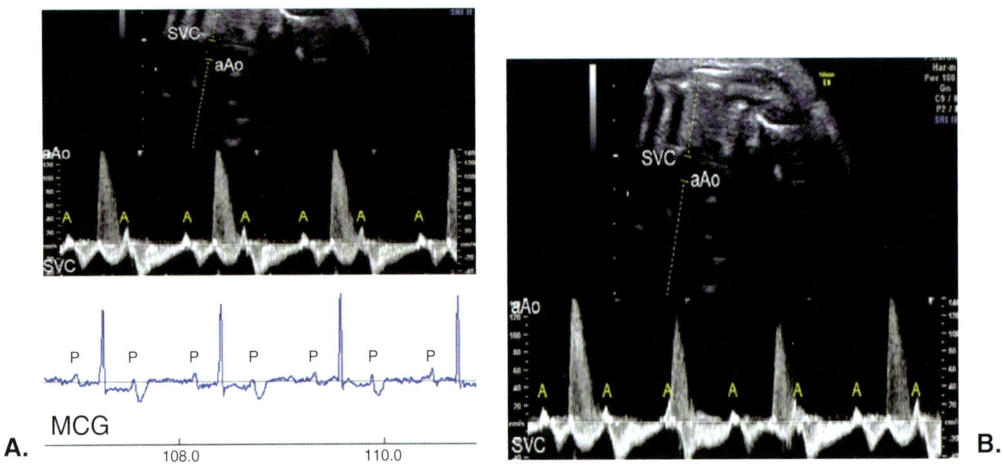

FIGURE 4.2.2 Simultaneous Doppler registrations from the superior vena cava (SVC) and ascending aorta (aAo), with corresponding fetal magnetocardiogram (MCG) recorded from a 28-week fetus with long QT syndrome type 2. **A:** 2:1 AV block with a ventricular rate of 60/min and an atrial rate of 120/min. **B:** After IV magnesium sulfate infusion, AV-dissociation (ventricular rate of 56 bpm and atrial rate of 105 bpm). a, atrial contraction; P, P-wave. (Adapted from Miyoshi T, Sakaguchi H, Shiraishi I, Yoshimatsu J, Ikeda T. Potential utility of pulsed-wave Doppler for prenatal diagnosis of fetal ventricular tachycardia secondary to long QT syndrome. *Ultrasound Obstet Gynecol*. 2018;51(5):697-699.)

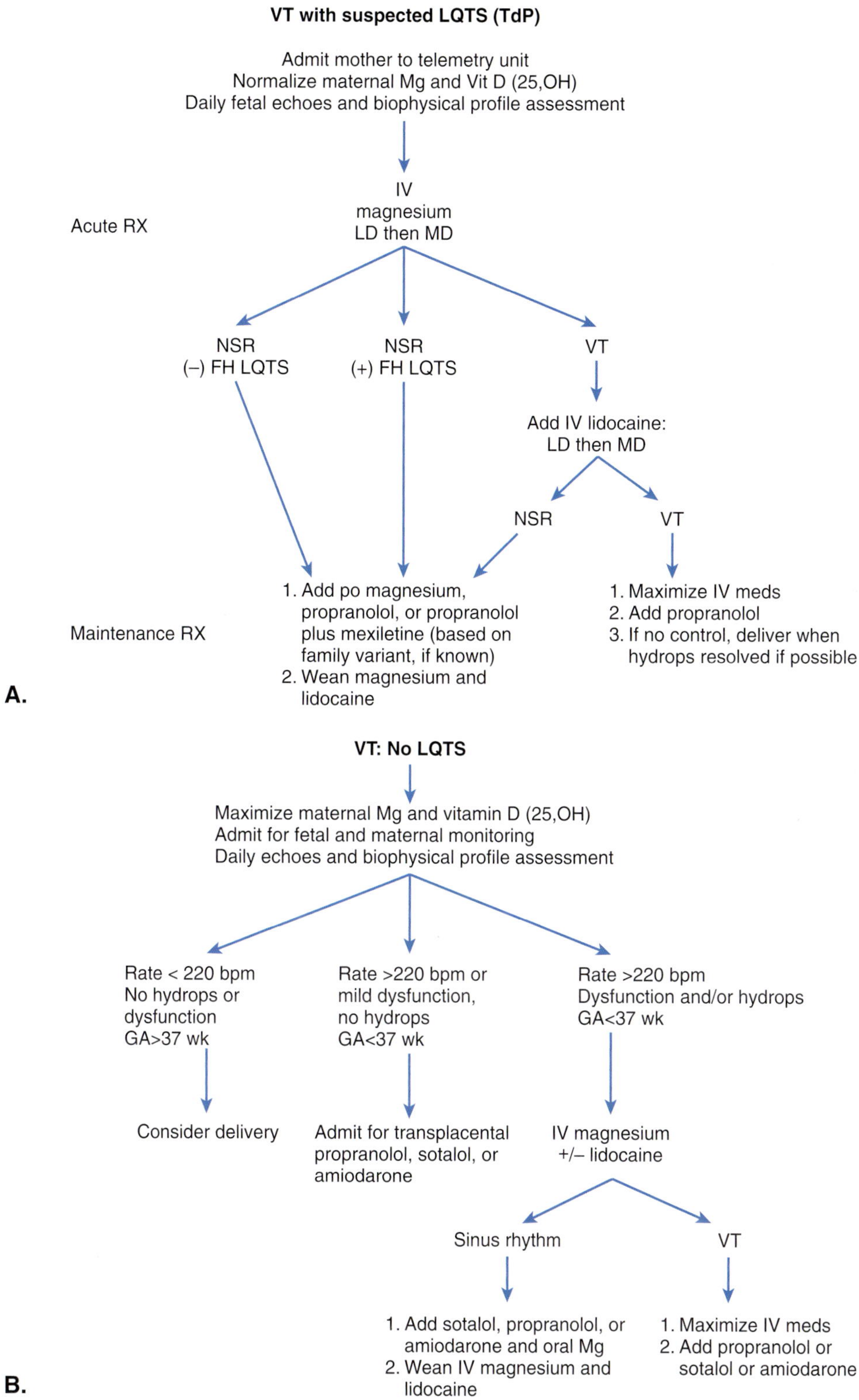

FIGURE 4.2.3 Treatment strategy for management of ventricular tachycardia. **A:** Fetal torsades de pointes and long QT syndrome. **B:** Fetal ventricular tachycardia without long QT syndrome. FH, family history; GA, gestational age; IV, intravenous; LD, loading dose; LQTS, long QT syndrome; MD, maintenance dose; Mg, magnesium; NSR, normal sinus rhythm; TdP, torsades de pointes; VT, ventricular tachycardia.

References

1. Strasburger JF, Cheulkar B, Wichman HJ. Perinatal arrhythmias: diagnosis and management. *Clin Perinatol.* 2007;34(4):627-652.
2. Hondeghem LM. Classification of antiarrhythmic agents and the two laws of pharmacology. *Cardiovasc Res.* 200l;45(1):57-60.
3. Burgada J, Blom N, Sarquella-Brugada G, et al. Pharmacological and non-pharmacological therapy for arrhythmias in the pediatric population. EHRA and AEPC=Arrhythmia Working Group joint consensus statement. *Europace.* 2013;15(9):1337-1382.
4. Sherer DM, Sadovksy E, Menashe M, et al. Fetal ventricular tachycardia associated with non-immune hydrops fetalis. A case report. *J Reprod Med.* 1990;335(3):292-294.
5. Polak PE, Stewart PA, Hess J. Complete AV dissociation and HS bundle tachycardia in a newborn: problems in prenatal diagnosis and postnatal management. *Int J Cardiol.* 1989;22(2):269-271.
6. Fouron JC, McNeal-Davidson A, Abadir S, et al. Prenatal diagnosis and prognosis of accelerated idioventricular rhythm. *Ultrasound Obstet Gynecol.* 2017;50(5):624-631.
7. Simpson JM, Maxwell D, Rosenthal E, et al. Fetal ventricular tachycardia secondary to long QT syndrome treated with maternal intravenous magnesium: case report and review of the literature. *Ultrasound Obstet Gynecol.* 2009;34(4):475-480.
8. Ueda K, Maeno Y, Miyoshi T, et al. The impact of intrauterine treatment of fetal tachycardia: a nationwide survey in Japan. *J Matern Fetal Neonatal Med.* 2018;31(19):2605-2610.
9. Oudijk MA, Gooskens RH, Stoutenbeek P, et al. Neurological outcome of children who were treated for fetal tachycardia complicated by hydrops. *Ultrasound Obstet Gynecol.* 2004;24(2):154-158.
10. Bhuiyan ZA, Momenah TS, Gong Q, et al. Recurrent intrauterine fetal loss due to near absence of HERG: clinical and functional characterization of a homozygous nonsense HERG Q1070X mutation. *Heart Rhythm.* 2008;5(4):5553-5561.
11. van Engelen AD, Weijtens O, Brenner JL, et al. Management, outcome and follow-up of fetal tachycardia. *J Am Coll Cardiol.* 1994;24(5):1371-1375.
12. Ohkuchi A, Shiraishi H, Minakami H, et al. Fetus with long QT syndrome manifested by tachyarrhthymia: a case report. *Prenat Diagn.* 1999;19(10):990-992.
13. Fouron JC. Fetal arrhythmias: the Saint Justine hospital experience. *Prenat Diagn.* 2004;24(13):1068-1080.
14. Schleich JM, Bernard Dur Haut Cilly F, Laurent MC, et al. Early prenatal management of a fetal ventricular tachycardia treated in utero by amiodarone with long term follow-up. *Prenat Diagn.* 2000;20(6):449-452.
15. Cuneo BF, Strasburger JF. Management strategy for fetal tachycardia. *Obstet Gynecol.* 2000;96(4):575-581.
16. Cuneo BF, Ovadia M, Strasburger JF, et al. Prenatal diagnosis and in utero treatment of torsades de pointes associated with congenital long QT syndrome. *Am J Cardiol.* 2003;91(11):1395-1398.
17. Cuneo BF, Etheridge SP, Horigome H, et al. Arrhythmia phenotype during fetal life suggests long QT syndrome genotype: risk stratification of perinatal long QT syndrome. *Circ Arrhythm Electrophysiol.* 2013;6(5):946-951.
18. Horigome H, Iwashita H, Yoshinaga M, et al. Magnetocardiographic demonstration of torsade de pointes in a fetus with congenital long QT syndrome. *J Cardiovasc Electrophysiol.* 2008;19(3):334-335.
19. Crimmins S, Vashit S, Doyle L, et al. A multidisciplinary approach to prenatal treatment of congenital long QT syndrome. *J Clin Ultrasound.* 2017;45(3):168-170.
20. Mioshi T, Sakaguchi H, Shiraishi I, et al. Potential utility of pulsed-wave Doppler for prenatal diagnosis of fetal ventricular tachycardia secondary to long QT syndrome. *Ultrasound Obstet Gynecol.* 2018;51(5):697-699.
21. Cuneo BF, Strasburger JF, Yu S, et al. In utero diagnosis of long QT syndrome by magnetocardiography. *Circulation.* 2013;128(20):2183-2191.
22. Blais BA, Satou G, Sklansky MS, Madnawat H, Moore JP. The diagnosis and management of long QT syndrome based on fetal echocardiography. *Heart Rhythm Case Rep.* 2017;3(9):407-410.
23. Miyake A, Sakaguchi H, Miyazaki A, Miyoshi T, Aiba T, Shiraishi I. Successful prenatal management of ventricular tachycardia and second-degree atrioventricular block in fetal long QT syndrome. *Heart Rhythm Case Rep.* 2016;3(1):53-57.
24. Hofbeck M, Ulmer H, Beinder E, et al. Prenatal findings in patients with prolonged QT interval in the neonatal period. *Heart.* 1997;77(3):198-204.

25. Horigome H, Nagashima M, Sumitomo N, et al. Clinical characteristics and genetic background of congenital long-QT syndrome diagnosed in fetal, neonatal and infantile life: a nationwide questionnaire survey in Japan. *Circ Arrhythm Electrophysiol.* 2010;3(1):10-17.
26. Beckermann TM, McLeod K, Murday V, et al. Novel SCN5A mutation in amiodarone-responsive multifocal ventricular ectopy associated cardiomyopathy. *Heart Rhythm.* 2014;11(8):1446-1453.
27. Mitchell JL, Cuneo BF, Etheridge SO, et al. Fetal heart rate predictors of long QT syndrome. *Circulation.* 2012;126(23):2688-2695.

Treatment of Immune-Mediated Atrioventricular Block

Helena M. Gardiner • Bettina F. Cuneo

INTRODUCTION

Among mothers with anti-Ro/SSA antibodies, fetal atrioventricular (AV) block is rare; the AV block phenotype and natural history are variable; and data on outcomes are scant, anecdotal, and retrospective. Not surprisingly, practice variation is considerable, and there are no evidence-based guidelines to direct treatment strategies. Thus, questions remain as to whether treatment can prevent AV block, alter the progression of 1° or 2° AV block to 3° AV block, or decrease the likelihood of dilated cardiomyopathy.[1-8] What is known is that 3° AV block is immutable, fetuses with 3° AV block are at high risk for perinatal demise, and survivors face lifelong cardiac pacing. This chapter will summarize published data on both prophylaxis of anti-Ro/SSA antibody–positive pregnancies and the treatment of 1°, 2°, and 3° fetal AV block.

STRATEGIES TO PREVENT FETAL AV BLOCK

Several prophylactic strategies have been proposed including administration of transplacental fluorinated steroids, plasmapheresis, and intravenous immune globulin (IVIG, 1 gram (g)/kilogram (kg) at 14 and 18 weeks or 0.4 g/kg 3×/wk from 12 to 24 weeks). However, these therapies have not been successful in preventing AV block.[2,9-12] In fact, due to duration of continuous treatment (from 16 weeks of gestation onward), prophylactic steroids have profound side effects including intrauterine growth restriction, hypoadrenalism, and oligohydramnios. Furthermore, they may worsen maternal diabetes mellitus.

The only prophylactic treatment shown to reduce recurrence of anti-Ro/SSA–mediated AV block is hydroxychloroquine (HCQ). HCQ inhibits activation of toll-like receptors, a class of transmembrane proteins that initiate the cellular immune response. By inhibiting ligation of toll-like receptors, the pathogenesis of immune-mediated damage to the fetal cardiac tissue is interrupted, lowering the risk of conduction system and myocardial (dilated cardiomyopathy) disease.[13]

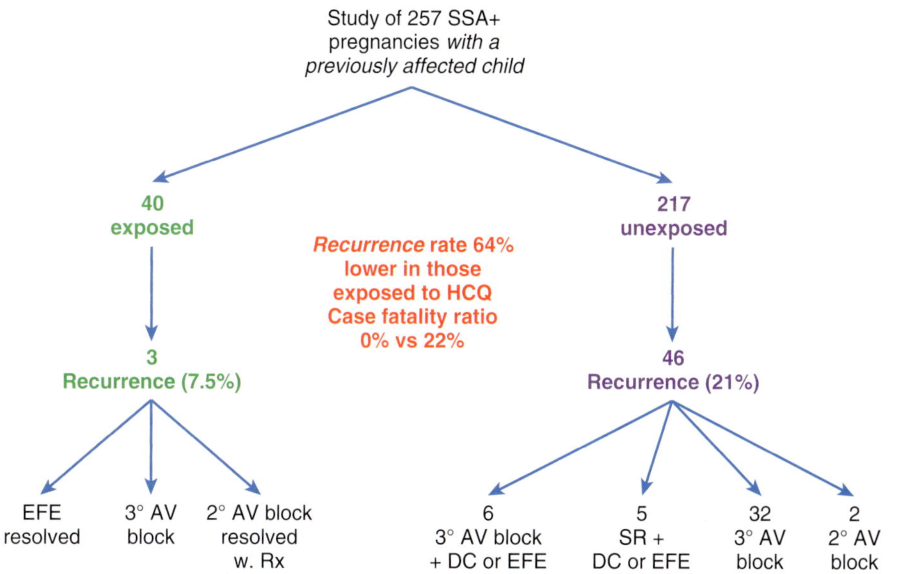

FIGURE 4.3.1 Results of a retrospective study of hydroxychloroquine prophylaxis to prevent recurrence of atrioventricular (AV) block in pregnancies with offspring previously affected with AV block. DC, dilated cardiomyopathy; EFE, endocardial fibroelastosis; SR, sinus rhythm; Rx, treatment. (Adapted from Izmirly PM, Costedoat-Chalumeau N, Pisoni CN, et al. Maternal use of hydroxychloroquine is associated with a reduced risk of recurrent anti-SSA/Ro-antibody-associated cardiac manifestations of neonatal lupus. *Circulation*. 2012;126(1):76-82.)

In retrospective studies, HCQ (200 mg twice a day), initiated before 11 weeks of gestation and continued throughout pregnancy, reduced the recurrence of fetal AV block from 18% to about 9%[14,15] (FIG. 4.3.1). These results were confirmed in PATCH (Preventive Approach to Congenital Heart Block with Hydroxychloroquine), a prospective study in which 5/63 (7.9%) mothers with a previously affected offspring had recurrence of fetal AV block.[16] Thus, in both prospective and retrospective studies, HCQ significantly reduced the recurrence rate of AV block in anti-Ro/SSA–positive mothers, with no evidence of cardiac toxicity in the newborns.[17] Currently, there are only limited data supporting the role of HCQ in mothers with no previously affected offspring.[18]

STRATEGIES TO TREAT ANTI-RO/SSA–MEDIATED FETAL AV BLOCK

Based on a hypothesis that inflammation is the basis of the cardiac manifestations of maternal anti-Ro/SSA antibodies, two approaches have been implemented. Therapeutic effects of both dexamethasone and IVIG treatment have been judged in two categories: restoring normal rhythm and improving outcomes. With regard to the effects of treatment on conduction system disease, treatment advocates believe dexamethasone can halt disease progression from 1° to 2° or 2° to 3° AV block or restore 1:1 AV conduction from 2° AV block. Improved treatment outcomes would include fewer fetuses with 3° AV block, fewer fetuses with dilated cardiomyopathy or cardiac dysfunction, and fewer premature deliveries. For example, some clinicians use dexamethasone only if cardiac dysfunction, AV valve regurgitation, pericardial effusion, or hydrops is present, regardless of conduction system disease, in the belief that treatment will prevent or improve myocardial disease.

Dexamethasone

From an immunologic perspective, elimination of candidate maternal autoantibodies and reduction of a generalized inflammatory response is the logical approach to the treatment of fetal AV block. Relevant to treating fetal disease, dexamethasone, a glucocorticoid agonist which crosses cell membranes, is only partially metabolized by placental 11β-hydroxysteroid dehydrogenase (11β-OHSD) with the remainder available to the fetus in an active form. The same is not true of prednisone, which does not transfer to the fetus. Dexamethasone binds with high affinity to specific cytoplasmic receptors which modify transcription and resultant protein synthesis to inhibit leukocyte infiltration at the site of inflammation. Dexamethasone thus interferes in the function of the mediators of the inflammatory response.[19]

Intravenous Immune Globulin

IVIG treatment has been of benefit in a variety of immune-mediated and inflammatory diseases in pregnant women and pediatric patients.[20] It is approved by the Federal Drug Administration for primary immunodeficiency, idiopathic thrombocytopenia purpura, Kawasaki disease, B cell-chronic lymphocytic leukemia with hypogammaglobulinemia, pediatric HIV infection, and allogenic bone marrow transplant in adults.[20] The major rationale for IVIG in the treatment of AV block was initially based on elimination of anti-Ro antibodies: "no antibody, no disease."[21,22] However, it remains highly speculative whether IVIG can effectively lower the level below the threshold needed to result in cardiac injury. We know that replacement doses of IVIG at 400 mg/kg do not prevent recurrence of fetal AV block.[2] However, in mice at doses of 1 gm/kg, IVIG is immunomodulatory via IgG-Fc sialylation and increased surface expression of the inhibitory FcγRIIb receptor on macrophages.[23] Data in humans support that IVIG inhibits phagocytosis of IgG-opsonized blood cells (in the case of AV block predicted to be cardiocytes opsonized by anti-Ro independent of Ig-Fc sialylation).[22,23] Clinical results in anecdotal reports have suggested IVIG improves outcome in cardiomyopathy[24] (TABLE 4.3.1), but it has not been evaluated as an adjunct treatment with dexamethasone for AV block with normal cardiac function.

Although expensive, IVIG may be an effective drug if used in treatment of emerging 3° AV block, especially in combination with dexamethasone.[25-29] However, whether monthly doses during pregnancy or postnatal treatment is required, is unknown and proof for any rationale is lacking. We await the results of future prospective studies to develop an evidence-based treatment plan for these high-risk fetuses.

TABLE 4.3.1 OUTCOME OF FETUSES TREATED WITH IVIG

Subject	AV Block Dx	IVIG, 70 g	Neonatal Rhythm	Outcome
1	3°	–	3°	VVI paced
2	3°	–	3°	VVI paced
3	3°	×1 (26 wk)	3°	Not paced
4	3°	–	3°	Postnatal death
5	3°	–	1°	2° AV block not paced
6	3°	–	3°	VVI paced
7	3°	×2 (23 and 26 wk)	–	IUFD
8	1°	q 2 wk (23-36 wk	NSR	NSR
9	None	q 2 wk (26-39 wk)	NSR	NSR
10	2°	–	2° and 3°	DDD paced
11	3°	–	3°	VVI paced
12	3°	–	3°	VVI paced
13	3°	–	3°	VVI paced
14	3°	×2 (25 and 28 wk)	3°	Postnatal death
15	3°	×3 (20, 23 and 28 wk)	3°	Postnatal death
16	None	×1 (21 wk)	NSR	NSR
17	3°	×2 (25 and 30 wk)	3°	DDD paced
18	3°	–	3°	DDD biV paced
19	None	–	1°	1° AV block
20	3°	×1 (25 wk)	3°	DDD paced

AV, atrioventricular; biV, biventricular pacing; DDD, ventricular sensed and paced; DX, diagnosed; IUFD, in utero fetal demise; IVIG, intravenous immune globulin; NSR, normal sinus rhythm; VVI, ventricular sensed and paced, inhibited; wks, weeks; ×, times.
Adapted from Trucco SM, Jaeggi E, Cuneo B, et al. Use of intravenous gamma globulin and corticosteroids in the treatment of maternal autoantibody-mediated cardiomyopathy. *J Am Coll Cardiol*. 2011;57(6):715-723

Treatment of 1° AV Block

True 1° AV block is probably a mitral inflow/aortic outflow Doppler AV interval of 170 milliseconds (ms) or greater[30-32] (see Part 3, Chapter 6). The false-positive diagnosis of 1° AV block with resultant unnecessary treatment of normal fetuses can occur because the current definition of 1° AV block assumes the echo AV intervals to be equivalent to ECG or fetal magnetocardiography PR intervals, when in fact the latter are 20 to 30 ms shorter. The findings that so many fetuses with untreated "1° AV block" (AV intervals 135-150 ms) have normal PR intervals at birth or within the first year of life[33,34] suggest that the risk/benefit of treatment is most favorable for AV intervals at least >170 ms. However, even with dexamethasone treatment in some cases the AV interval duration can shorten, but 1° AV block can persist in utero and after birth.[26,30,31,33,34]

Treatment of 2° AV Block (Fig. 4.3.2)

Unfortunately, a review of the literature on treatment of 2° AV block is more confusing than helpful as often timing, dose and frequency of medications, or the time between the last normal fetal heart rate and 2° AV block is often not included. Anecdotally, treatment given within 6 to 8 hours of an abnormal fetal heart rhythm has restored normal conduction (TABLE 4.3.2), and based on a recent meta-analysis, 2° AV block is potentially reversible.[4] Overall regression from 2° AV block to 1:1 AV conduction was reported in 24% of subjects, irrespective of treatment with dexamethasone (TABLE 4.3.3).[4]

There are other difficulties in assessing treatment effect in 2° AV block. First, it is rarely specified if the 2° AV block is type 1 or type 2, and preliminary data suggest that type 1 is more likely to regress to 1:1 AV conduction than is type 2. Second, there is often insufficient information on the atrial coupling intervals and isovolumic contraction times. Thus, one cannot exclude the possibility that some reported cases may have been blocked atrial bigeminy rather than 2° AV block.[35] Third, 3° AV block with accrochage, a rhythm that occurs when the dissociated atrial and ventricular beats synchronize may be mistaken for 2° AV block and interpreted to be a treatment failure when the infant is born with 3° AV block.[36]

The timing of treatment, especially for 2° AV block, appears to be important in success of treatment. Treatment within 2 to 4 hours of confirming 2° AV block by echo and 4 to 6 hours after auscultation of an irregular rhythm, has reestablished 1:1 AV conduction.[28,29,37] In contrast, in fetuses where treatment was delayed beyond 12 hours, fetuses progressed to 3° AV block or showed a transient response but progressed to 3° AV block either in utero or after birth.[29,33,34] The duration of treatment may also play a role in maintaining 1:1 AV conduction: in one case of 2° AV block, steroids were discontinued after conversion to normal rhythm and 2° AV block returned and progressed to 3° AV block by birth.[28] Finally, the treatment dose may have an effect on the outcome: reversal of 2° AV block was confirmed by a normal postnatal ECG in a fetus given 6 mg/day, rather than the usual dose of 4 mg/day.[35]

Thus, lack of proven treatment efficacy for restoring normal rhythm may be due to several methodological problems, including the power being too low to address the study hypothesis, the dosage of dexamethasone and/or IVIG being too low, or administration too late to be effective.[38] Further studies are clearly indicated, but based on limited data, it is worthwhile to treat 2° AV block when it is identified. If there is progression, to 3° AV block, discussion with the parents to continue therapy is warranted.

Treatment of 3° AV Block

Some investigators have reported conversion of fetal 3° to 2° AV block or 3° AV block to sinus rhythm following steroid treatment, but these reports require careful interpretation, and the consensus is that 3° AV block is irreversible. There is little agreement as to whether overall outcomes with 3° AV block improve with treatment largely because data are retrospective and not randomized.[1-8] One study found dexamethasone did not

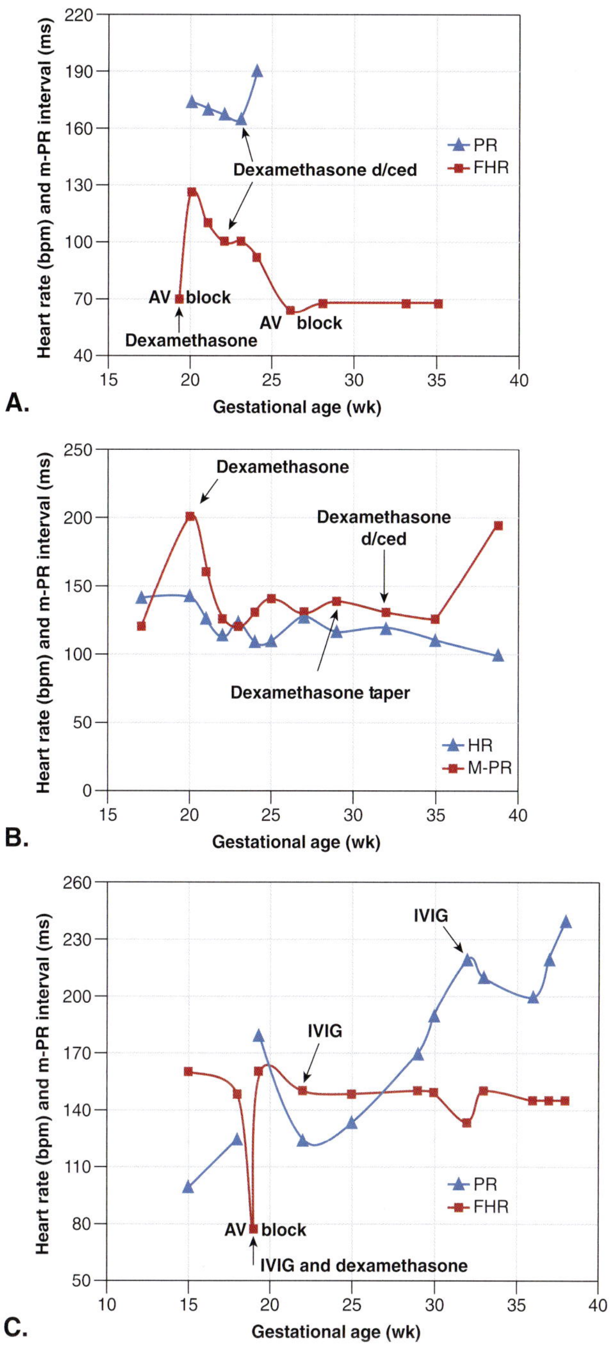

FIGURE 4.3.2 Results of treatment with dexamethasone **(A)** or dexamethasone and intravenous immune globulin (IVIG) **(B and C)** on heart rate (red line) and atrioventricular (AV) interval (blue line). **A:** Fetus with 2° AV block treated with dexamethasone at 19 weeks. The rhythm initially improved to 1° AV block (heart rate 130 beats per minute and AV interval ~170 ms, which further improved to 160 ms). Treatment was discontinued at 24 weeks: by the following week the AV interval increased to 190 ms and by 26 weeks the fetus was again in 2° AV block. No additional treatment was given, and at birth, the rhythm was 3° AV block. **B:** 20-week fetus with 1° AV block (AV interval 200 ms) treated with dexamethasone and IVIG. The AV interval normalized, but despite continued dexamethasone, the fetal heart rate (FHR) slowly fell to 100 beats per minute. The AV interval increased after dexamethasone was stopped at 32 weeks. The neonatal rhythm was sinus bradycardia with 1° AV block. **C:** 19-week fetus with type 1°, 2° AV block successfully treated with dexamethasone and IVIG. 1:1 AV conduction was restored, and neonatal ECG revealed 1° AV block. (Reprinted from Cuneo BF, Ambrose SE, Tworetzky W. Detection and successful treatment of emergent anti-SSA-mediated fetal atrioventricular block. *Am J Obstet Gynecol*. 2016;215(4):527-528.)

TABLE 4.3.2 TIME FROM DETECTION OF IRREGULAR RHYTHM TO CONFIRMATORY ECHO AND TREATMENT

GA (wk)	Detection to Echo (h)	Echo	Rx	Birth Rhythm
18.9[28]	≥24	3° AV block	Dex + IVIG	3° AV block
22.9[29]	≥24	3° AV block	Dex + IVIG	3° AV block
19.5[29]	≥24	3° AV block	Dex + IVIG	3° AV block
21[34]	<12	2°AV block	Dex + IVIG	1:1 AV
19[34]	<12	2°AV block	Dex + IVIG	1:1 AV
19[§]	<12	2°AV block	Dex	1:1 AV
19[34]	<24	2°AV block	Dex + IVIG	1:1 AV
18[34]	<18	2°/3° AV block	Dex + IVIG	1:1 AV

AV, atrioventricular; Dex, dexamethasone; GA, gestational age; h, hours; IVIG, intravenous immune globulin; wk, weeks.
[§]Buyon J.MD, personal communication.

TABLE 4.3.3 OUTCOME OF 2° AV BLOCK

Result	Fetuses Treated	Fetuses Not Treated
Overall *Progression*	17/31 (54%)	8/11 (73%)
2° AV block to 3° AV block		
Overall *Regression*	9/38 (24%)	4/19 (21%)
2° AV block to 1° AV block	6/31 (19%)	1/11 (9%)
2° AV block to NSR		
Stable rhythm	4/38 (11%)	0/19 (0%)

AV, atrioventricular; NSR, normal sinus rhythm.
Modified from Ciardulli A, D'Antonio F, Magro-Malosso ER, et al. Maternal steroid therapy for fetuses with second-degree immune-mediated congenital atrioventricular block: a systematic review and meta-analysis. *Acta Obstet Gynecol Scand*. 2018;97(7):787-794.

restore sinus rhythm but did resolve hydrops in 3/5 fetuses with 3° AV block. Since the outcome of hydrops and 3° AV block is so dismal, a short course of dexamethasone may improve or resolve the hydrops but should be given with no expectation of improved rhythm. Based on a single retrospective study,[25] IVIG may be a better choice than dexamethasone if there is cardiac dysfunction with 3° AV block.

TREATMENT OF OTHER RHYTHMS ASSOCIATED WITH ANTI-RO/SSA AV BLOCK

While AV block is the signature rhythm of anti-Ro/SSA–mediated cardiac disease, sinus bradycardia, atrial flutter, ventricular ectopy, and junctional ectopic tachycardia (JET) have been reported[39,40] alone or in combination with AV block. In the few published cases, sinus bradycardia has not improved with dexamethasone treatment. On the other hand, the rate and duration of JET in association with 3° AV block have decreased in some treated cases but not in others.[36] Thus, it is not known if the natural history of anti-Ro/SSA mediated JET is persistence or if treatment influences outcome. In contrast to congenital JET,40 few cases of anti-Ro/SSA mediated JET without AV block have been reported.

SIDE EFFECTS OF THERAPIES

Dexamethasone Treatment

The safety of administering high-dose dexamethasone therapy to the fetus has been questioned and neurodevelopmental concerns have been raised, particularly in view of its questionable efficacy. Studies of its chronic use in anti-Ro/SSA pregnancies are scarce, but animal studies have reported that high-dose steroids administered to the developing fetal brain may be associated with abnormal brain maturity and cystic lesions. Recent small studies of medium-term neurodevelopmental outcomes in human fetuses treated with dexamethasone appear reassuring, but large, blinded studies have not been completed to confirm these data.[41,42] Growth restriction and oligohydramnios appear to be more common in fetuses with AV block treated with dexamethasone. However, a high proportion of unaffected and untreated fetuses of mothers with connective tissue disease are small: ranging from 15% to 38%.[43,44] A study in Sweden found that compared to the normal population, infants of mothers with Sjogren syndrome or systemic lupus erythematosus were four times more likely to be growth restricted.[34] A second study looking at growth in siblings with maternal rheumatologic disorders and fetal AV block (n = 72) or with normal rhythm found that children with AV block are smaller than siblings but only until 11 years of age.[45] The incidence of growth restriction was highest (30%) in mothers with systemic lupus erythematosus (SLE) regardless of fetal AV block. Two studies evaluating side effects of dexamethasone on 71 fetuses found oligohydramnios (14%), maternal hypertension (3%), insulin-dependent diabetes (3%), insomnia, or mood changes (7%).[3,26] Three infants in these studies were delivered because of severe oligohydramnios. Lastly, hypoaldosteronism is a complication of prolonged steroid use; thus cortisol levels in mother and baby should be followed after birth and stress dose steroids given as indicated. In one study, the incidence of hypoaldosteronism fell to zero after the treatment protocol changed from treatment until birth to weaning dexamethasone after 28 weeks of gestation.[26]

Before dexamethasone treatment for any degree of AV block, it is imperative to discuss risks, potential benefits, and lack of evidence-based data with the family. In cases of progression to 3° AV block with treatment but without extranodal disease or hydrops, discontinuing dexamethasone is probably the best option. Weaning the dexamethasone dose after 28 weeks should be strongly considered in cases where treatment has restored 1:1 AV conduction.

Intravenous Immune Globulin

Unlike fluorinated steroids, IVIG's only side effects are exposure to pooled blood products and a possible maternal allergic reaction. It is therefore given over several hours and in a monitored setting. Pretreatment with diphenhydramine can reduce the risk of an allergic reaction but is rarely necessary. IVIG is expensive, and at this time in the United States, insurance may not pay for treatment in all cases.

SUMMARY

Recent large but retrospective studies have shown no difference in outcome between fetus with 3° AV block treated and not treated with dexamethasone. Until further studies say differently, it appears treatment should be reserved for fetuses with 2° AV block or an AV interval >170 ms since, in some cases, normal AV conduction has been restored. Recommendations for the type and duration of treatment are based on a few case series and include dexamethasone and/or IVIG. Because of successful treatment of some cases, equipoise is difficult, and with the rarity of AV block, a randomized controlled study will be difficult to perform. At this time, the risks and benefits of each treatment must be discussed with families and the limited data acknowledged. As a recent Swedish study reported that subjects with antibody-mediated 3° AV block have an increased risk of dilated cardiomyopathy, myocardial and cerebral infarction, as well as a range of autoimmune disorders.[46] Thus, the urgency to develop effective treatment protocols to prevent progression to 3° AV block and the development of cardiomyopathy has never been greater.

References

1. Kuleva M, Le Bidois J, Decaudin A, et al. Clinical course and outcome of antenatally detected atrioventricular block: experience of a single tertiary centre and review of the literature. *Prenat Diagn.* 2015;35(4):354-361.
2. Van den Berg NW, Slieker MG, van Beynum IM, et al. Fluorinated steroids do not improve outcome of isolated atrioventricular block. *Int J Cardiol.* 2016;225:167-171.
3. Hutter D, Silverman ED, Jaeggi ET. The benefits of transplacental treatment of isolated congenital complete heart block associated with maternal anti-Ro/SSA antibodies: a review. *Scand J Immunol.* 2010;72(3):235-241.
4. Ciardulli A, D'Antonio F, Magro-Malosso ER, et al. Maternal steroid therapy for fetuses with second-degree immune-mediated congenital atrioventricular block: a systematic review and meta-analysis. *Acta Obstet Gynecol Scand.* 2018;97(7):787-794.
5. Fesslova V, Vignati G, Brucato A, et al. The impact of treatment of the fetus by maternal therapy on the fetal and postnatal outcomes for fetuses diagnosed with isolated complete atrioventricular block. *Cardiol Young.* 2009;19(3):282-290.
6. Izmirly PM, Saxena A, Sahl SK, et al. Assessment of fluorinated steroids to avert progression and mortality in anti-SSA/Ro-associated cardiac injury limited to the fetal conduction system. *Ann Rheum Dis.* 2016;75(6):1161-1165.
7. Lopes LM, Tavares GM, Damiano AP, et al. Perinatal outcome of fetal atrioventricular block: one-hundred-sixteen cases from a single institution. *Circulation.* 2008;118(12):1268-1275.
8. Jaeggi ET, Fouron JC, Silverman ED, Ryan G, Smallhorn J, Hornberger LK. Transplacental fetal treatment improves the outcome of prenatally diagnosed complete atrioventricular block without structural heart disease. *Circulation.* 2004;110(12):1542-1548.
9. Friedman DM, Llanos C, Izmirly PM, et al. Evaluation of fetuses in a study of intravenous immunoglobulin as preventive therapy for congenital heart block: results of a multicenter, prospective, open-label clinical trial. *Arthritis Rheum.* 2010;62(4):1138-1146.
10. Pisoni CN, Brucato A, Ruffatti A, et al. Failure of intravenous immunoglobulin to prevent congenital heart block: findings of a multicenter, prospective, observational study. *Arthritis Rheum.* 2010;62(4):1147-1152.
11. Miyakata S, Takeuchi K, Yamaji K, Kanai Y, Tsuda H, Takasaki Y. Therapeutic plasmapheresis for the prevention of congenital complete heart block associated with anti-SS-A/Ro antibody and anti-SS-B/La antibody. *Ryumachi.* 2001;41(4):726-735.
12. Makino S, Yonemoto H, Itoh S, Takeda S. Effect of steroid administration and plasmapheresis to prevent fetal congenital heart block in patients with systemic lupus erythematosus and/or Sjögren's syndrome. *Acta Obstet Gynecol Scand.* 2007;86(9):1145-1146.
13. Costedoat-Chalumeau N, Amoura Z, Le Thi Hong D, et al. Questions about dexamethasone use for the prevention of anti-SSA related congenital heart block. *Ann Rheum Dis.* 2003;62(10):1010-1012.

14. Izmirly PM, Costedoat-Chalumeau N, Pisoni CN, et al. Maternal use of hydroxychloroquine is associated with a reduced risk of recurrent anti-SSA/Ro-antibody–associated cardiac manifestations of neonatal lupus. *Circulation.* 2012;126:76-82.
15. Izmirly PM, Kim MY, Llanos C, et al. Evaluation of the risk of anti-SSA/Ro-SSB/La antibody associated cardiac manifestations of neonatal lupus in fetuses of SLE mothers exposed to hydroxychloroquine. *Ann Rheum Dis.* 2010;69:1827-1830.
16. Izmirly P, Kim M, Friedman DM, et al. Efficacy of hydroxychloroquine on the recurrence of congenital heart block in pregnancies of anti-SSA/Ro-Positive mothers. *J Am Coll Cardiol.* 2020. In press.
17. Barsalou J, Jaeggi E, Laskin CA, et al. Prenatal exposure to antimalarials decreases the risk of cardiac but not non-cardiac neonatal lupus: a single-centre cohort study. *Rheumatology (Oxford).* 2017;56(9):1552-1559.
18. Friedman D, Lovig L, Halushka M, Clancy RM, Izmirly PM, Buyon JP. No histologic evidence of foetal cardiotoxicity following exposure to maternal hydroxychloroquine. *Clin Exp Rheumatol.* 2017;35(5):857-859.
19. Alvarez D, Briassouli P, Clancy RM, et al. A novel role of endothelin-1 in linking Toll-like receptor 7-mediated inflammation to fibrosis in congenital heart block. *J Biol Chem.* 2011;286:3044-54.
20. Vandevyer S, Dejager L, Tuckerman J, Liebert C. New insights into the anti-inflammatory mechanisms of glucocorticoid: an emerging role for glucocorticoid-receptor-mediated transactivation. *Endocrinology.* 2013;154(3):993-1007.
21. Looney RJ, Huggins J. Use of intravenous immunoglobulin G (IVIG). *Best Pract Res Clinc Haematol.* 2006;19(1):3-25.
22. Anthony RM, Wermeling F, Karlsson MC, Ravetch JV. Identification of a receptor required for the anti-inflammatory activity of IVIG. *Proc Natl Acad Sci USA.* 2008;105(50):1957-1958.
23. Schwab I, Nimmerjahn F. Intravenous immunoglobulin therapy: how does IgG modulate the immune system? *Nat Rev Immunol.* 2013;13(3):176-189.
24. Nagelkerke SQ, Dekkers G, Kustiawan I, et al. Inhibition of FcγR-mediated phagocytosis by IVIG is independent of IgG-Fc sialylation and FcγRIIb in human macrophages. *Blood.* 2014;124(25):3709-3718.
25. Trucco SM, Jaeggi E, Cuneo B, et al. Use of intravenous gamma globulin and corticosteroids in the treatment of maternal auto antibody mediated cardiomyopathy. *J Am Coll Cardiol.* 2011;57(6):715-723.
26. Cuneo BF, Lee M, Roberson D, et al. A management strategy for fetal immune-mediated atrioventricular block. *J Matern Fetal Neonatal Med.* 2010;23(12):1400-1405.
27. David AL, Ataullah I, Yates R, Sullivan I, Charles P, Williams D. Congenital fetal heart block: a potential therapeutic role for intravenous immunoglobulin. *Obstet Gynecol.* 2010;116(suppl 2):543-547.
28. Cuneo BF, Ambrose SE, Tworetzky W. Detection and successful treatment of emergent anti-SSA-mediated fetal atrioventricular block. *Am J Obstet Gynecol.* 2016;215(4):527-528.
29. Cuneo BF, Sonesson SE, Levasseur S, et al. Home monitoring for fetal heart rhythm during anti-Ro pregnancies. *J Am Coll Cardiol.* 2018;72(16):1940-1951.
30. Jaeggi ET, Silverman ED, Laskin C, Kingdom J, Golding F, Weber R. Prolongation of the atrioventricular conduction in fetuses exposed to maternal anti-Ro/SSA and anti-La/SSB antibodies did not predict progressive heart block. A prospective observational study on the effects of maternal antibodies on 165 fetuses. *J Am Coll Cardiol.* 2011 29;57(13):1487-1492.
31. Cuneo BF, Bitant S, Strasburger JF, Kaizer AM, Wakai RT. Assessment and outcome of AV conduction in normal and anti-Ro/SSA antibody positive pregnancies evaluated by echocardiography and magnetocardiography. *Ultrasound Obstet Gynecol.* 2019;54(5):625-633.
32. Van Bergen AH, Cuneo BF, Davis N. Prospective echocardiographic evaluation of atrioventricular conduction in fetuses with maternal Sjögren's antibodies. *Am J Obstet Gynecol.* 2004;191(3):1014-1018.
33. Sonesson SE, Ambrosi A, Wahren-Herlenius M. Benefits of fetal echocardiographic surveillance in pregnancies at risk of congenital heart block: single-center study of 212 anti-Ro52-positive pregnancies. *Ultrasound Obstet Gynecol.* 2019;54(1):87-95.
34. Skog A, Lagnefeldt L, Conner P, Wahren-Herlenius M, Sonesson SE. Outcome in 212 anti-Ro/SSA-positive pregnancies and population-based incidence of congenital heart block. *Acta Obstet Gynecol Scand.* 2016;95(1):98-100.
35. Sonesson SE, Eliasson H, Conner P, Wahren-Herlenius M. Doppler echocardiographic isovolumetric time intervals in diagnosis of fetal blocked atrial bigeminy and 2:1 atrioventricular block. *Ultrasound Obstet Gynecol.* 2014;44(2):171-175.
36. Zhao H, Cuneo BF, Strasburger JF, Huhta JC, Gotteiner NL, Wakai RT. Electrophysiological characteristics of fetal atrioventricular block. *J Am Coll Cardiol.* 2008;51(1):77-84.
37. Kan N, Silverman ED, Kingdom J, Dutil N, Laskin C, Jaeggi E. Serial echocardiography for immune-mediated heart disease in the fetus: results of a risk-based prospective surveillance strategy. *Prenat Diagn.* 2017;37(4):375-382.

38. Pike JI, Donofrio MT, Berul CI. Ineffective therapy, underpowered studies, or merely too little, too late? Risk factors and impact of maternal corticosteroid treatment on outcome in antibody-associated fetal heart block. *Circulation*. 2011;124:1927-1935.
39. Cuneo BF, Strasburger JF, Niksch A, Ovadia M, Wakai RT. An expanded phenotype of maternal SSA/SSB antibody-associated fetal cardiac disease. *J Matern Fetal Neonatal Med*. 2009;22(3):233-238.
40. Dubin AM, Cuneo BF, Strasburger JF, Wakai RT, Van Hare GF, Rosenthal DN. Congenital junctional ectopic tachycardia and congenital complete atrioventricular block: a shared etiology? *Heart Rhythm*. 2005;2(3):313-315.
41. Brucato A, Astori MG, Cimaz R, et al. Normal neuropsychological development in children with congenital complete heart block who may or may not be exposed to high-dose dexamethasone in utero. *Ann Rheum Dis*. 2006;65(11):1422-1426.
42. Kelly EN, Sananes R, Chiu-Man C, Silverman ED, Jaeggi E. Prenatal anti-Ro antibody exposure, congenital complete atrioventricular heart block, and high-dose steroid therapy: impact on neurocognitive outcome in school-age children. *Arthritis Rheumatol*. 2014;66(8):2290-2296.
43. Chen D, Lao M, Zhany J. Fetal and maternal outcomes of planned pregnancy in patients with systemic lupus erythematosus: a retrospective multicenter study. *J Immunol Res*. 2018;2018:2413637.
44. Tardif ML, Mahone M. Mixed connective tissue disease inpregnancy: a case series and systematic literature review. *Obstet Med*. 2019;12(1):31-37.
45. Skog A, Eliasson H, Tingström J, et al. Long-term growth of children with autoantibody-mediated congenital heart block. *Acta Paediatr*. 2013;102(7):718-726.
46. Mofors J, Eliasson H, Ambrosi A, et al. Comorbidity and long-term outcome in patients with congenital heart block and their siblings exposed to Ro/SSA autoantibodies in utero. *Ann Rheum Dis*. 2019;78(5):696-703.

PART 5

Care of the Pregnancy at Risk for Maternal or Fetal Arrhythmia

The Inherited Arrhythmia Syndromes

Danna Spears

INTRODUCTION

The Inherited arrhythmia syndromes are relatively uncommon, but their true prevalence is difficult to accurately quantify, as gene carriers may not manifest disease. Reported prevalence ranges from 1/2000 in long QT syndrome (LQTS)[1] and Brugada syndrome[2] to 1/10,000 for catecholaminergic polymorphic ventricular tachycardia (CPVT).[3] This chapter will summarize the experience of pregnant women with the above disorders, as well as mothers with inheritable cardiomyopathies who are also at risk of ventricular arrhythmias. There are no formal guidelines for management of these pregnancies, rather suggestions to consider based on limited data. The general approach to management of these disorders during pregnancy includes identification of high-risk features, avoidance of arrhythmia provocation, arrhythmia prophylaxis when possible, and appropriate neonatal screening.

GENERAL STRATEGY

Creating an individualized labor and delivery plan with multidisciplinary input from electrophysiology, genetics, maternal fetal medicine, and anesthesiology should improve outcome for the pregnant woman and her baby. Maternal risk factors and history of cardiac "events" (cardiac arrest, ventricular arrhythmia, or syncope) should be taken into consideration when determining intrapartum monitoring and the method of delivery. For example, maternal cardiac telemetry should be considered when the mother has a history of cardiac dysfunction or cardiac events. Ideally, genetic testing of the affected mother should be completed prior to delivery to allow for the option of cord blood testing for the family variant in the offspring at the time of delivery. The mother should avoid all medications with the potential to provoke arrhythmia-related events and continue the most protective antiarrhythmic treatment such as beta-adrenergic blocking agent[4] (discussed below). Anesthetic planning should include review of all maternal medications to avoid inadvertently putting the mother at greater than a priori risk.[5,6]

In general, for a woman with a primary arrhythmia disorder and normal cardiac function, unassisted vaginal delivery is not contraindicated.[7] However, in some arrhythmia disorders, adverse outcomes are more likely during exertion or emotional stress, that is, when the heart rate is elevated.[8] Because the mother's heart rate increases significantly in the active pushing phase of labor, and ~20% of women achieve 100% of their maximum age-predicted heart rate at this time,[9] higher-risk women may benefit from epidural anesthesia, and assisted or operative delivery. However, the impact of mode of delivery and anesthesia on sympathetic activation and circulating maternal and fetal catecholamine levels is not well studied. In fact, there is little agreement between small published studies.[9-12] TABLE 5.1.1 summarizes the suggestions for management of the pregnant woman with an inherited arrhythmia.

After delivery, the mother's prophylactic antiarrhythmic medications should be continued as the postpartum time is especially high risk for certain inherited arrhythmias. The infant should have a 12-lead ECG and consultation with a pediatric cardiologist and geneticist prior to hospital discharge. Experienced clinicians and genetic counselors can provide subsequent recommendations for family screening[13,14] (see Part 1, Chapter 3) and ongoing cardiology care if the infant carries the family variant.

TABLE 5.1.1 MANAGEMENT OF THE PREGNANT WOMAN WITH INHERITED ARRHYTHMIA

Inherited Arrhythmia	Increased Risk during Pregnancy	Arrhythmia Triggers	Peripartum Monitoring?	Indications for Cesarean Delivery	Fetal Phenotype?
LQTS	Yes, postpartum esp. LQT2	QT prolonging medications	With oxytocin	Obstetrical	Yes
CPVT (AD RyR2) (AR CASQ2)	No	Ectopy	Yes	Hx of cardiac arrest or unstable rhythm	No
Brugada (AD SCN5A and others)	No	Fever, bupivacaine, lidocaine, propofol	No	Obstetrical	No
ARVC AD, VP	No		Yes	Heart failure or unstable arrhythmias	Yes
HOCM (AD)	No	Vasodilation, hypotension	Yes	Obstetrical	Yes

AD, autosomal dominant; AR, autosomal recessive; ARVC, arrhythmogenic right ventricular cardiomyopathy; CPVT, catecholaminergic polymorphic ventricular tachycardia; esp, especially; HOCM, hypertrophic obstructive cardiomyopathy; Hx, history; LQTS, long QT syndrome; VP, variable penetrance.

LONG QT SYNDROME

LQTS is a disorder of myocardial repolarization associated with a prolonged QT interval on the surface ECG and usually inherited in an autosomal dominant fashion.[15] Torsades de pointes (TdP) is the form of polymorphic ventricular tachycardia (VT) classically described in LQTS and is the triggered arrhythmia that leads to syncope and sudden death.[16] There are at least 15 genetically distinct subtypes of LQTS, but the three most commonly encountered forms are due to mutations in KCNQ1 (LQT1), KCNH2 (LQT2), and SCN5A (LQTS3).[17] The diagnosis of LQTS and its association with some fetal and neonatal losses are discussed in Part 3, Chapter 7.

Pregnancy is a significant modulator of outcome in LQTS.[18-20] There is some heterogeneity in the literature regarding risk of arrhythmia during pregnancy, but the bulk of data suggests that there is likely no significant increase in risk until after delivery.[21-23] Prior to commercial genetic testing, the incidence of syncope and sudden death in mothers with LQTS was 3.8% prior to pregnancy and 9.0% during pregnancy. The event rate increased substantially to 23.4% in the first 9 months postpartum.[18] Even in a low-risk cohort, that is, mothers with no events prior to pregnancy, the risk of postpartum events remained significantly elevated (9%).[18] In these early studies, only a minority of women were using a beta-blocker at the time of their event; since then beta-blocking agents have been found to protect against cardiac events.[24,25]

In the genomic era, it has become evident that the genetic LQT subtype is also an important modulator of pregnancy-related arrhythmia risk.[21,26] For example, postpartum cardiac event rates are <1% in LQT1, 16% in LQT2, and have not been reported in LQT3.[20,21]

The factors responsible for the increase in cardiac events during the postpartum period are not well understood. After birth, estrogen levels fall, and oxytocin and prolactin levels increase. Falling levels of estrogen may increase the expression of myocardial adrenergic receptors[27] and may also influence mechanisms regulating intracellular calcium balance, predisposing to afterdepolarizations and arrhythmogenesis.[28-30] In female transgenic rabbits with a KCNH2 G628S pathogenic variant, prolactin and oxytocin were found to increase QT interval and action potential duration and predispose to ventricular arrhythmia.[31] Environmental factors that abruptly increase maternal heart rate such as sudden acoustic stimuli or sudden intense emotion may also be important arrhythmia triggers, especially for LQT2 mothers because of the pronounced failure of repolarization to accommodate to rapid increases in heart rate.

Beta-Adrenergic Blocking Agents in LQTS

Beta-adrenergic blocking agents are highly effective in the prevention of maternal arrhythmia events in LQTS and are the first-line therapy for arrhythmia prophylaxis in this condition.[4] Beta-blockade is most effective in patients with LQT1 and LQT2 and advocated by most in LQT3.[9,32] There is strong evidence to support the efficacy of beta-blockade in preventing pregnancy-related arrhythmia events: beta-blocker use significantly reduces postpartum major cardiac event rates from 3.7% to 0.8%.[19,20] There are abundant data supporting the safety of commonly used beta-blockers in pregnancy.[1,33] The beta-blockers with proven efficacy in LQTS include nadolol, propranolol, metoprolol, and atenolol; however, atenolol should not be used in pregnancy, as it is associated with significant intrauterine growth restriction (pregnancy class D).[34-38] Of the beta-blockers with demonstrated efficacy in LQTS, nadolol, propranolol, and metoprolol are pregnancy risk Category C. There is some evidence that metoprolol, particularly the shorter acting formulation with twice-a-day dosing, is inferior to nadolol or propranolol, particularly in individuals with a prior history of arrhythmia events.[39] Overall, nadolol was found to be most effective and is considered the beta-blocker of choice overall, but especially in higher risk patients, including LQT2 mothers, women with QTc >500 ms, and individuals with a prior history of syncope or cardiac arrest.[32,35-37,39] Nadolol dosing up to 1 to 1.5 mg/kg/d is the typical dose used in LQTS. If nadolol is poorly tolerated or not available, propranolol, another noncardioselective beta-blocker, can be considered.

Data on the use of nadolol in pregnancy are limited. However, nadolol has a long half-life and is excreted in the breast milk to a greater degree than propranolol or metoprolol[40,41]; thus it is likely to accumulate to some degree in the nursing infant. Although the American Academy of Pediatrics classified nadolol as compatible with breast-feeding,[42] nursing infants of mothers consuming nadolol should be closely observed for symptoms of beta-blockade including bradycardia and hypotension. It is estimated that the neonate would receive about 5.1% of the maternal weight-adjusted dose. Propranolol, on the other hand, shows a low risk for accumulation in a breastfeeding infant.[42] There is increasing experience with the use of bisoprolol, particularly in LQT1; however, small sample size and lack of data supporting its safe use in pregnancy preclude its routine use in this population.[43]

Gestational Surveillance of LQTS

There are no clear guidelines for surveillance of LQTS over the course of pregnancy, but important principles include confirmation of the diagnosis, treatment with beta-blocker for arrhythmia prophylaxis, and realization that the fetus has a 50% chance of carrying the family variant. Beta-blockers should blunt the maximum maternal heart rate, with the dose adjusted to ensure resting heart rate <100 bpm during pregnancy. Periodic Holter monitoring may be useful as a guide to heart rate trends over the course of 24 to 48 hours. Although maximal, symptom-limited treadmill testing is not routinely performed in pregnancy, a modified treadmill test may be useful to ensure adequate beta-blockade in high-risk LQTS mothers.

Labor and Delivery Plan for LQTS

The plan for labor and delivery should be individualized. Low-risk women (no history of arrhythmia events) who are adequately treated with beta-blocker can safely proceed with spontaneous vaginal delivery unless maternal or fetal indications for assisted or cesarean delivery are present. Although active pushing is expected to increase the maximal heart rate, it is expected that the heart rate response would be blunted in a woman with adequate beta-blockade.[8] Maternal intrapartum rhythm monitoring is not necessary, as event rates are extremely low.

Any pharmacologic therapy in an individual with LQTS should be reviewed for potential QT prolongation.[6] Oxytocin, commonly used during labor and delivery, has some potential for QT prolongation, but this should not preclude its use when indicated.[44-46] A reasonable approach to oxytocin use is to optimize serum potassium and magnesium levels and to obtain an ECG at baseline, and then 1 to 2 hours after oxytocin is initiated. The drug should be discontinued if the QTc exceeds 500 ms or increases by 60 ms from baseline.[45,46] Theoretically oxytocin may also predispose the LQT-positive fetus to QT prolongation and ventricular arrhythmias, but this has not been reported. Decisions regarding analgesia, including neuronal axial blockade, should be made according to maternal preference and estimated obstetric risk.

Maternal TdP requires immediate recognition and treatment, including defibrillation for sustained arrhythmia.[47] Pharmacotherapy should be reviewed for potentially QT-prolonging drugs, and they should be immediately discontinued. Electrolyte imbalance, particularly hypokalemia or hypomagnesemia, should be corrected. Treatment of bradycardia or frequent pauses with temporary pacing followed by beta-blockade, and addition of lidocaine if needed, may be required for management of ongoing ventricular arrhythmias.

There is evidence that fetal loss, both miscarriage and stillbirth, is increased with familial LQTS compared to the general population.[48] These findings are irrespective of fetus genotype and occur to a greater extent when the mother, not the father, has LQTS.[48] Any fetal loss should be tested for the family variant.

Neonatal screening by cord-blood genetic testing for the family pathogenic variant can be performed. Given the potential for arrhythmia events (as high as 4% in the first year of life) and sudden infant death,[49-52] such testing is recommended. Since the QT interval is often prolonged in normal newborns, 12-lead ECG screening of the neonate is unreliable. If a variant of unknown significance is detected on genetic screening or if genetic screening of the neonate cannot be offered, an ongoing clinical screening with serial ECGs is indicated.[53]

CATECHOLAMINERGIC POLYMORPHIC VENTRICULAR TACHYCARDIA

Catecholaminergic polymorphic ventricular tachycardia (CPVT) is a rare genetic arrhythmia disorder with an estimated prevalence of 1 in 10,000[3]. The diagnosis is made by identification of heterozygous pathogenic variants in the myocardial calcium-handling genes RYR2 or CASQ2, which are inherited in an autosomal dominant (RYR2) or autosomal recessive (CASQ2) fashion.[54] In CPVT, arrhythmia occurs typically in the absence of structural heart disease or prolonged QT.[55] This condition is characterized by the onset of ventricular arrhythmias with increasing exertion or emotional stress, beginning with isolated premature ventricular complexes (PVCs) with predictable progression to bidirectional couplets and nonsustained ventricular tachycardia to more complex ventricular arrhythmias and ventricular fibrillation (FIG. 5.1.1). Women who may be at higher risk for arrhythmia events include those with a history of cardiac arrest prior to diagnosis, and women who were diagnosed in childhood.[56] Genetic variants have been identified in the myocardial calcium-handling genes RYR2 and CASQ2.[54]

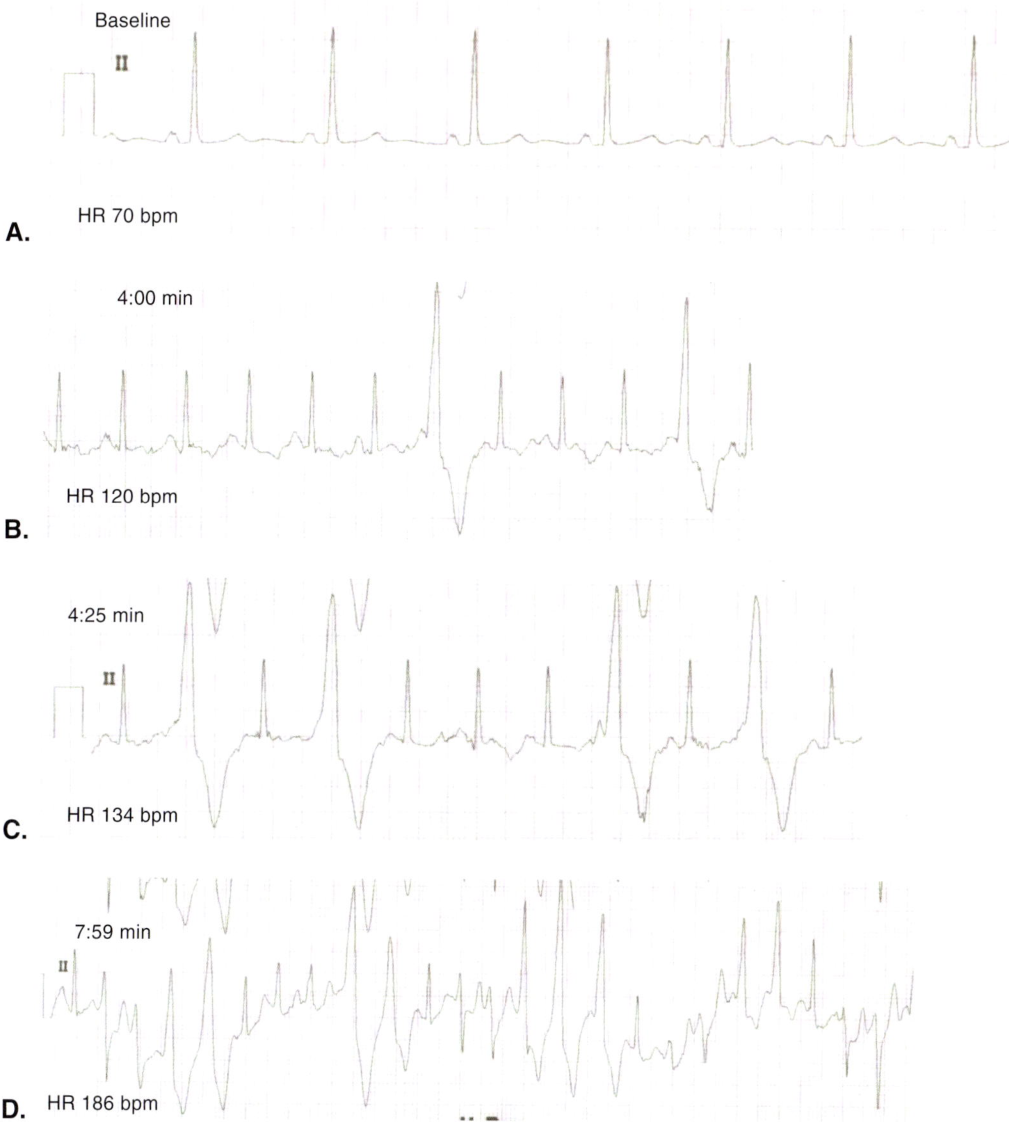

FIGURE 5.1.1 Rhythm tracings from the exercise-stress test of an adolescent with syncope upon exertion. **A:** Baseline. Normal heart rate and cardiac intervals. **B:** Four minutes after exercise, premature ventricular contractions are seen. **C:** Six minutes after exercise, the rhythm changes to ventricular bigeminy. **D:** At almost 8 min, sustained bidirectional ventricular tachycardia at a rate of 186 bpm is seen and the patient reported dizziness. The test was stopped and the rhythm normalized during recovery. She is currently treated with nadolol and flecainide and is doing well.

Data regarding CPVT in pregnancy are sparse, and there are no clear guidelines for management of women with CPVT in pregnancy.[57,58] Beta-blockers are highly effective in reducing arrhythmia events from 58% to 27% over an 8-year period in one study[55]; in a second study, cardiac events occurred only in pregnant women not on beta-blockers.[58] Nadolol is the recommended beta-blocking agent with the most significant risk reduction in cardiac events and exertional ventricular arrhythmias.[59] Women breakthrough ventricular arrhythmia despite beta-blockade may benefit from additional therapies, including addition of flecainide, sympathectomy, or implantable cardioverter-defibrillator (ICD) implantation in select cases.[4,60,61]

The approach to surveillance during pregnancy should focus on adequate beta-blockade and monitoring for breakthrough arrhythmia and symptoms such as syncope or presyncope. Holter monitoring can guide beta-blocker titration, and in high-risk women, modified exercise stress testing should be considered. The target dose of nadolol in CPVT is higher than that for LQTS and may be as high as 2 mg/kg/d.[59]

The labor and delivery plan should include maternal cardiac telemetry. This is advisable as the onset of arrhythmia typically follows a stepwise progression from isolated PVCs to more complex and unstable ventricular arrhythmias. The optimal mode of delivery is dictated by a woman's prior history of arrhythmia and adequacy of medical therapy. Women with poorly controlled arrhythmias or a history of cardiac arrest should be considered for operative delivery, as this is likely associated with the least adrenergic stimulation.[12] Beta-blockade should not be interrupted at any time.[61] Neonatal screening should include cord-blood genetic testing if a familial pathogenic variant has been identified and a 12-lead ECG. If a variant of unknown significance has been detected, or if genetic screening of the neonate cannot be offered, ongoing clinical screening is indicated.

BRUGADA SYNDROME

Brugada syndrome is an autosomal dominant inherited mutation in any of at least 16 genes, most commonly the SCN5A gene.[62] Brugada syndrome may also be acquired, that is, not inherited. The hallmark of Brugada syndrome is the ECG finding of >2 mm coved ST segment elevation in at least one of the right precordial leads (V1-3), which may be transient **(FIG. 5.1.2)**.[63] Brugada syndrome may be complicated by arrhythmias, which can result in syncope or sudden death.[64] Events typically occur during sleep, with fever, or after exposure to provocative agents, which interfere with the first phase of cardiac depolarization. Women with high-risk features such as a history of cardiac arrest or syncope of likely arrhythmic origin should be considered for ICD implantation.[65]

The labor and delivery plan for Brugada syndrome requires few considerations. Fortunately, event rates in women with Brugada syndrome do not appear to be elevated during pregnancy.[66,67] Management of Brugada syndrome in pregnancy is otherwise conservative, with aggressive fever management and avoidance of medications that may provoke arrhythmias. A list of these medications can be found at www.brugadadrugs.org.[5] These medications include many antiarrhythmic medications and anesthetic drugs such as bupivacaine, lidocaine, and propofol. There is no cardiovascular contraindication to unassisted vaginal delivery in mothers with Brugada syndrome.

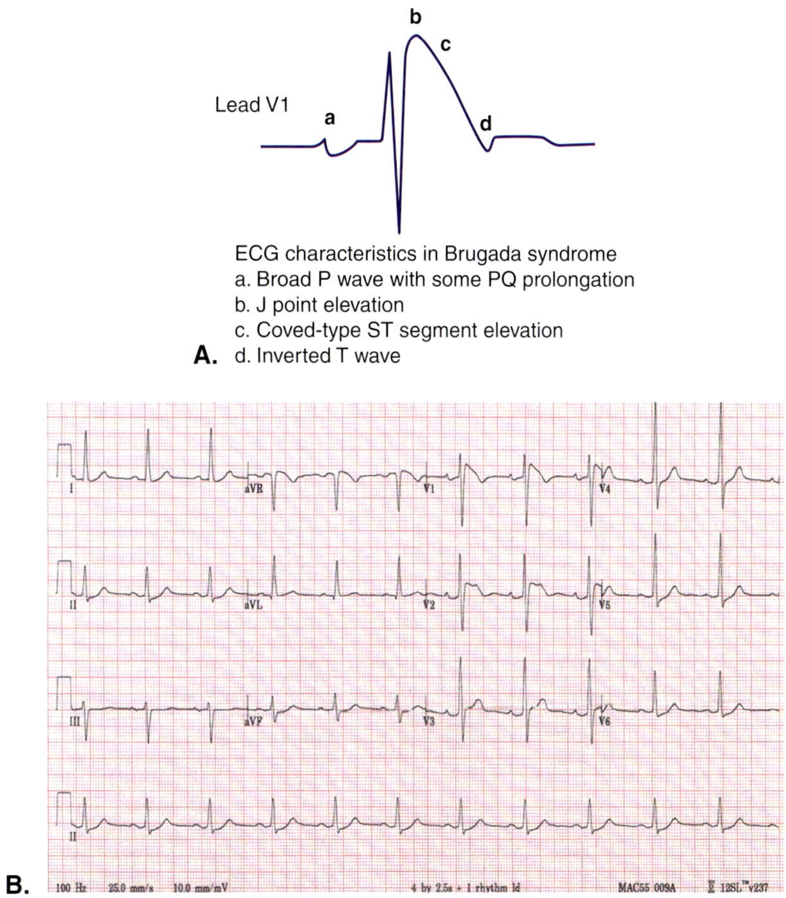

FIGURE 5.1.2 Brugada syndrome ECG. **A:** Typical findings seen in lead 2 in Brugada syndrome. **B:** 12-Lead ECG in a patient with Brugada syndrome. (A, Reprinted from Brugada Syndrome. ECGpedia. https://en.ecgpedia.org/wiki/Brugada_Syndrome. B, Reprinted from Steinberg JS, Mittal S. *Electrophysiology: The Basics*. Philadelphia, PA: Wolters Kluwer; 2017.)

Unfortunately, there are presently no recognized features to suggest a fetal Brugada phenotype. However, pathogenic SCN5A gene variants can have multiple modes of fetal presentation, including sinus bradycardia,[68] abnormal repolarization, and ventricular arrhythmias leading to hydrops or fetal loss[69] and high-grade AV block.[70] As with any of the inherited arrhythmia disorders, genetic testing should be offered to any affected parent, to facilitate family screening if a pathogenic mutation is found. If genetic testing is not possible, clinical neonatal screening is recommended.

INHERITED CARDIOMYOPATHIES WITH A RISK OF ARRHYTHMIA

Arrhythmogenic Right Ventricular Cardiomyopathy

Arrhythmogenic right ventricular cardiomyopathy (ARVC) is one of the heritable cardiomyopathies with risk of arrhythmia.[71-73]

In ARVC, five pathogenic desmosomal gene variants have been identified, with autosomal dominant inheritance and variable penetrance. Although a single gene variant may be causative, subjects with ARVC frequently carry more than one pathogenic variant in the same gene (compound heterozygosity), while only 30% to 50% of phenotype positive patients do not carry any of the pathologic variants (see Part 1, Chapter 3). In the setting of ARVC, major maternal cardiac events including ventricular arrhythmia or heart failure are reported in 3% to 18% of pregnancies.[73-76] The incidence of ventricular arrhythmia recurrence is not increased in pregnancy, in women already taking a beta-blocker.[77] Some women will have their first arrhythmia presentation during pregnancy, but overall, the risk of a first arrhythmia or heart failure event is not significantly increased in pregnancy.[78,79] Disease progression and severity are associated with increasing cumulative levels of physical exertion,[80] but pregnancy does not appear to have a detrimental effect on the clinical course of ARVC. Worsening of right ventricular morphological or electrical parameters after one or more pregnancies has not been demonstrated.[81] Women with ARVC who are at the highest risk of complications are those having major right ventricular structural abnormalities prior to conception[78,82] (FIG. 5.1.3).

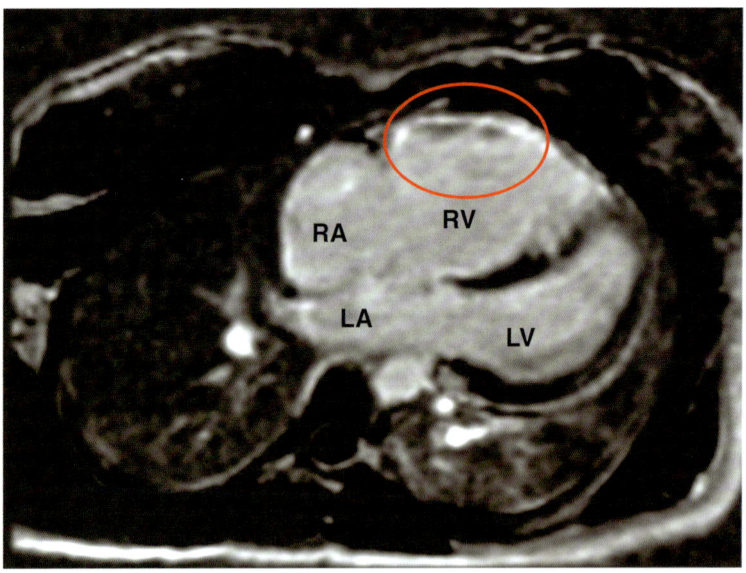

FIGURE 5.1.3 Magnetic resonance imaging of arrhythmogenic right ventricular cardiomyopathy. The fatty infiltrate is seen on the anterior free wall of the RV (red circle). LA, left atrium; LV, left ventricle; RA, right atrium; RV, right ventricle.

The optimal mode of delivery in ARVC is driven by underlying ventricular function and arrhythmia stability. In general, the cesarean delivery rates in ARVC are not different from those in the general population but should be considered in the setting of symptomatic ventricular failure, unstable arrhythmia, or for obstetric indications.[78,79] Peripartum cardiac rhythm monitoring is recommended, given the inherent risk of arrhythmia in this population.

There are published case reports of ARVC presenting in fetal life with morphologic right ventricular changes and arrhythmia[83-85] (FIG. 5.1.4). Fetal onset of disease appears to have a poor prognosis, although early medical therapy can be useful to stabilize ventricular arrhythmias.[84] The importance of pediatric follow-up cannot be understated. There have been many reports of ARVC manifesting in very early childhood.[86-90] Significant cardiac events have been reported in up to 14% of offspring of affected mothers, justifying screening and close cardiac monitoring from early childhood.[89]

Hypertrophic Cardiomyopathy

Hypertrophic cardiomyopathy (HCM) is a more common inherited cardiomyopathy with frequent arrhythmia complications, inherited in autosomal dominant fashion[91-93] (FIG. 5.1.5). Preconception management of any woman with familial cardiomyopathy should be optimized, including risk stratification based on history and symptoms, arrhythmia prophylaxis with beta-adrenergic blocking agents, genetic counseling, and, if the mother is high risk, defined as a family or personal history of cardiac arrest, discussion of an ICD placement. Verapamil, a calcium channel blocking agent used in HCM, should be avoided during pregnancy because it crosses the placenta and can affect atrioventricular conduction in the fetus.

Several reports outline the care and outcome of pregnant women with HCM.[94-103] In a recent study of women with cardiomyopathy followed through pregnancy, major maternal cardiac events and neonatal events were observed in 35%.[96] High-risk mothers benefit from close peripartum monitoring, especially if they develop palpitations or presyncope. Beta-blocker treatment is recommended for mothers with more than mild left ventricular outflow obstruction and/or maximal left ventricular wall thickness of ≥15 mm.[100] A planned (induced) vaginal delivery is the delivery of choice in the low-risk mother. Since reduced preload can exacerbate left ventricular tract obstruction, anesthetic agents causing vasodilation and hypotension should be avoided.

Inherited HCM can be detected during fetal life[103-106] (FIG. 5.1.6). Fetuses with HCM are at risk for intrauterine demise due to heart failure: in one study, 8/21 died in utero.[103] The phenotype of heritable HCM may not be the same as other family members, for example, pathogenic MYH7 variants can result in both dilated and hypertrophic cardiomyopathy.[105] Since HCM is characterized by an autosomal dominant inheritance pattern, such that the risk of transmission from either parent to offspring is 50%, genetic testing should be offered to the affected parent to facilitate family screening if a pathogenic mutation is found. If genetic testing is not possible, clinical neonatal screening is recommended. All infants at risk for heritable arrhythmia syndromes should have a 12-lead ECG and consultation with a pediatric cardiologist prior to hospital discharge.

(text continued on page 232)

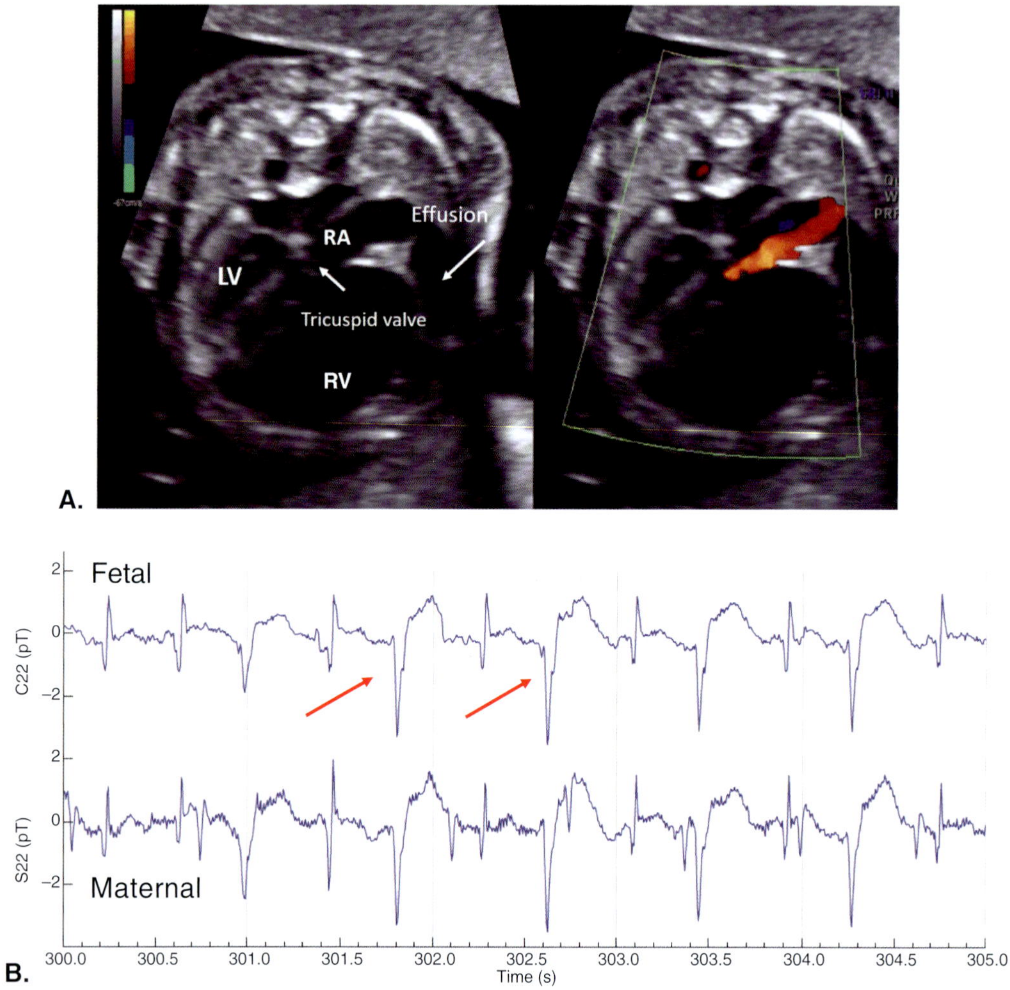

FIGURE 5.1.4 A 19-week fetus with arrhythmogenic right ventricular cardiomyopathy and ventricular bigeminy. **A:** Two-dimensional echo image showing dilated right ventricle (RV) compressing the left ventricle (LV). A pericardial effusion is also present. Color Doppler in the next frame shows tricuspid insufficiency. **B:** Fetal magnetocardiogram of ventricular bigeminy. RA, right atrium.

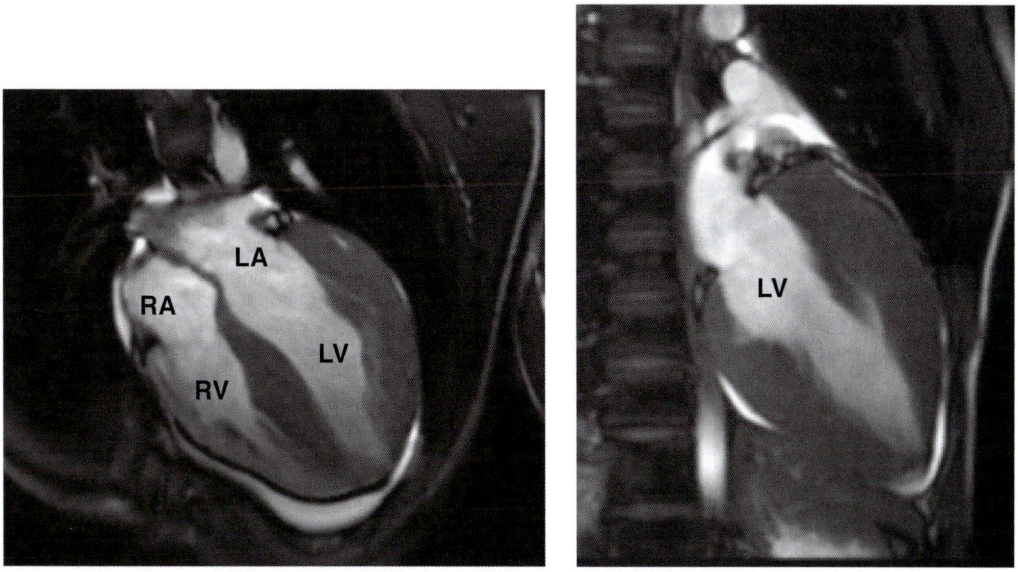

FIGURE 5.1.5 MRI of a patient with hypertrophic obstructive cardiomyopathy. The thickened free walls and septum are dark and the blood pool is light. LA, left atrium; LV, left ventricle; RA, right atrium; RV, right ventricle.

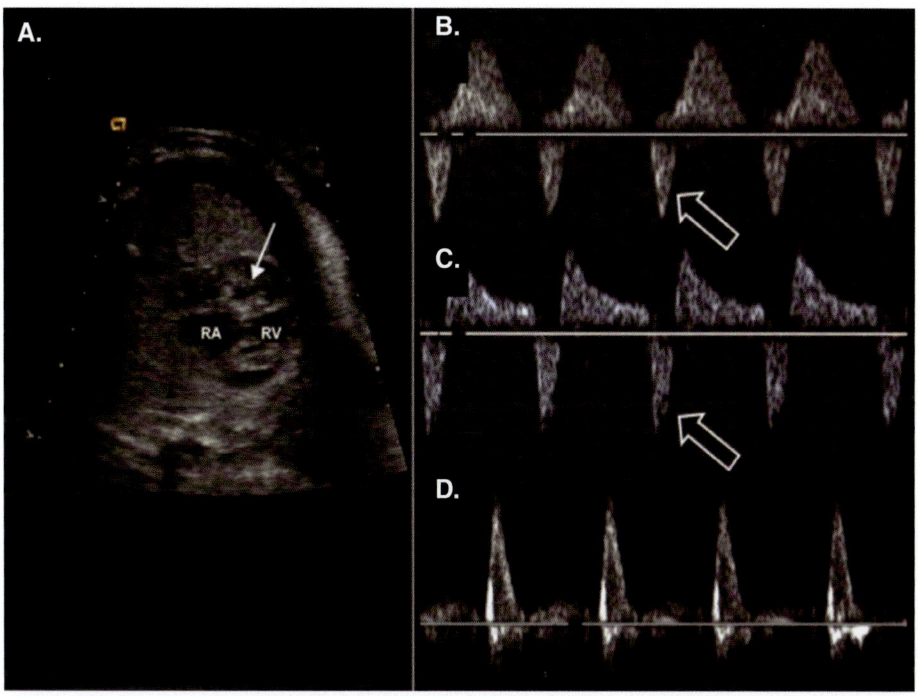

FIGURE 5.1.6 Echocardiographic findings in a fetus with hypertrophic obstructive cardiomyopathy. **A:** Two-dimensional image showing biventricular hypertrophy. The LV cavity is almost completely obliterated (Arrow). **B** to **D:** Spectral Doppler consistent with diastolic dysfunction and reduced ventricular compliance. Reverse flow during atrial systole (arrows) in the ductus venosus **(B)** and the pulmonary vein **(C)**, and tricuspid valve Doppler showing monophasic filling of the right ventricle. (Reprinted from Hinton RB, Michelfelder EC, Marino BS, Bove KE, Ware SM. A fetus with hypertrophic cardiomyopathy, restrictive, and single-ventricle physiology, and a beta-myosin heavy chain mutation. *J Pediatr*. 2010;157(1):164-166.)

SUMMARY

Successful pregnancy management of the mother with inherited arrhythmia syndrome begins before birth. First, it is important to establish appropriate treatment for primary prevention of maternal arrhythmias and continue that treatment throughout and after the pregnancy. In majority of affected women, treatment is appropriate doses of beta-adrenergic blocking agents, with nadolol being the most effective. Additional treatment with flecainide or an ICD may be necessary in some high-risk women. Second, genetic testing of the mother should be strongly considered so if a pathogenic mutation is found, it can be tested for in the infant by cord blood analysis. Third, assembling an experienced multidisciplinary team to care for the mother during pregnancy, labor and delivery, and after birth will increase the likelihood of a good outcome for mother and baby. The need for intrapartum monitoring, type of delivery and anesthetic management, and cord blood testing can all be discussed in prenatal counseling. Once the pregnancy is established, arrhythmia triggers should be avoided, and prophylactic arrhythmia treatment continued. After birth, management of the infant includes 12-lead ECG and consultation with a pediatric cardiologist for ongoing surveillance and possibly treatment if cord blood testing results are positive for the inherited pathogenic variant.

References

1. Schwartz PJ, Stramba-Badiale M, Crotti L, et al. Prevalence of the congenital long-QT syndrome. *Circulation*. 2009;120(18):1761-1767.
2. Vutthikraivit W, Rattanawong P, Putthapiban P, et al. Worldwide prevalence of brugada syndrome: a systematic review and meta-analysis. *Zhonghua Minguo Xin Zang Xue Hui Za Zhi*. 2018;34(3):267-277.
3. Imberti JF, Underwood K, Mazzanti A, Priori SG. Clinical challenges in catecholaminergic polymorphic ventricular tachycardia. *Heart Lung Circ*. 2016;25(8):777-783.
4. Priori SG, Wilde AA, Horie M, et al. Executive summary: HRS/EHRA/APHRS expert consensus statement on the diagnosis and management of patients with inherited primary arrhythmia syndromes. *Europace*. 2013;15(10):1389-1406.
5. Postema PG, Neville J, de Jong JSSG, Romero K, Wilde AAM, Woosley RL. Safe drug use in long QT syndrome and brugada syndrome: comparison of website statistics. *Europace*. 2013;15(7):1042-1049.
6. Fazio G, Vernuccio F, Grutta G, Re GL. Drugs to be avoided in patients with long QT syndrome: focus on the anaesthesiological management. *World J Cardiol*. 2013;5(4):87-93.
7. Committee on Obstetric Practice. Committee opinion no. 687: approaches to limit intervention during labor and birth. *Obstet Gynecol*. 2017;129(2):e20-e28.
8. Söhnchen N, Melzer K, de Tejada BM, et al. Maternal heart rate changes during labour. *Eur J Obstet Gynecol Reprod Biol*. 2011;158(2):173-178.
9. Pohjavuori M, Rovamo L, Laatikainen T, Kariniemi V, Pettersson J. Stress of delivery and plasma endorphins and catecholamines in the newborn infant. *Biol Res Pregnancy Perinatol*. 1986;7(1):1-5.
10. Westgren M, Lindahl SG, Nordén NE. Maternal and fetal endocrine stress response at vaginal delivery with and without an epidural block. *J Perinat Med*. 1986;14(4):235-241.
11. Ochedalski T, Lachowicz A. Maternal and fetal hypothalamo-pituitary-adrenal axis: different response depends upon the mode of parturition. *Neuro Endocrinol Lett*. 2004;25(4):278-282.
12. Vogl SE, Worda C, Egarter C, et al. Mode of delivery is associated with maternal and fetal endocrine stress response. *Br J Obstet Gynecol*. 2006;113(4):441-445.
13. Ingles J, Zodgekar PR, Yeates L, et al. Guidelines for genetic testing of inherited cardiac disorders. *Heart Lung Circ*. 2011;20(11):681-687.
14. Care M, Chauhan V, Spears D. Genetic testing in inherited heart diseases: practical considerations for clinicians. *Curr Cardiol Rep*. 2017;19(9):88.
15. Schwartz PJ, Moss AJ, Vincent GM, Crampton RS. Diagnostic criteria for the long QT syndrome. An update. *Circulation*. 1993;88(2):782-784.

16. Roden DM. Torsade de pointes. *Clin Cardiol.* 1993;16(9):683-686.
17. Splawski I, Shen J, Timothy KW, et al. Spectrum of mutations in long-qt syndrome genes. KVLQT1, HERG, SCN5A, KCNE1, and KCNE2. *Circulation.* 2000;102(10):1178-1185.
18. Rashba EJ, Zareba W, Moss AJ, et al. Influence of pregnancy on the risk for cardiac events in patients with hereditary long QT syndrome. *Circulation.* 1998;97(5):451-456.
19. Seth R, Moss AJ, McNitt S, et al. Long QT syndrome and pregnancy. *J Am Coll Cardiol.* 2007;49(10):1092-1098.
20. Heradien MJ, Goosen A, Crotti L, et al. Does pregnancy increase cardiac risk for LQT1 patients with the KCNQ1-A341V mutation?. *J Am Coll Cardiol.* 2006;48(7):1410-1415.
21. Khositseth A, Tester DJ, Will ML, Bell CM, Ackerman MJ. Identification of a common genetic substrate underlying postpartum cardiac events in congenital long QT syndrome. *Heart Rhythm.* 2004;1(1):60-64.
22. Garg L, Garg J, Krishnamoorthy P, et al. Influence of pregnancy in patients with congenital long QT syndrome. *Cardiol Rev.* 2017;25(4):197-201.
23. Schwartz PJ, Priori SG, Spazzolini C, et al. Genotype-phenotype correlation in the long-qt syndrome: gene-specific triggers for life-threatening arrhythmias. *Circulation.* 2001;103(1):89-95.
24. Kim JA, Lopes CM, Moss AJ, et al. Trigger-specific risk factors and response to therapy in long QT syndrome type 2. *Heart Rhythm.* 2010;7(12):1797-1805.
25. Priori SG, Napolitano C, Schwartz PJ, et al. Association of long QT syndrome loci and cardiac events among patients treated with beta blockers. *J Am Med Assoc.* 2004;292(11):1341-1344.
26. Tuveng JM, Berling BM, Bunford G, et al. Long QT syndrome KCNH2 mutation with sequential fetal and maternal sudden death. *Forensic Sci Med Pathol.* 2018;14(3):367-371.
27. Dent MR, Tappia PS, Dhalla NS. Gender related alterations of β-adrenoceptor mechanisms in heart failure due to arteriovenous fistula. *J Cell Physiol.* 2012;227(8):3080-3087.
28. Odening KE, Choi B-R, Liu GX, et al. Estradiol promotes sudden cardiac death in transgenic long QT type 2 rabbits while progesterone is protective. *Heart Rhythm.* 2012;9(5):823-832.
29. Chen J, Weber M, Um SY, Walsh CA, Tang Y, McDonald TV. A dual mechanism for I(ks) current reduction by the pathogenic mutation KCNQ1-S277L. *Pacing Clin Electrophysiol.* 2011;34(12):1652-1664.
30. Yan C, Yu Y-H, Ou Yang S-Y, et al. Perinatal management and outcome of different types of fetal arrhythmia. *Nan Fang Yi Ke Da Xue Xue Bao.* 2011;31(6):987-990.
31. Bodi I, Sorge J, Castiglione A, et al. Postpartum hormones oxytocin and prolactin cause pro-arrhythmic prolongation of cardiac repolarization in long QT syndrome type 2. *Europace.* 2019;21(7):1126-1138.
32. Moss AJ. Long QT syndromes. *Curr Treat Options Cardiovasc Med.* 2000;2(4):317-322.
33. Chow T, Galvin J, McGovern B. Antiarrhythmic drug therapy in pregnancy and lactation. *Am J Cardiol.* 1998;82(4A):58I-62I.
34. Ackerman MJ, Priori SG, Dubin AM, et al. Beta-blocker therapy for long QT syndrome and catecholaminergic polymorphic ventricular tachycardia: are all beta-blockers equivalent?. *Heart Rhythm.* 2017;14(1):e41-e44.
35. Abu-Zeitone A, Peterson DR, Polonsky B, McNitt S, Moss AJ. Efficacy of different beta-blockers in the treatment of long QT syndrome. *J Am Coll Cardiol.* 2014;64(13):1352-1358.
36. Ackerman MJ, Priori SG, Dubin A, et al. Beta blocker therapy for long QT syndrome and catecholaminergic polymorphic ventricular tachycardia: are all beta blockers equivalent?. *Heart Rhythm.* 2016;14(1):e41-e44.
37. Mazzanti A, Maragna R, Vacanti G, et al. Interplay between genetic substrate, qtc duration, and arrhythmia risk in patients with long QT syndrome. *J Am Coll Cardiol.* 2018;71(15):1663-1671.
38. Duan L, Ng A, Chen W, Spencer HT, Lee M-S. Beta-blocker subtypes and risk of low birth weight in newborns. *J Clin Hypertens (Greenwich).* 2018;20(11):1603-1609.
39. Chockalingam P, Crotti L, Girardengo G, et al. Not all beta-blockers are equal in the management of long QT syndrome types 1 and 2: higher recurrence of events under metoprolol. *J Am Coll Cardiol.* 2012;60(20):2092-2099.
40. Sandström B, Regårdh CG. Metoprolol excretion into breast milk. *Br J Clin Pharmacol.* 1980;9(5):518-519.
41. Thorley KJ, McAinsh J. Levels of the beta-blockers atenolol and propranolol in the breast milk of women treated for hypertension in pregnancy. *Biopharm Drug Dispos.* 1983;4(3):299-301.
42. American Academy of Pediatrics Committee on Drugs. Transfer of drugs and other chemicals into human milk. *Pediatrics.* 2001;108(3):776-789.
43. Steinberg C, Padfield GJ, Al-Sabeq B, et al. Experience with bisoprolol in long-qt1 and long-qt2 syndrome. *J Interv Card Electrophysiol.* 2016;47(2):163-170.
44. Charbit B, Funck-Brentano C, Samain E, Jannier-Guillou V, Albaladejo P, Marty J. QT interval prolongation after oxytocin bolus during surgical induced abortion. *Clin Pharmacol Ther.* 2004;76(4):359-364.

45. Martillotti G, Talajic M, Rey E, Leduc L. Long QT syndrome in pregnancy: are vaginal delivery and use of oxytocin permitted? A case report. *J Obstet Gynaecol Can.* 2012;34(11):1073-1076.
46. Yap YG, Camm AJ. Drug induced QT prolongation and torsades de pointes. *Heart.* 2003;89(11):1363-1372.
47. Drew BJ, Ackerman MJ, Funk M, et al. Prevention of torsade de pointes in hospital settings: a scientific statement from the American Heart Association and the American College of Cardiology Foundation. *J Am Coll Cardiol.* 2010;55(9):934-947.
48. Cuneo B, Swan H, Clur SA, et al. Incidence of stillbirth is increased in familial long QT syndrome: a retrospective study from 8 international centers. *Ultrasound Obstet Gynecol.* 2017;50(suppl 1):1-47.
49. Schulze-Bahr E, Fenge H, Etzrodt D, et al. Long QT syndrome and lifethreatening arrhythmia in a newborn: molecular diagnosis and treatment response. *Heart.* 2004;90(1):13-16.
50. Tester DJ, Wong LCH, Chanana P, et al. Cardiac genetic predisposition in sudden infant death syndrome. *J Am Coll Cardiol.* 2018;71(11):1217-1227.
51. Tester DJ, Medeiros-Domingo A, Will ML, Haglund CM, Ackerman MJ. Cardiac channel molecular autopsy: insights from 173 consecutive cases of autopsy-negative sudden unexplained death referred for postmortem genetic testing. *Mayo Clin Proc.* 2012;87(6):524-539.
52. Ioakeimidis NS, Papamitsou T, Meditskou S, Iakovidou-Kritsi Z. Sudden infant death syndrome due to long QT syndrome: a brief review of the genetic substrate and prevalence. *J Biol Res (Thessalon).* 2017;24:6.
53. Philip Saul J, Schwartz PJ, Ackerman MJ, Triedman JK. Rationale and objectives for ECG screening in infancy. *Heart Rhythm.* 2014;11(12):2316-2321.
54. Priori SG, Napolitano C, Memmi M, et al. Clinical and molecular characterization of patients with catecholaminergic polymorphic ventricular tachycardia. *Circulation.* 2002;106(1):69-74.
55. Sumitomo N, Harada K, Nagashima M, et al. Catecholaminergic polymorphic ventricular tachycardia: electrocardiographic characteristics and optimal therapeutic strategies to prevent sudden death. *Heart.* 2003;89(1):66-70.
56. Lieve KV, van der Werf C, Wilde AA. Catecholaminergic polymorphic ventricular tachycardia. *Circ J.* 2016;80(6):1285-1291.
57. Romagano MP, Quiñones JN, Ahnert A, Martinez R, Smulian JC. Catecholaminergic polymorphic ventricular tachycardia in pregnancy. *Obstet Gynecol.* 2016;127(4):735-739.
58. Cheung CC, Lieve KV, Roston TM, et al. Pregnancy in catecholaminergic polymorphic ventricular tachycardia. *JACC Clin Electrophysiol.* 2019;5(3):387-394.
59. Leren IS, Saberniak J, Majid E, Haland TF, Edvardsen T, Haugaa KH. Nadolol decreases the incidence and severity of ventricular arrhythmias during exercise stress testing compared with β1-selective β-blockers in patients with catecholaminergic polymorphic ventricular tachycardia. *Heart Rhythm.* 2016;13(2):433-440.
60. Kannankeril PJ, Moore JP, Cerrone M, et al. Efficacy of flecainide in the treatment of catecholaminergic polymorphic ventricular tachycardia: a randomized clinical trial. *JAMA Cardiol.* 2017;2(7):759-766.
61. van der Werf C, Zwinderman AH, Wilde AAM. Therapeutic approach for patients with catecholaminergic polymorphic ventricular tachycardia: state of the art and future developments. *Europace.* 2012;14(2):175-183.
62. Hosseini SM, Kim R, Udupa S, et al. Reappraisal of reported genes for sudden arrhythmic death: an evidence-based evaluation of gene validity for brugada syndrome. *Circulation.* 2018;138(12):1195-1205.
63. Savastano S, Rordorf R, Vicentini A, et al. A comprehensive electrocardiographic, molecular, and echocardiographic study of brugada syndrome: validation of the 2013 diagnostic criteria. *Heart Rhythm.* 2014;11(7):1176-1183.
64. Brugada J, Brugada R, Brugada P. Right bundle-branch block and st-segment elevation in leads V1 through V3: a marker for sudden death in patients without demonstrable structural heart disease. *Circulation.* 1998;97(5):457-460.
65. Priori SG, Gasparini M, Napolitano C, et al. Risk stratification in brugada syndrome: results of the PRELUDE (programmed electrical stimulation predictive value) registry. *J Am Coll Cardiol.* 2012;59(1):37-45.
66. Rodríguez-Mañero M, Casado-Arroyo R, Sarkozy A, et al. The clinical significance of pregnancy in brugada syndrome. *Rev Esp Cardiol (Engl Ed).* 2014;67(3):176-180.
67. Giambanco L, Incandela D, Maiorana A, Alio W, Alio L. Brugada syndrome and pregnancy: highlights on antenatal and prenatal management. *Case Rep Obstet Gynecol.* 2014;2014:531648.
68. Benson DW, Wang DW, Dyment M, et al. Congenital sick sinus syndrome caused by recessive mutations in the cardiac sodium channel gene (SCN5A). *J Clin Invest.* 2003;112(7):1019-1028.

69. Miller TE, Estrella E, Myerburg RJ, et al. Recurrent third-trimester fetal loss and maternal mosaicism for long QT syndrome. *Circulation.* 2004;109(24):3029-3034.
70. Lin L, Takahashi-Igari M, Kato Y, et al. Prenatal diagnosis of atrioventricular block and QT interval prolongation by fetal magnetocardiography in a fetus with trisomy 18 and SCN5AR1193Q variant. *Case Rep Pediatr.* 2017;2017:6570465.
71. Marcus FI, Edson S, Towbin JA. Genetics of arrhythmogenic right ventricular cardiomyopathy: a practical guide for physicians. *J Am Coll Cardiol.* 2013;61(19):1945-1948.
72. Leren IS, Saberniak J, Haland TF, Edvardsen T, Haugaa KH. Combination of ECG and echocardiography for identification of arrhythmic events in early ARVC. *JACC Cardiovasc Imaging.* 2017;10(5):503-513.
73. Fontaine G, Fontaliran F, Frank R. Arrhythmogenic right ventricular cardiomyopathies: clinical forms and main differential diagnoses. *Circulation* 1998;97(16):1532-1535.
74. Bauce B, Daliento L, Frigo G, Russo G, Nava A. Pregnancy in women with arrhythmogenic right ventricular cardiomyopathy/dysplasia. *Eur J Obstet Gynecol Reprod Biol.* 2006;127:186-189.
75. Murray B, Tichnell C, James C, Tandi H, Calkins H. Pregnancy in arrhythmogenic right ventricular dysplasia/cardiomyopathy. *J Am Coll Cardiol.* 2013;62(20):191-192.
76. Iriyama T, Kamei Y, Kozuma S, Taketani Y. Management of patient with arrhythmogenic right ventricular cardiomyopathy during pregnancy. *J Obstet Gynaecol Res.* 2013;39(1):390-394.
77. Wang W, Cadrin-Tourigny J, Bhonsale A, et al. Arrhythmic outcome of arrhythmogenic right ventricular cardiomyopathy patients without implantable defibrillators. *J Cardiovasc Electrophysiol.* 2018;29:1396.
78. Cozzolino M, Perelli F, Corioni S, Carpinella G, Mecacci F. Successful obstetric management of arrhythmogenic right ventricular cardiomyopathy. *Gynecol Obstet Invest.* 2014;78(4):266-271.
79. Hodes AR, Tichnell C, Te Riele ASJM, et al. Pregnancy course and outcomes in women with arrhythmogenic right ventricular cardiomyopathy. *Heart.* 2016;102(4):303-312.
80. Gandjbakhch E, Varlet E, Duthoit G, et al. Pregnancy and newborn outcomes in arrhythmogenic right ventricular cardiomyopathy/dysplasia. *Int J Cardiol.* 2018;258:172-178.
81. Ruiz Salas A, Barrera Cordero A, Navarro-Arce I, et al. Impact of dynamic physical exercise on high-risk definite arrhythmogenic right ventricular cardiomyopathy. *J Cardiovasc Electrophysiol.* 2018;29(11):1523-1529.
82. Castrini AI, Lie H, Leren IS, et al. Number of pregnancies and subsequent phenotype in a cross-sectional cohort of women with arrhythmogenic cardiomyopathy. *Eur Heart J Cardiovasc Imaging.* 2019;20(2):192-198.
83. Anouar J, Mohamed S, Kamel K. Management of a rare case of arrhythmogenic right ventricular dysplasia in pregnancy: a case report. *Pan Afr Med J.* 2014;19:246.
84. Lopes LM, Pacheco T. A prenatal case of arrhythmogenic right ventricular dysplasia. *Arq Bras Cardiol.* 2018;110(2):201-202.
85. Honda T, Kanai Y, Ohno S, et al. Fetal arrhythmogenic right ventricular cardiomyopathy with double mutations in TMEM43. *Pediatr Int.* 2016;58(5):409-411.
86. Matsuoka Y, Kawaguchi K, Okishima T, Hayakawa K. An infant with suspected right ventricular dysplasia presenting unique ventriculograms. 1988;11(1):55-58.
87. Makanda A, Trémouroux-Wattiez M, Stijns-Cailteux M, de Jonghe D, Moretto M, Vliers A. Arrhythmogenic dysplasia of the right ventricle in a 16-month-old child. *Arch Mal Coeur Vaiss.* 1989;82(5):811-814.
88. Patterson MW, De Souza E. Two-dimensional echocardiographic diagnosis of arrhythmogenic right ventricular dysplasia presenting as frequent ventricular extrasystoles in a child. *Pediatr Cardiol.* 1988;9(1):41-43.
89. Tomisawa M, Onouchi Z, Goto M, Nakata K, Mizukawa K, Kusunoki T. Right ventricular aneurysm with ventricular premature beats. *Br Heart J.* 1974;36(12):1182-1185.
90. Nava A, Thiene G, Canciani B, et al. Clinical profile of concealed form of arrhythmogenic right ventricular cardiomyopathy presenting with apparently idiopathic ventricular arrhythmias. *Int J Cardiol.* 1992;35(2):195-206; discussion 207.
91. Kuck KH. Arrhythmias in hypertrophic cardiomyopathy. *Pacing Clin Electrophysiol.* 1997;20(10 pt 2):2706-2713.
92. Monserrat L, Elliott PM, Gimeno JR, Sharma S, Penas-Lado M, McKenna WJ. Non-sustained ventricular tachycardia in hypertrophic cardiomyopathy: an independent marker of sudden death risk in young patients. *J Am Coll Cardiol.* 2003;42(5):873-879.
93. Zipse MM, Tzou WS. Sudden cardiac death in nonischemic cardiomyopathy: refining risk assessment. *J Cardiovasc Electrophysiol.* 2017;28(11):1361-1366.

94. Goland S, van Hagen IM, Elbaz-Greener G, et al. Pregnancy in women with hypertrophic cardiomyopathy: data from the European Society of Cardiology initiated Registry of Pregnancy and Cardiac disease (ROPAC). *Eur Heart J*. 2017;38(35):2683-2690.
95. Billebeau G, Etienne M, Cheikh-Khelifa R, et al. Pregnancy in women with a cardiomyopathy: outcomes and predictors from a retrospective cohort. *Arch Cardiovasc Dis*. 2018;111(3):199-209.
96. haman R, Varnava A, Hamid MS, et al. Pregnancy related complications in women with hypertrophic cardiomyopathy. *Heart*. 2003;89(7):752-756.
97. Pieper PG, Walker F. Pregnancy in women with hypertrophic cardiomyopathy. *Neth Heart J*. 2013;21(1):14-18.
98. Autore C, Conte MR, Piccininno M, et al. Risk associated with pregnancy in hypertrophic cardiomyopathy. *J Am Coll Cardiol*. 2002;40(10):1864-1869.
99. Tanaka H, Kamiya C, Katsuragi S, et al. Cardiovascular events in pregnancy with hypertrophic cardiomyopathy. *Circ J*. 2014;78(10):2501-2506.
100. Ashikhmina E, Farber MK, Mizuguchi KA. Parturients with hypertrophic cardiomyopathy: case series and review of pregnancy outcomes and anesthetic management of labor and delivery. *Int J Obstet Anesth*. 2015;24(4):344-355.
101. Regitz-Zagrosek V, Blomstrom Lundqvist C, Borghi C, et al. ESC guidelines on the management of cardiovascular diseases during pregnancy: the task force on the management of cardiovascular diseases during pregnancy of the European Society of Cardiology (ESC). *Eur Heart J*. 2011;32(24):3147-3197.
102. Elliott PM, Anastasakis A, Borger MA, et al. 2014 ESC guidelines on diagnosis and management of hypertrophic cardiomyopathy: the task force for the diagnosis and management of hypertrophic cardiomyopathy of the European Society of Cardiology (ESC). *Eur Heart J*. 2014;35(39):2733-2779.
103. Weber R, Kantor P, Chitayat D, et al. Spectrum and outcome of primary cardiomyopathies diagnosed during fetal life. *JACC Heart Fail*. 2014;2(4):403-411.
104. Hinton RB, Michelfelder EC, Marino BS, Bove KE, Ware SM. A fetus with hypertrophic cardiomyopathy, restrictive, and single-ventricle physiology, and a beta-myosin heavy chain mutation. *J Pediatr*. 2010;157(1):164-166.
105. Hill MG, Sekhon MK, Reed KL, et al. Intrauterine treatment of a fetus with familial hypertrophic cardiomyopathy secondary to MYH7 mutation. *Pediatr Cardiol*. 2015;36(8):1774-1777.
106. Lee TM, Hsu DT, Kantor P, et al. Pediatric cardiomyopathies. *Circ Res*. 2017;121(7):855-873.

The Anti-Ro/SSA Positive Pregnancy

Helena M. Gardiner • Bettina F. Cuneo

INTRODUCTION

This chapter focuses on aspects of pregnancy related to anti-Ro/SSA antibody–associated fetal cardiac diseases collectively known as cardiac neonatal lupus erythematosus (NLE). The cardiac manifestations include fetal atrioventricular (AV) block and myocardial disease.

The population prevalence of fetal AV block is approximately 1:15,000 live births.[1,2] Fetal AV block, a disease of the second trimester, develops in 2% to 3% of mothers who carry anti-Ro/SSA antibodies.[3-7] Although anti-Ro/SSA antibodies are present in various rheumatologic disorders including Sjogren syndrome and systemic lupus erythematosus, many of the mothers whose fetuses develop AV block are clinically asymptomatic.[8,9] Furthermore, in rheumatologic disorders, the risk of fetal AV block is independent of maternal disease severity.

Although rare, the burden of anti-Ro/SSA antibody–mediated fetal AV block is considerable as the perinatal mortality of 17% exceeds that for all noncardiac congenital anomalies combined. Furthermore, almost all survivors require lifelong cardiac pacing with its associated complications.[10] In addition, dilated cardiomyopathy, which occurs in 7% to 19% of AV block cases and can present in the perinatal period or in childhood, has a very poor prognosis[11-16] (see Part 3, Chapter 5).

It has been hypothesized that 3° AV block is the endpoint of sequential progression from normal rhythm to 1° then 2° AV block and culminating in 3° AV block **(FIG. 5.2.1)**. Once 3° AV block occurs, it is irreversible and normal rhythm cannot be restored. However, anti-inflammatory treatment during 1° or 2° AV block has, in some cases, restored normal rhythm.[12,17-23]

These findings have formed the basis for the multidisciplinary care of the anti-Ro/SSA antibody positive pregnant woman. Such care begins with the rheumatologist identifying mothers with anti-Ro/SSA antibodies and referring them to an obstetrician or maternal fetal medicine specialist for prenatal counseling. The goal of prenatal counseling is first, to identify mothers at high risk for fetal cardiac NLE either by anti-Ro/SSA antibody titers (see below) or by history of a previously affected fetus or child, and second, to formulate a surveillance plan with a maternal fetal medicine specialist or pediatric cardiologist that is cost-effective and clinically effective and identifies a window of opportunity for treatment that can be effective.

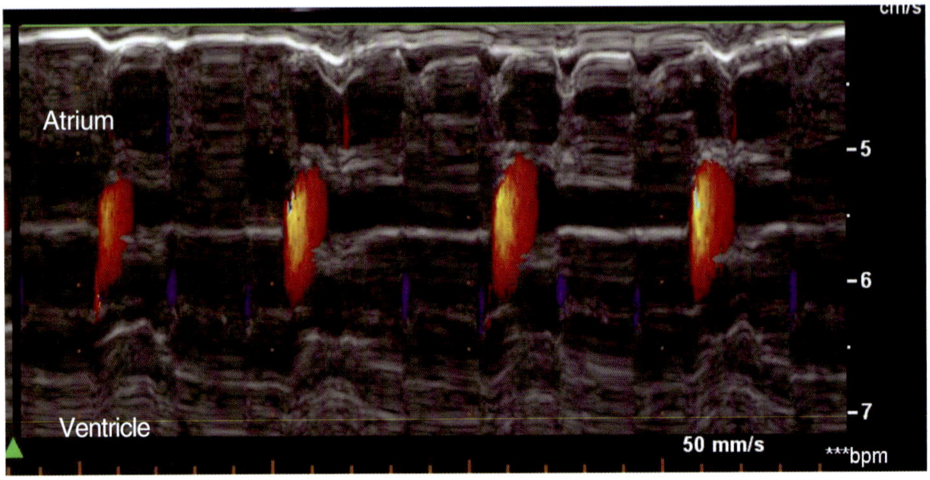

FIGURE 5.2.1 Color M-mode of 3° AV block. Atrial contractions (blue) occur regularly and independently of ventricular contractions (orange). AV, atrioventricular.

CARE OF THE ANTI-RO/SSA ANTIBODY POSITIVE MOTHER WITH NO PRIOR AFFECTED CHILD

While the risk of fetal anti-Ro/SSA–mediated disease increases after one affected child, the risk does not decrease after an unaffected child. Published recommendation for fetal surveillance is weekly or biweekly echoes on all anti-Ro/SSA antibody positive pregnancies from 17 to 26 weeks, in order to detect 1° or 2° AV block or early myocardial dysfunction (endocardial fibroelastosis or atrioventricular valve insufficiency).[24] However, recent fetal echo guidelines from the American Institute of Ultrasound in Medicine recommend fetal echo surveillance to be "considered" in anti-Ro/SSA positive pregnancies, and "indicated" only with a history of a cardiac NLE in a previous offspring.[25] In reality, clinical practice varies widely. Some obstetricians and pediatric cardiologist will not begin surveillance until after 18 weeks (when 3° AV block may already be established), some will perform weekly or biweekly ultrasounds/echoes, and some combine ultrasounds with home or office Doppler monitoring, while others have concluded surveillance is not helpful in preventing AV block and do nothing at all.[26]

CARE OF THE ANTI-RO/SSA ANTIBODY POSITIVE MOTHER WITH A PRIOR AFFECTED CHILD

The risk of recurrence with one affected child with either cardiac or cutaneous manifestations of NLE is as high as 18%.[3,4,10,27] Hydroxychloroquine has shown great promise in reducing the recurrence of fetal AV block[28] and is used by rheumatologists to prevent disease flare-up during pregnancy in women with systemic lupus erythematosus. It was recognized that women given this drug (400 mg/d) before 10 gestational weeks had a 10-fold reduction in recurrence of offspring affected with 3° AV block and zero fetal and childhood mortality compared to the 22% in those untreated.[29] A beneficial effect is supported by a lower prevalence of 3° AV block in current prospective studies in populations where this drug is in routine clinical use[30] and safety demonstrated in a histological report showing no cardiotoxicity in the fetal myocardium following its early administration.[31] These findings are encouraging and suggest prophylaxis with hydroxychloroquine may be the most effective drug with the lowest risk-benefit ratio to date.

In addition to prophylactic treatment with hydroxychloroquine, surveillance for the development of AV block in the pregnancy will still be needed, as in a prospective trial, the risk of recurrence is decreased, but not eliminated (J Buyon, personal communication).

Limitations of Current Surveillance for AV Block

For those with limited experience Doppler/M-Mode tracings of diagnostic quality are not always easy to obtain or interpret **(FIGS. 5.2.2** and **5.2.3)**. In addition, AV block is a complicated rhythm, and it is not always easy to distinguish 2° from 3° AV block, even with fetal magnetocardiogram (fMCG) **(FIG. 5.2.4)**. Errors in the interpretation of Doppler and M-mode traces reduce confidence in the results produced from some studies that have analyzed retrospective tracings without independent assessment of their quality. Weekly Doppler ultrasound screening of anti-Ro52 antibody–exposed fetuses has reported prolonged values of the AV interval in up to one-third, many of which resolved spontaneously either during fetal surveillance or after delivery.[32,33] One plausible explanation for this is that the Doppler measurement of the AV time interval includes the isovolumic contraction time (ICT) and intra-atrial conduction time. A prolonged AV interval may be secondary to either a prolonged ICT or intra-atrial conduction delay rather than AV block **(FIG. 5.2.5)**.[5,34] Furthermore, it may be difficult to measure an accurate AV interval if the mitral E- and A-waves are fused, which occurs in several clinical situations **(FIG. 5.2.2)**. This is supported by the results of a study that recorded Doppler AV time intervals and fetal ECG (fECG) PR intervals in a cohort of fetuses exposed to anti-Ro/SSA antibodies. In this study, a proportion of the fetuses with prolonged Doppler AV intervals had normal PR intervals measured by fECG and later confirmed on neonatal ECG.[35] In another study, fMCG PR intervals were on average 20 ms shorter than echo Doppler AV intervals in the same patient on the same day.[36]

Another limitation of the recommended weekly fetal echocardiograms is that they occur too infrequent to detect AV block, except serendipitously. In fact, weekly or biweekly echo surveillance, even in expert centers, has not been able to prevent the development of 3° AV block occurring between visits.[35,37,38] It seems that more frequent than once-a-week evaluation of fetal heart rate and rhythm is warranted. One option is fetal heart rate and rhythm (FHR) monitoring by the mother in the ambulatory setting, with confirmation of abnormal monitoring by echocardiography. Preliminary results suggest good maternal compliance and that very early administration of fluorinated steroids after maternal reporting may prevent progression to 3° AV block, while treatment delay of more than 24 to 36 hours appeared to be ineffective.[21,22,37] However, an irregular or slow fetal heart rate is not always the first presenting feature of cardiac NLE, and while FHR monitoring is feasible and well accepted by mothers, it has altered outcome in only a few cases.[21,22]

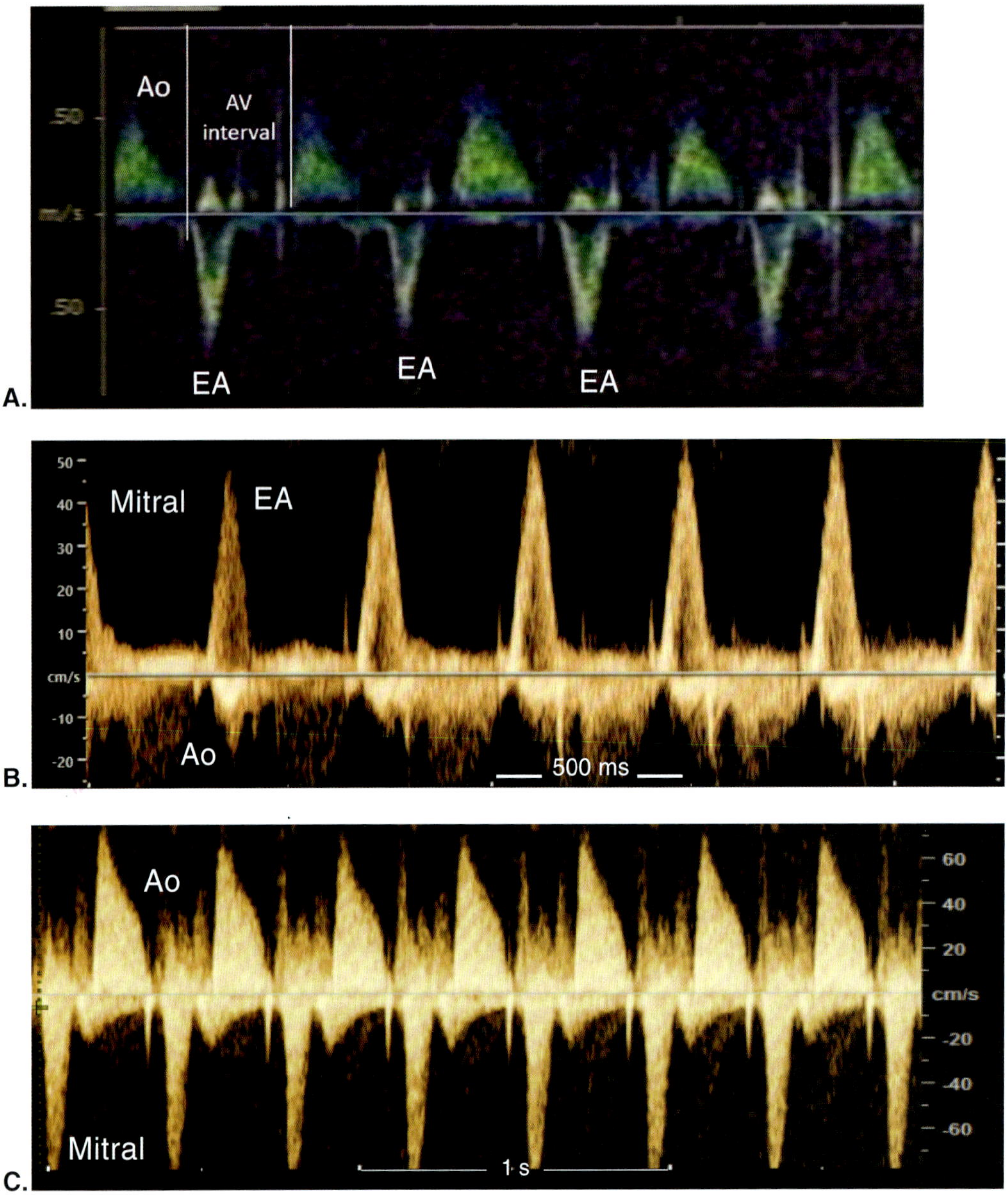

FIGURE 5.2.2 Three reasons for fused (or single) mitral inflow E- and A-waves. **A:** First-degree AV block. We suspect this occurs because as the AV interval prolongs the mitral A-wave moves toward the E-wave until they fuse. **B:** Fetal heart rates >160 beats per minute. Filling becomes biphasic when the fetal heart rate and rhythm slows. **C:** Severe LV dysfunction, for example in the recipient twin with twin to twin transfusion syndrome. Inflow time is reduced, resulting in fusion of the E- and A-waves. Ao, aorta; AV, atrioventricular; LV, left ventricle.

Therefore, the role of echocardiography in surveillance of anti-Ro/SSA antibody positive pregnancies may not be for arrhythmias, but to detect the early extra-nodal inflammatory response in cardiac NLE, including atrioventricular valve regurgitation, myocardial brightness, and endocardial fibroelastosis (FIG. 5.2.6) involving the atrial walls, atrioventricular junction, and the ventricles (FIG. 5.2.7). In fact, endocardial fibro-

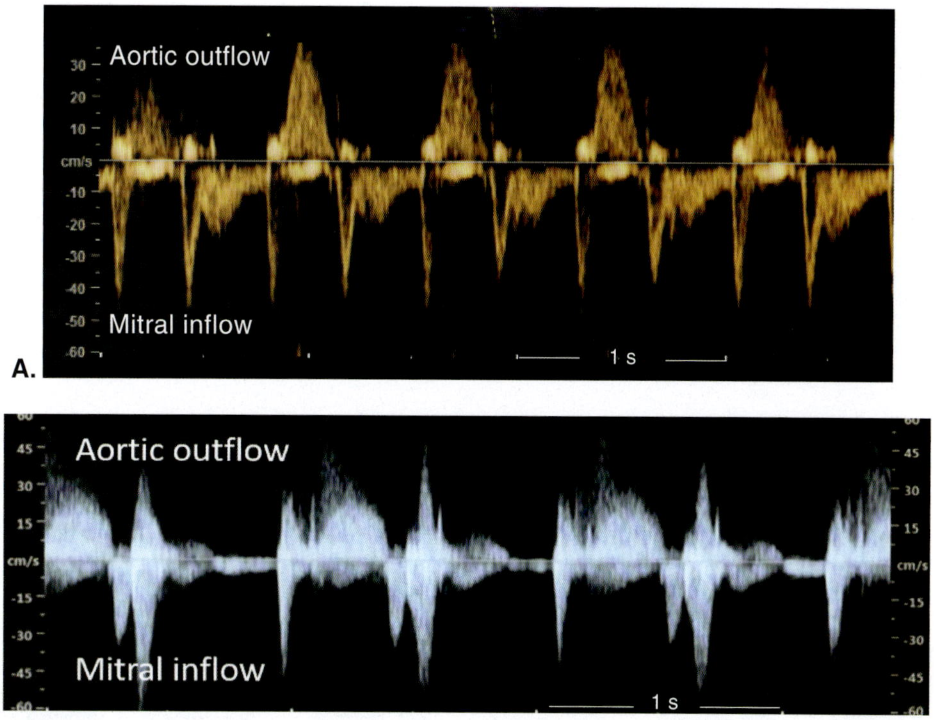

FIGURE 5.2.3 **A:** Blocked atrial bigeminy can be easily mistaken for **(B)** type 2, 2° AV block.

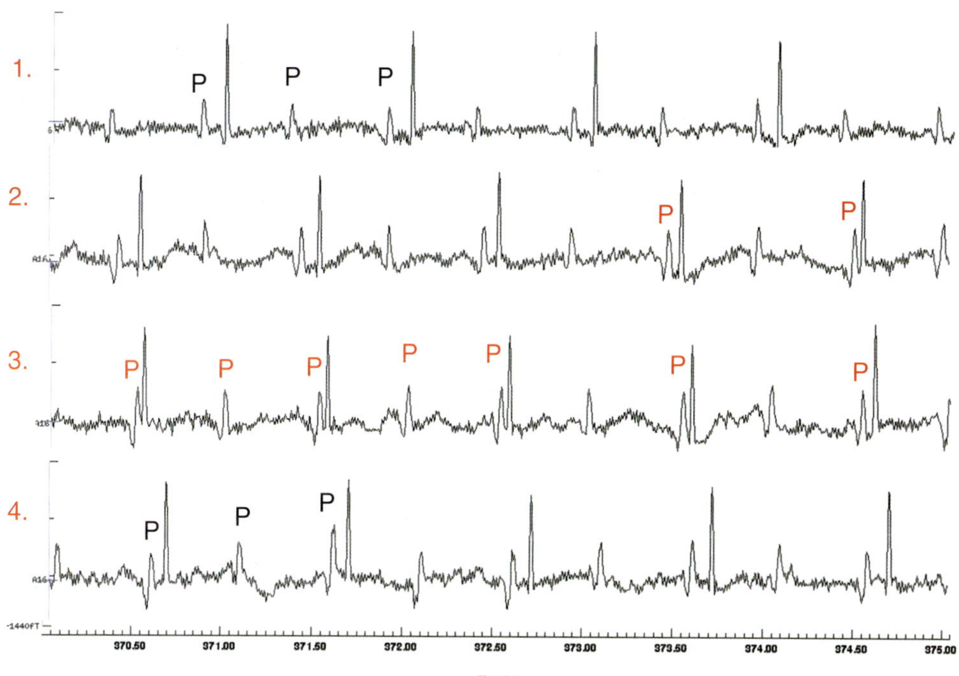

FIGURE 5.2.4 Fetal magnetocardiogram (fMCG) of a fetus with 2° AV block (black P-waves) and intermittent 3° AV block with accrochage (red P-waves). Accrochage refers to the tendency of dissociated atrial and ventricular rhythms to synchronize, and could be mistaken for 2° AV block. AV, atrioventricular.

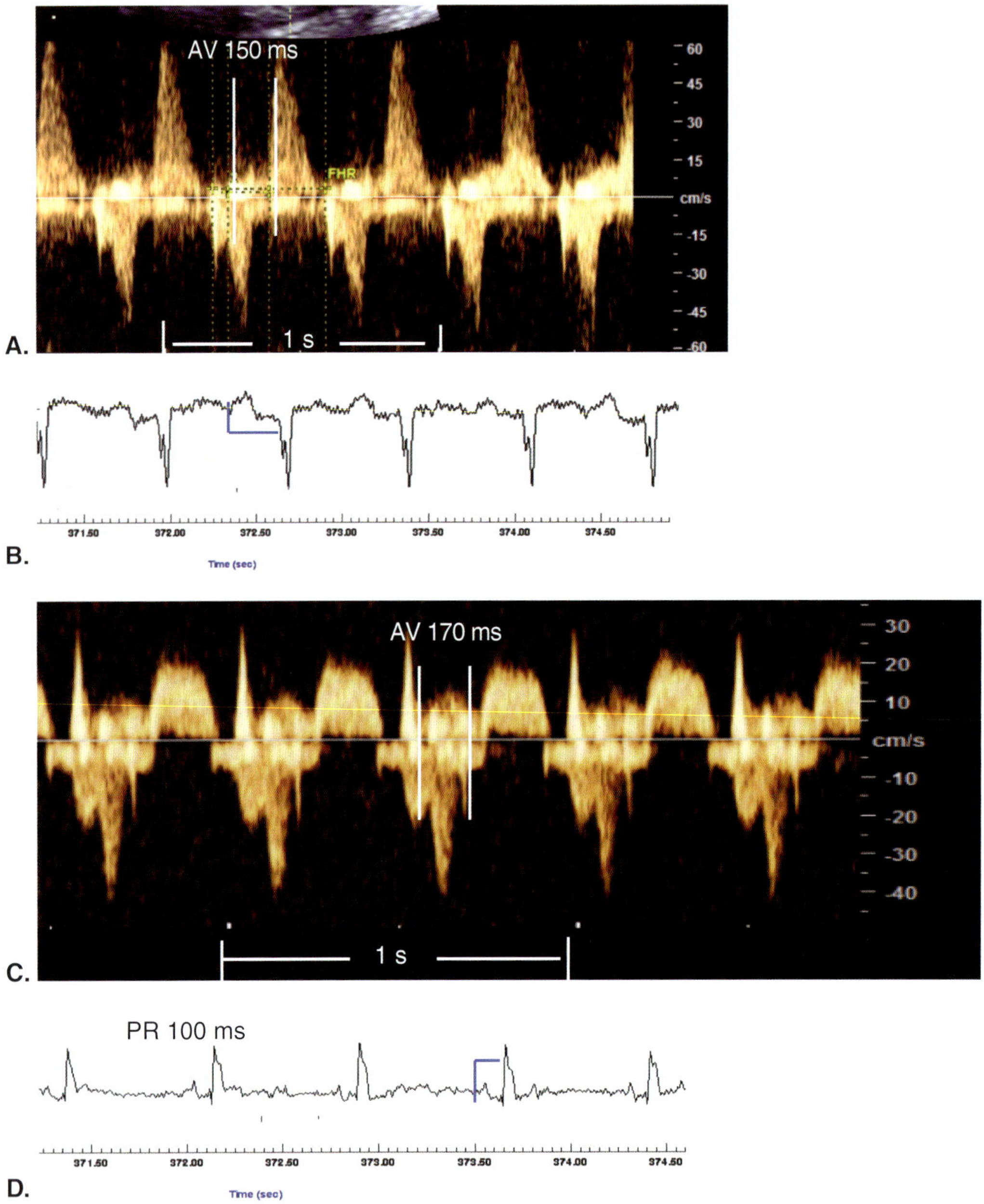

FIGURE 5.2.5 Mitral inflow and aortic outflow Doppler tracings of two fetuses with prolonged AV intervals and their respective fetal magnetocardiograms (fMCGs). **A** and **B:** The echo AV interval is 170 ms, but the fMCG PR interval is normal (100 ms). This fetus had ventricular dysfunction, and the prolonged echo AV intervals were due to a prolonged isovolumic contraction time, not conduction system disease. **C** and **D:** The prolonged echo AV interval (150 ms) was due to intra-atrial conduction delay as seen by the wide P-wave on the fMCG. AV, atrioventricular; FHR, fetal heart rate and rhythm.

elastosis and poor ventricular function have been reported at early fetal echocardiography, in combination with increased AV Doppler intervals (160-200 ms) preceding 3° AV block.[26] Extra-nodal (myocardial) disease and 1° AV block cannot be detected by home Doppler monitoring.

A.

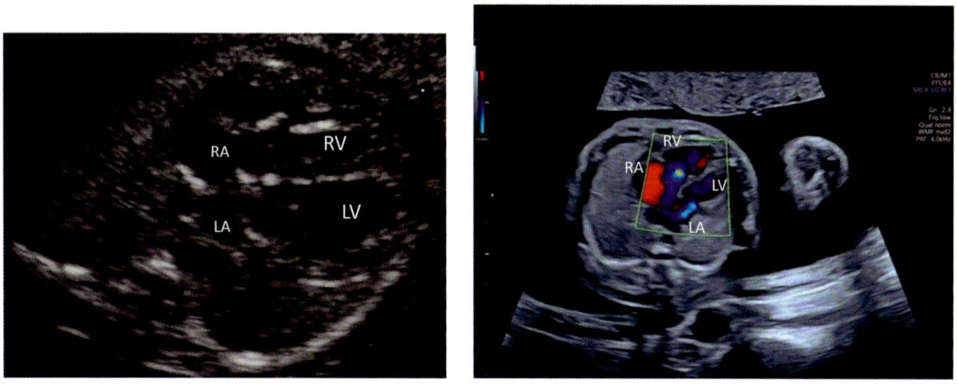

B.

FIGURE 5.2.6 Extra-nodal findings in NLE. **A:** Four chamber view showing patchy endocardial fibroelastosis in the atrial septum, the chordae of the mitral and tricuspid valves, and the intraventricular septum. **B:** Tricuspid and mitral insufficiency (blue color in the right atrium and left atrium, respectively. LA, left atrium; LV, left ventricle; RA, right atrium; RV, right ventricle.

Risk stratification by maternal anti-Ro/SSA antibody level may guide the need for surveillance regardless of the method.[37,39] A protocol surveilling only mothers with antibody titers ≤50 U/mL did not miss any cases of AV block, since all were found in the high-titer (>50 U/mL) group. A combination of limited echoes to detect myocardial NLE and frequent home Doppler monitoring to detect conduction system disease only in high-titer mothers may identify the optimal period for treatment to reverse disease and reduce costs of unnecessary surveillance **(FIG. 5.2.5)**. Further data are needed to support these findings in a larger population, but the early results are promising and may exclude a substantial number of pregnant anti-Ro/SSA positive women needing

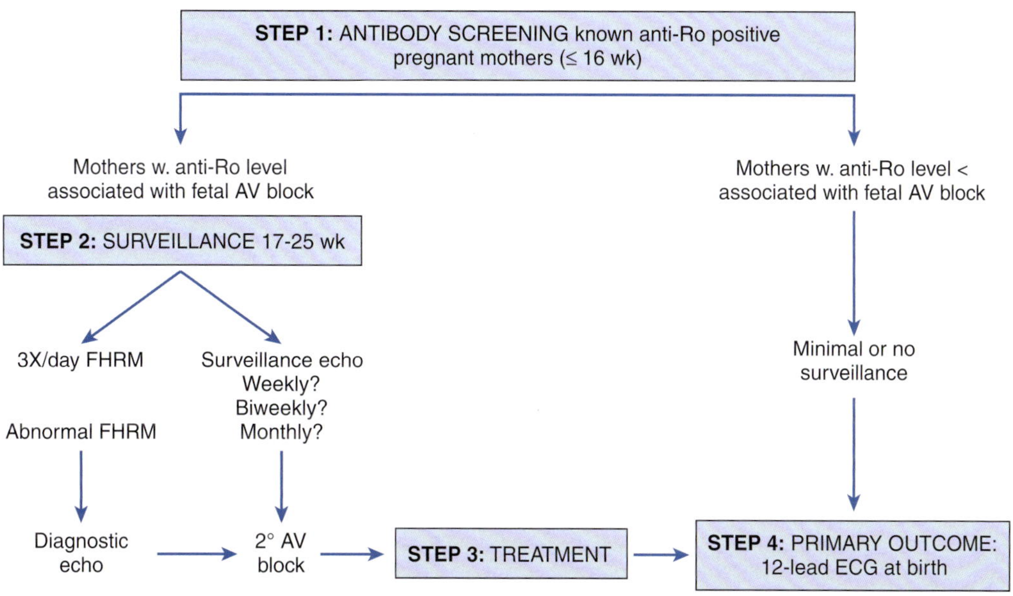

FIGURE 5.2.7 A protocol for management of the anti-Ro/SSA antibody positive pregnancy using antibody titers to risk stratify surveillance. The optimal frequency of echocardiograms in high-titer mothers is still in question. FHRM, fetal heart rate and rhythm monitoring.

surveillance. In recent single center study surveilling mothers from 18 weeks onward, not only was 3° AV block not prevented, but one case presented at 17 weeks. The authors concluded that they could not support the expense and efficacy of weekly surveillance of at-risk pregnancies.[38]

SUMMARY

Currently, optimal surveillance for fetal cardiac NLE has not been established by evidence-based protocols. Limiting surveillance to high-antibody-titer (≥50 U/mL) mothers, employing a combination of ambulatory Doppler monitoring with echo confirmation of abnormal FHR, and a minimum number of surveillance echocardiograms to detect myocardial disease during the risk period of 18 to 25 weeks seem like a reasonable approach, but only further studies can establish order from chaos.

References

1. Serdoz LV, Cappato R. Congenital complete atrioventricular block in the early pediatric population. *Heart Int.* 2006;2(1):1.
2. Siren MK, Julkunen H, Kaaja R. The increasing incidence of isolated congenital heart block in Finland. *J Rheumatol.* 1998;25(9):1862-1864.
3. Brucato A, Frassi M, Franceschini F, et al. Risk of congenital complete heart block in newborns of mothers with anti-Ro/SSA antibodies detected by counterimmunoelectrophoresis: a prospective study of 100 women. *Arthritis Rheum.* 2001;44(8):1832-1835.
4. Cimaz R, Spence DL, Hornberger L, Silverman ED. Incidence and spectrum of neonatal lupus erythematosus: a prospective study of infants born to mothers with anti-Ro autoantibodies. *J Pediatr.* 2003;142(6):678-683.
5. Costedoat-Chalumeau N, Amoura Z, Lupoglazoff JM, et al. Outcome of pregnancies in patients with anti-SSA/Ro antibodies: a study of 165 pregnancies, with special focus on electrocardiographic variations in the children and comparison with a control group. *Arthritis Rheum.* 2004;50(10):3187-3194.
6. Friedman DM, Kim MY, Copel JA, et al. Utility of cardiac monitoring in fetuses at risk for congenital heart block: the PR Interval and Dexamethasone Evaluation (PRIDE) prospective study. *Circulation.* 2008;117(4):485-493.
7. Gladman G, Silverman ED, Yuk L, et al. Fetal echocardiographic screening of pregnancies of mothers with anti-Ro and/or anti-La antibodies. *Am J Perinatol.* 2002;19(2):73-80.
8. Rivera TL, Izmirly PM, Birnbaum BK, et al. Disease progression in mothers of children enrolled in the Research Registry for Neonatal Lupus. *Ann Rheum Dis.* 2009;68(6):828-835.
9. Waltuck J, Buyon JP. Autoantibody-associated congenital heart block: outcome in mothers and children. *Ann Intern Med.* 1994;120(7):544-551.
10. Izmirly PM, Saxena A, Kim MY, et al. Maternal and fetal factors associated with mortality and morbidity in a multi-racial/ethnic registry of anti-SSA/Ro-associated cardiac neonatal lupus. *Circulation.* 2011;124(18):1927-1935.
11. Fredi M, Andreoli L, Bacco B, et al. First report of the Italian registry on immune-mediated congenital heart block (Lu.Ne Registry). *Front Cardiovasc Med.* 2019;6:11.
12. Levesque K, Morel N, Maltret A, et al. Description of 214 cases of autoimmune congenital heart block: results of the French neonatal lupus syndrome. *Autoimmun Rev.* 2015;14(12):1154-1160.
13. Mofors J, Eliasson H, Ambrosi A, et al. Comorbidity and long-term outcome in patients with congenital heart block and their siblings exposed to Ro/SSA autoantibodies in utero. *Ann Rheum Dis.* 2019;78(5):696-703.
14. Morel N. Incidence, risk factors, and mortality of neonatal and late onset dilated cardiomyopathy associated with cardiac neonatal lupus. *Int J Cardiol.* 2017;248:263-269.
15. Moak JP, Barron KS, Hougen TJ, et al. Congenital heart block: development of late-onset cardiomyopathy, a previously underappreciated sequela. *J Am Coll Cardiol.* 2001;37(1):238-242.
16. Nield LE, Silverman ED, Smallhorn JF, et al. Endocardial fibroelastosis associated with maternal anti-Ro and anti-La antibodies in the absence of atrioventricular block. *J Am Coll Cardiol.* 2002;40(4):796-802.

17. Doti PI, Escoda O, Cesar-Diaz S, et al. Congenital heart block related to maternal autoantibodies: descriptive analysis of a series of 18 cases from a single center. *Clin Rheumatol.* 2016;35(2):351-356.
18. Eliasson H, Sonesson SE, Sharland G, et al. Isolated atrioventricular block in the fetus: a retrospective, multinational, multicenter study of 175 patients. *Circulation.* 2011;124(18):1919-1926.
19. Friedman DM, Kim MY, Copel JA, Llanos C, Davis C, Buyon JP. Prospective evaluation of fetuses with autoimmune-associated congenital heart block followed in the PR Interval and Dexamethasone Evaluation (PRIDE) Study. *Am J Cardiol.* 2009;103(8):1102-1106.
20. Askanase AD, Friedman DM, Copel J, et al. Spectrum and progression of conduction abnormalities in infants born to mothers with anti-SSA/Ro-SSB/La antibodies. *Lupus.* 2002;11(3):145-151.
21. Cuneo BF, Ambrose SE, Tworetzky W. Detection and successful treatment of emergent anti-SSA-mediated fetal atrioventricular block. *Am J Obstet Gynecol.* 2016;215(4):527-528.
22. Cuneo BF, Sonesson SE, Levasseur S, et al. Home monitoring for fetal heart rhythm during anti-Ro pregnancies. *J Am Coll Cardiol.* 2018;72(16):1940-1951.
23. Saleeb S, Copel J, Friedman D, Buyon JP. Comparison of treatment with fluorinated glucocorticoids to the natural history of autoantibody-associated congenital heart block: retrospective review of the research registry for neonatal lupus. *Arthritis Rheum.* 1999;42(11):2335-2345.
24. Donofrio MT, Moon-Grady AJ, Hornberger LK, et al. Diagnosis and treatment of fetal cardiac disease: a scientific statement from the American Heart Association. *Circulation.* 2014;129(21):2183-2242.
25. AIUM practice parameter for the performance of fetal echocardiography. *J Ultrasound Med.* 2020; 39:E5-E15.
26. Carvalho JS, Chaour R, Copel J, et al. Management of anti-Ro/anti-LA affected pregnancies: is there a consensus? Results international survey. *Ultrasound Obstet Gynecol.* 2018;52:25-26.
27. Izmirly PM, Llanos C, Lee LA, Askanase A, Kim MY, Buyon JP. Cutaneous manifestations of neonatal lupus and risk of subsequent congenital heart block. *Arthritis Rheum.* 2010;62(4):1153-1157.
28. Costedoat-Chalumeau N, Amoura Z, Duhaut P, et al. Safety of hydroxychloroquine in pregnant patients with connective tissue diseases: a study of one hundred thirty-three cases compared with a control group. *Arthritis Rheum.* 2003;48(11):3207-3211.
29. Izmirly PM, Costedoat-Chalumeau N, Pisoni CN, et al. Maternal use of hydroxychloroquine is associated with a reduced risk of recurrent anti-SSA/Ro-antibody-associated cardiac manifestations of neonatal lupus. *Circulation.* 2012;126(1):76-82.
30. Izmirly PM, Kim MY, Llanos C, et al. Evaluation of the risk of anti-SSA/Ro-SSB/La antibody associated cardiac manifestations of Neonatal lupus in fetuses of SLE mothers exposed to hydroxychloroquine. *Ann Rheum Dis.* 2010;69:1827-1830.
31. Friedman D, Lovig L, Halushka M, Clancy RM, Izmirly PM, Buyon JP. No histologic evidence of foetal cardiotoxicity following exposure to maternal hydroxy chroloquine. *Clin Exp Rheumatol.* 2017;35(5):857-859.
32. Sonesson SE, Salomonsson S, Jacobsson LA, Bremme K, Wahren-Herlenius M. Signs of first-degree heart block occur in one-third of fetuses of pregnant women with anti-SSA/Ro 52-kd antibodies. *Arthritis Rheum* 2004;50:1253-1261.
33. Jaeggi ET, Silverman ED, Laskin C, Kingdom J, Golding F, Weber R. Prolongation of the atrioventricular conduction in fetuses exposed to maternal anti-Ro/SSA and anti-La/SSB antibodies did not predict progressive heart block. A prospective observational study on the effects of maternal antibodies on 165 fetuses. *J Am Coll Cardiol.* 2011;57:1487-1492.
34. Bergman G, Eliasson H, Bremme K, Wahren-Herlenius M, Sonesson SE. Anti-Ro52/SSA antibody-exposed fetuses with prolonged atrioventricular time intervals show signs of decreased cardiac performance. *Ultrasound Obstet Gynecol.* 2009;34(5):543-549.
35. Sonesson SE, Eliasson H, Conner P, Wahren-Herlenius M. Doppler echocardiographic isovolumetric time intervals in diagnosis of fetal blocked atrial bigeminy and 2:1 atrioventricular block. *Ultrasound Obstet Gynecol.* 2014;44(2):171-175.
36. Gardiner HM, Belmar C, Pasquini L, et al. Fetal ECG: a novel predictor of atrioventricular block in anti-Ro positive pregnancies. *Heart.* 2007;93:1454-1460.
37. Kan N, Silverman ED, Kingdom J, Dutil N, Laskin C, Jaeggi E. Serial echocardiography for immune-mediated heart disease in the fetus: results of a risk-based prospective surveillance strategy. *Prenat Diagn.* 2017;37(4):375-382.
38. Krishnan A, Arya B, Moak JP, Donofrio MT. Outcomes of fetal echocardiographic surveillance in anti-SSA exposed fetuses at a large fetal cardiology center. *Prenat Diagn.* 2014;34(12):1207-1212.
39. Jaeggi E, Laskin C, Hamilton R, Kingdom J, Silverman E. The importance of the level of maternal anti-Ro/SSA antibodies as a prognostic marker of the development of cardiac neonatal lupus erythematosus a prospective study of 186 antibody-exposed fetuses and infants. *J Am Coll Cardiol.* 2010;55(24):2778-2784.

Delivery Planning

Mary T. Donofrio • Alfred Abuhamad

INTRODUCTION

The prenatal diagnosis of fetal arrhythmias has improved perinatal outcomes in several ways (TABLE 5.3.1). First, treatment of incessant arrhythmias can decrease the risk of anticipated intrauterine heart failure. Second, risk stratification of arrhythmias optimizes several vital aspects of care, including delivery timing, mode and location, and postnatal management. Third, intrapartum care can be coordinated among obstetric, neonatal, and cardiology services, including pediatric electrophysiologists, cardiac intensivists, and cardiac surgeons as deemed appropriate by the risk and severity of the fetal condition (FIG. 5.3.1). Finally, delivery of a critical patient can be organized around a multidisciplinary call tree which is sent to the team when the fetus reaches a viable gestational age and then is activated when delivery is imminent. This type of communication ensures all key players are present, and care is coordinated at the time of delivery (FIG. 5.3.2).

TABLE 5.3.1 BENEFITS OF FETAL ARRHYTHMIA DIAGNOSIS

Rhythm	Action	In Utero Benefits	Delivery Time/ Location	Postnatal Care
Incessant SVA without hydrops	Rx	Reduce risk of hydrops	Term NSVD at cardiac center	Observation ± Rx
Incessant SVA with hydrops	Rx ± direct Rx	Reverse hydrops	Term NSVD at cardiac center	Observation ± Rx
VT or VT + 2° AV block	Rx Postnatal channelopathy testing	Reduce risk or reverse hydrops Identify affected family members	Term NSVD at cardiac center	Observation + Rx; consider device
Intermittent SVA	Observation	Reduce proarrhythmic risk from unnecessary Rx	Term NSVD at local site	Observation
Ectopy	Observation	Reduce family and provider anxiety	Term NSVD at local site	Observation
Evolving AV block, normal heart	Rx	May prevent progression to complete AV block or restore NSR	Term NSVD at local site	± continued Rx
CHB, normal heart	Rx	May prevent or improve DCM	Term CD at cardiac center	Consider device
CHB, CHD with heterotaxy	Rx	Postpone delivery until term or near term	Term delivery at cardiac center	Consider palliative care or device and palliation/repair

AV block, atrioventricular block; CAV block, congenital atrioventricular block; CHB, complete heart block; CHD, congenital heart disease; CS, caesarian delivery; NSVD, normal spontaneous vaginal delivery; NSR, normal sinus rhythm; Rx, treatment; SVA, supraventricular arrhythmia (tachycardia and atrial flutter); VT, ventricular tachycardia.

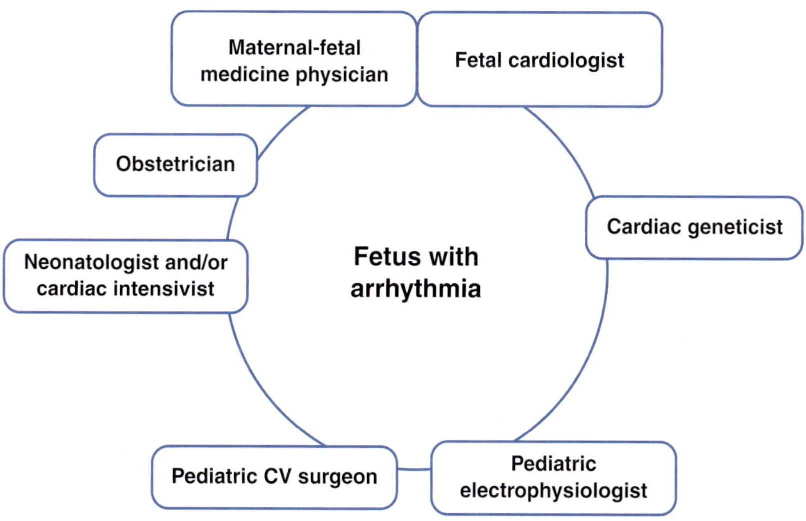

FIGURE 5.3.1 Team of physicians caring pre- and postoperatively for the fetus and neonate with arrhythmia. In addition to interacting with the mother and fetus, the team must cooperate and communicate with each other. CV, cardiovascular.

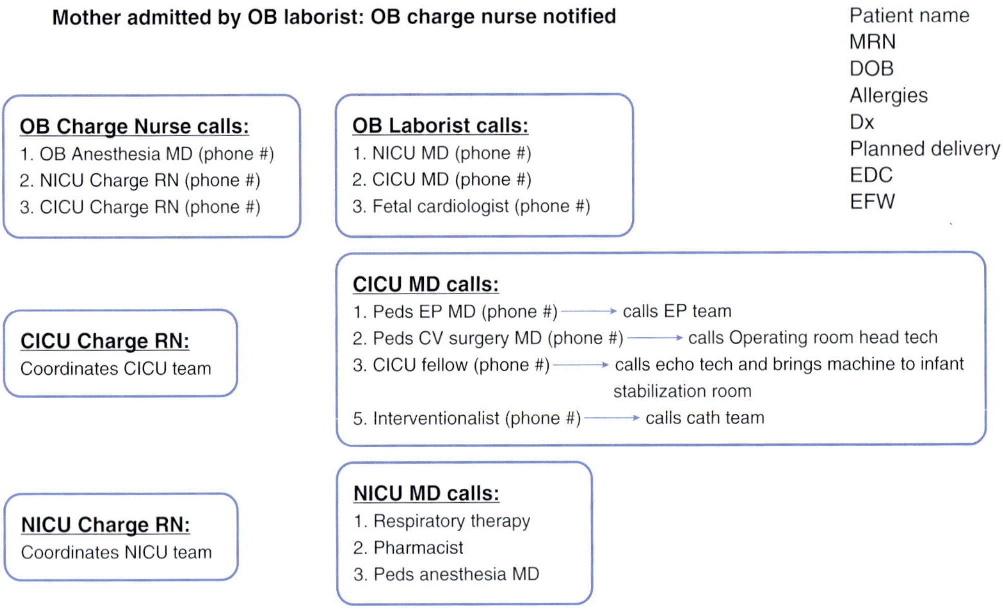

FIGURE 5.3.2 An example of a "call" or "phone tree" from a fetal care center with in-house laborists, obstetric and pediatric anesthesiology, and neonatal and cardiac ICU attendings. Details of the call tree will vary between institutions. Cath, cardiac catheterization; CICU, cardiac intensive care unit; CV, cardiovascular; DOB, date of birth, Dx, diagnosis, EDC, estimated date of confinement; EFW, estimated fetal weight; EP, electrophysiologist; MD, medical doctor; NICU, neonatal intensive care unit; OB, obstetrician; Peds, pediatric; RN, registered nurse.

INTRAPARTUM AND DELIVERY CONSIDERATIONS

Delivery Timing

The main goal of fetal arrhythmia management is to achieve a term delivery of a nonhydropic fetus in sinus rhythm. The timing of delivery must be balanced between the risks of prematurity and those associated with continuing the pregnancy, that is, the on-going risks of heart failure, potential adverse effects of medication, and the possibility of intrauterine demise. In general, delay of delivery until 39 completed weeks of gestation is desirable as neonatal outcomes are improved in both low-risk pregnancies and in those complicated by fetal cardiac abnormalities.[1-6] Even for the late preterm fetus with tachycardia-induced heart failure, in utero treatment may still be the best course of action, given that resuscitation of a hydropic newborn is challenging, and outcomes are poor. If heart failure progresses despite treatment, delivery should be considered.[7] Indications for an urgent delivery, regardless of gestational age, include an abnormal modified biophysical profile score (fetal tone, breathing, movement) (see Part 2, Chapter 1) or if the mother's health is at risk from HELLP syndrome (hemolysis, elevated liver enzymes, and low platelet count) or preeclampsia.

Assessment of fetal wellness is an important consideration for timing of delivery. Unfortunately, arrhythmias render the often used "cardiovascular profile score" (CVPS)[8] (TABLE 5.3.2) of limited usefulness as Doppler flow characteristics are abnormal

TABLE 5.3.2 CARDIOVASCULAR PROFILE SCORE

	Normal 2 Points	-1 Point	-2 Points
Hydrops	None	Ascites or pleural effusion or pericardial effusion	Skin edema
Venous Doppler (umbilical vein and ductus venosus)	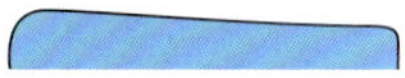 UV 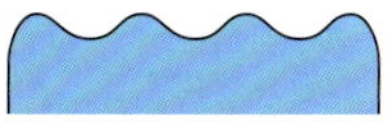 DV	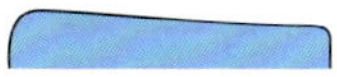 UV 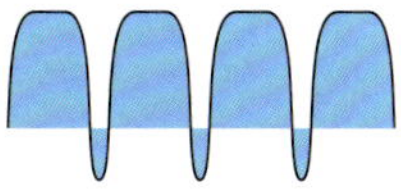 DV	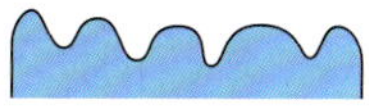 UV pulsations
Heart size (heart area/chest area)	>0.20 and <0.35	0.35-0.50	>0.50 or <0.20
Cardiac function	Normal TV and MV RV/LV FS > 0.28 Biphasic diastolic filling	Holosystolic TR or RV/LV S.F. < 0.28	Holosystolic MR or TR *dP/dt* < 400 or Monophasic filling
Arterial Doppler (umbilical artery)	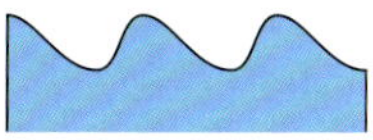 UA	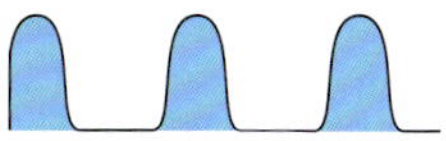 UA (AEDV)	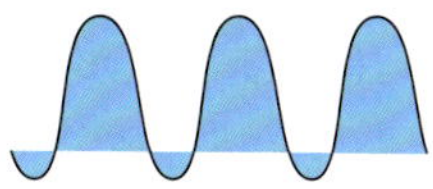 UA (REDV)

AEDV, absent end-diastolic velocity; *dP/dt*, change in pressure over time of TR jet; DV, ductus venosus; FS, ventricular fractional shortening; LV, left ventricle; MR, mitral valve regurgitation; MV, mitral valve; REDV, reversed end-diastolic velocity; RV, right ventricle; TR, tricuspid valve regurgitation; TV, tricuspid valve; UV, umbilical vein.
Note: CVP score is 10 if there are no abnormal signs and reflects two points for each of five categories: Hydrops, venous Doppler, heart size, cardiac function, and arterial Doppler.
Adapted from Hofstaetter C, Hansmann M, Eik-Nes SH, Huhta JC, Luther SL. A cardiovascular profile score in the surveillance of fetal hydrops. *J Matern Fetal Neonatal Med*. 2006;19(7):407-413.

with atrioventricular (AV) dissociation, AV block, or if the fetal heart rate (FHR) > 190 bpm (as seen in supraventricular and ventricular tachycardias). The CVPS can, however, be helpful in assessing cardiovascular well-being if there are brief periods of normal rhythm **(FIG. 5.3.3)**.

Delivery Mode

There are no studies evaluating the method of delivery and associated neonatal outcome for the nondistressed fetus with persistent arrhythmias; however, it is difficult to be assured of fetal well-being during labor in the presence of a sustained arrhythmia.[9] In addition, an already compromised fetus may become further distressed during labor because of reduced placental flow during uterine contractions.[10] Until other techniques of monitoring fetal well-being during labor are available, the preference will remain to deliver fetuses with persistent arrhythmias by cesarean delivery.[11-13] Thus, another impetus for pharmacologic conversion of near-term fetus with nonsinus tachycardia is to avoid an operative delivery. In a nationwide study of fetal arrhythmias in Japan, successful in utero treatment reduced the rate of cesarean delivery (30% vs. 71%), preterm birth (12% vs. 42%), and neonatal arrhythmias (49% vs. 78%).[13]

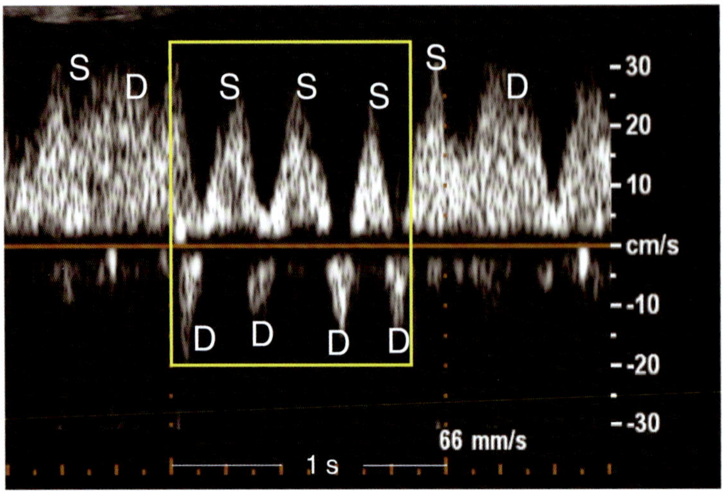

FIGURE 5.3.3 Pulsed Doppler tracing of the ductus venosus (DV) in a fetus with intermittent supraventricular tachycardia. During the brief period of normal rhythm, the DV flow pattern (both systolic [S] and diastolic [D]) is above baseline and is normal; though note that during tachycardia (yellow box), there is holodiastolic flow reversal.

Delivery Location

If postnatal treatment of a fetal arrhythmia is anticipated, delivery at or near a tertiary cardiac center should be considered as there is evidence that overall neonatal condition and outcomes are improved by delivery at centers with resources for monitoring, treatment, and intensive care for infants with rhythm disturbances.[12,14-16] Newborns with AV block and severe ventricular bradycardia have been shown to benefit from stabilization and isoproterenol infusion prior to neonatal pacing,[17-19] but even the neonate with AV block and a ventricular rate >70 bpm will need evaluation and monitoring. TABLE 5.3.3 shows the recommendations for delivery site location, timing of delivery, and recommended personnel in the delivery room. FIG. 5.3.4 is an example of a delivery setup anticipating the needs of a critically ill infant.

TABLE 5.3.3 DELIVERY RECOMMENDATIONS FOR THE FETUS WITH ARRHYTHMIA

LOC	Definition	Example CHD	Delivery Recommendations	Delivery Room Recommendations
P	Arrhythmia in which palliative care is planned	Fetus with arrhythmia and severe or fatal anomaly unlikely to survive	Arrange for family support/palliative care at local hospital	Normal delivery
1	Arrhythmia without predicted risk of hemodynamic instability	Atrial ectopy; ventricular ectopy with normal heart	Arrange cardiology consultation or outpatient evaluation at local hospital	Routine delivery room care, neonatal evaluation, and ECG
2	Arrhythmia with minimal risk of hemodynamic in delivery room but requiring postnatal cardiac care	Intermittent SVT, remote history of SVT on no meds and sinus bradycardia; all with structurally normal heart and no concern for channelopathy	Consider term (39 wk) induction at hospital with neonatologist and accessible cardiology consultation	Neonatologist in delivery room; postnatal rhythm monitoring and ECG
3	Arrhythmia with hemodynamic instability requiring specialty care for stabilization	Stable AV block with HR >60 bpm; recent SVT on treatment	Planned induction at 39 wk or cesarean delivery if AV block. Delivery at cardiac center	Neonatologist in the delivery room; cardiologist on site
4	Arrhythmia with expected immediate hemodynamic instability	Uncontrolled arrhythmias with hydrops, or severe ventricular dysfunction or abnormal BPP. Includes VT, SVT or AV block with HR < 50 bpm	Cesarean section at cardiac center with necessary specialists in delivery room	Immediate surgery for temporary pacing, electronic cardioversion, resuscitation, IV antiarrhythmic agents

AV block, atrioventricular block; bpm, beats per minute; BPP, biophysical profile score; ECG, electrocardiogram; IV, intravenous; SVT, supraventricular tachyarrhythmia; VT, ventricular tachycardia; wk, week. Modified from Donofrio MT, Moon-Grady AJ, Hornberger LT, et al. Diagnosis and treatment of fetal cardiac disease: a scientific statement from the American Heart Association. *Circulation*. 2014;129: 2183-2242.

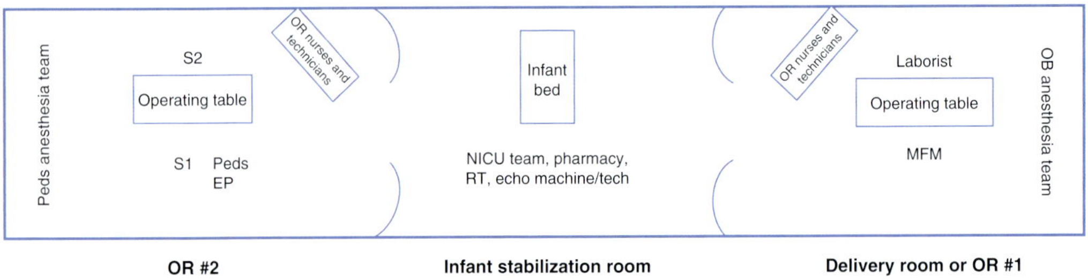

FIGURE 5.3.4 An example of the optimal delivery site for an infant anticipated to be critically ill with low cardiac output who will need immediate intervention. The infant is delivered by cesarean method in operating room #1 (which can also be a delivery room), then handed off to the neonatologist, evaluated briefly by the neonatal team and cardiologist in the infant stabilization room, then goes to operating room #2 where the surgical, anesthesia, and electrophysiology teams are waiting. Preparations should be made for resuscitation including managing the heart rate and improving cardiac output, including preparation for the use of extracorporeal membrane oxygenator (ECMO) if deemed appropriate. Based on the function and the heart rate, resuscitation should include medical treatment of the arrhythmia as well as low cardiac output. If the infant is in AV block with bradycardia that does not respond to isoproterenol, preparation should be made for placement of either a temporary or permanent epicardial pacemaker.

THE IMPORTANCE OF ACCURATE DIAGNOSIS

An accurate diagnosis of any arrhythmia is imperative before any considerations for delivery. Bradycardia can signify fetal hypoxia and acidosis, but it can also be a manifestation of long QT syndrome (LQTS) or benign and transient nonconducted premature atrial contractions. Typically, sinus bradycardia from hypoxia during labor is characterized by a 1:1 AV relationship and preceded by nonreassuring FHR patterns such as category 2 or 3 tracings[9,20] (see Part 2, Chapter 1). In contrast, sinus bradycardia noted early in gestation may suggest fetal LQTS or one of the inherited bradycardias. A history of an irregular rhythm preceding the bradycardia in the early third trimester suggests nonconducted premature atrial contractions, since new-onset bradycardia at this gestational age is unlikely to be AV block except with LQTS or in congenitally corrected transposition of the great arteries. In the case of tachycardia, delivery room care is more straightforward and successful if supraventricular arrhythmias (SVAs) with 1:1 AV conduction are differentiated from atrial flutter or ventricular tachycardia. The diagnosis, though not the etiology of the arrhythmia, can be made by echocardiography at the time the fetus presents.

Risk assessment for anticipated compromise in the delivery room is based largely on postnatal disease-specific clinical experience.[14] If it is expected that specialized delivery room care will be needed, planning of the delivery to include experienced specialists should be arranged to facilitate care with rapid intervention to control the rhythm and stabilize the circulation. Guidelines for pediatric cardiopulmonary resuscitation should be followed, including securing the airway and supporting ventilation and draining pleural and pericardial effusions that are hemodynamically significant.[21] Personnel at the delivery of an at-risk patient often include neonatologist(s) to resuscitate the infant, a pediatric cardiac intensivist, echocardiographer, and a pediatric electrophysiologist, along with their armamentarium.

Fetuses with arrhythmia benefit from intervention in the delivery room, particularly if delivery indications include impending heart failure, hydrops, or fetal distress.[11,12,15,16,22] Risks are high for the following:

1. The fetus with uncontrolled tachyarrhythmias
2. The fetus with AV block
3. The fetus with known or suspected channelopathy

In all three situations, a pediatric electrophysiologist is very helpful in the delivery planning.

Fetuses With Supraventricular Arrhythmias

Delivery Room Management

Supraventricular tachycardia (SVT) is the most common type of SVA. AV reciprocating (also called reentrant) tachycardia utilizing an accessory AV connection is the most common SVA mechanism[23,24] and results in a short RP tachycardia (FIG. 5.3.5A and Part 3, Chapter 3). Of note, unlike in childhood, atrial flutter (FIG. 5.3.5B) in the fetus and newborn may be due to an accessory AV connection and can occur with SVT in the same patient[23,24] (FIG. 5.3.6). Delivery discussion should include a plan for rhythm control in the delivery room, including options for electrical conversion to sinus rhythm

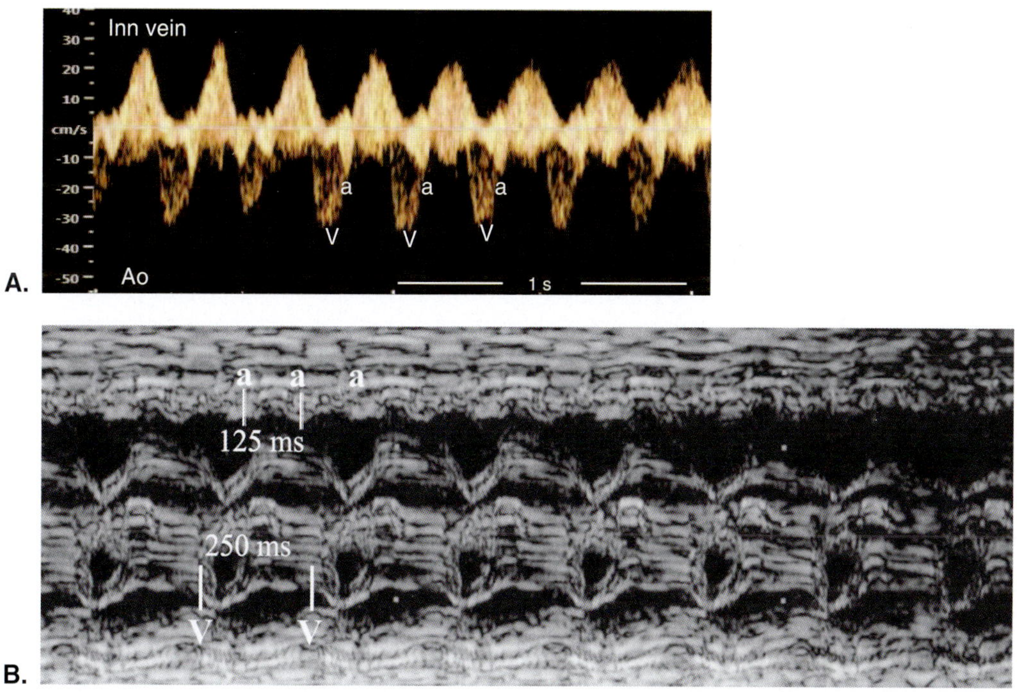

FIGURE 5.3.5 **A:** Spectral Doppler tracing of the innominate vein (Inn vein) and aorta (Ao) taken from the three-vessel tracheal view showing a short VA supraventricular tachycardia at a rate of 260 bpm. **B:** M-mode of ventricle (V) and atrium (a) of a fetus in atrial flutter. The atrial rate is 480 bpm and the ventricular rate is 240 bpm.

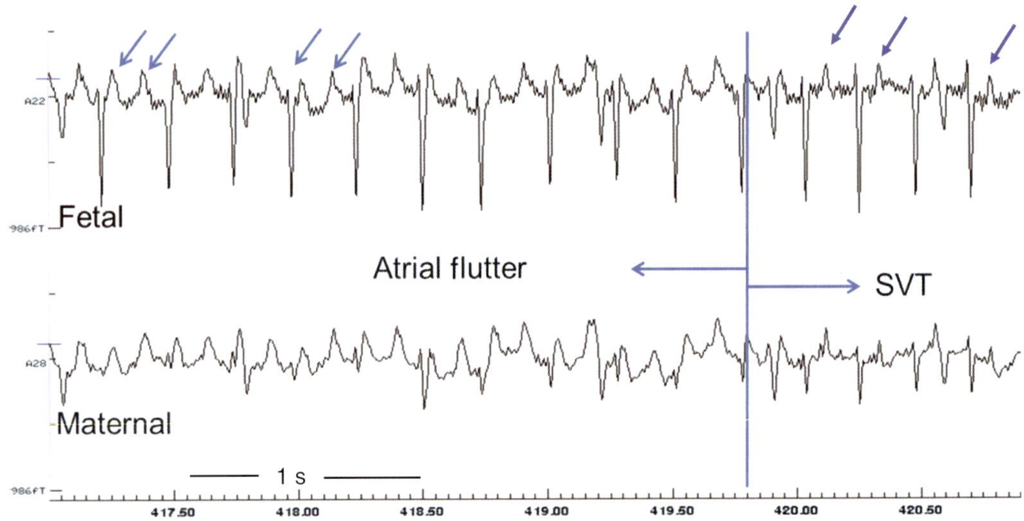

FIGURE 5.3.6 Continuous rhythm tracing from a fetal magnetocardiogram (fMCG) demonstrating a fetus with both atrial flutter with 2:1 conduction and supraventricular tachycardia (SVT) with 1:1 conduction. The atrial contractions are shown by the blue arrows.

or initiation of medications for rhythm control.[14] The urgency of intervention in the delivery room depends on the infant's hemodynamic condition. If the infant is hemodynamically stable, time should be taken to obtain an electrocardiogram (ECG) or rhythm tracing. Once intravenous access is obtained, adenosine can be given to terminate the SVA[25] **(FIG. 5.3.7)**. The baby should have ECG and blood pressure monitoring during drug administration to assess response. For SVA that is refractory to adenosine, intravenous esmolol may be used for a rapid beta-adrenergic blocking effect.[26]

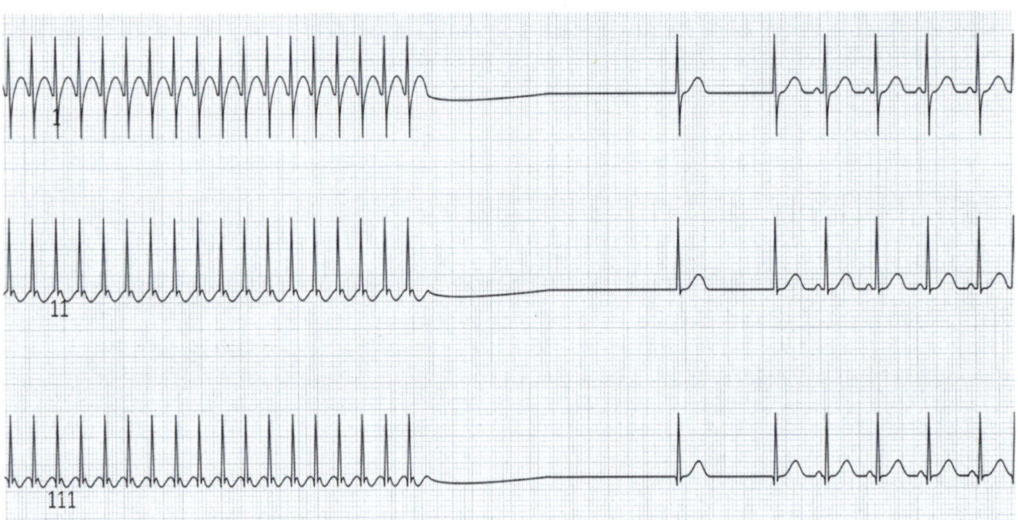

FIGURE 5.3.7 Postnatal rhythm tracing of an infant given adenosine in the delivery room. Note the period of asystole.

If medical treatment is unsuccessful, and particularly for the unstable neonate, synchronized DC cardioversion with 0.5 to 2 J/kg or transesophageal pacing can be considered, though for the latter, an electrophysiologist is needed to perform the procedure.[16,25] In rare instances, DC cardioversion may only result in temporary cessation of the tachyarrhythmia. If this occurs, medical treatment can be initiated, though consultation with a pediatric electrophysiologist is likely to result in more tailored management of the arrhythmia.

Once sinus rhythm has been restored, it is important to note that antiarrhythmic agents initiated in utero can lead to sinus node dysfunction either before delivery or following postnatal cardioversion. For this reason, some suggest that external pacing be available when a fetus with unsuccessfully in utero treatment of an SVA delivers.[16]

Postnatal Management

Admission for heart rhythm monitoring is recommended for newborns with a recent history of sustained tachyarrhythmias. Newborns may have depressed cardiac function even after conversion to sinus rhythm. Furthermore, most recurrences of fetal tachycardia are in the first 72 hours after delivery. However, there is no consensus regarding postnatal treatment after successful conversion of fetal tachycardia, given that a high percentage will not have recurrence.[16,25] Of note and a word of caution is that the postnatal arrhythmia diagnosis is not always the same as the prenatal diagnosis. In one study, the postnatal diagnosis was different than the presumed prenatal diagnosis in 14% of patients.[13] This suggests that confirmation of the arrhythmia mechanism by bedside monitoring or 12-lead ECG during tachycardia is needed before initiating postnatal treatment.

Fetuses With AV Block

Delivery Room Management

For fetuses with AV block (**FIG. 5.3.8**), planned intervention with chronotropic drug infusion and/or pacing in the immediate neonatal period or even in the delivery room has been shown to improve survival.[18,19,27] The management of AV block depends on multiple factors including whether there are associated fetal cardiac malformations which occur in ~40% of fetuses with AV block.[27,28] Fetuses with cardiac malformations, especially those with left atrial isomerism, are at significant risk of cardiac failure and hydrops, given their limited ability to maintain normal cardiac output (**FIG. 5.3.9**). Management of fetuses with AV block, with or without congenital heart disease, depends on the severity of bradycardia as well as the presence and severity of cardiac failure.[27-31] The risks of fetal compromise and hydrops are increased if the FHR is <55 bpm.[27,28,31] Newborns with AV block may be asymptomatic in utero and at birth or may present with symptoms of low cardiac output. Complications from premature delivery due to fetal compromise and hydrops in the presence of severe bradycardia increase the severity of illness, the complexity of management, and the likelihood of a poor outcome (see Part 3, Chapter 4).

Interventions in the delivery room for newborns with AV block with hydrops and/or FHRs <55 bpm include chronotropic and inotropic agents and preparation for temporary pacing. Central line placement and inotropic drug infusions, if necessary,

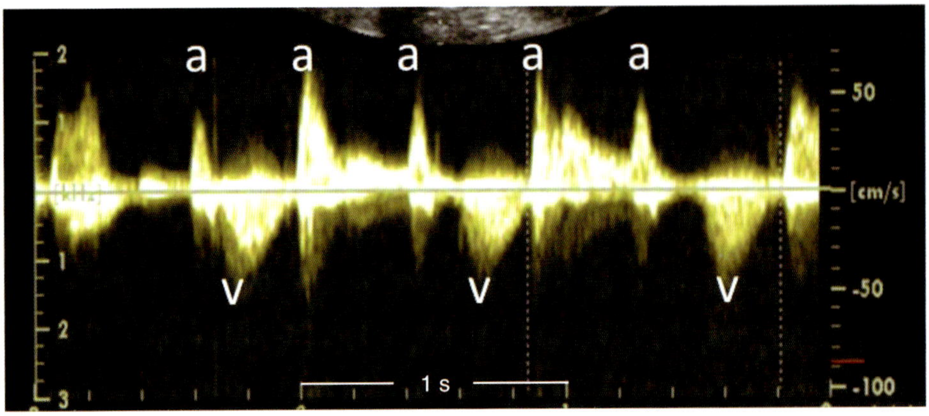

FIGURE 5.3.8 Mitral inflow and aortic outflow spectral Doppler of a fetus with complete AV block. Note the AV dissociation with a normal atrial rate (~150 bpm) that is faster than the ventricular rate (~60 bpm). a, atrial beat; v, ventricular beat.

should be started immediately, thus reducing the chances of hemodynamic instability. The beta-agonist isoproterenol, typically started at a dose of 0.1 µg/kg/min and titrated up for heart rate effect, is suggested to stabilize the infant. A left ventricle with endocardial fibroelastosis or a spongy myocardium does not always adapt to the rapid and sustained afterload increase when the umbilical cord is clamped, and if the heart rate cannot increase to compensate, cardiac output may fall. Once a profound metabolic acidosis develops from low cardiac output, effective myocardial stimulation for pacing may not be possible, thus it is suggested that pacing be available at the time of delivery. Temporary external pacing using defibrillator pads can be attempted for compromised newborns, though there may be technical difficulties, especially if the baby is premature and hydropic. Another potentially better option may be surgical placement of temporary pacing leads via either a small subxiphoid or anterior chest incision, performed in a second operating room adjacent to the obstetrical operating room (FIG. 5.3.4). If severe cardiac compromise is anticipated, the use of the ex utero intrapartum treatment (EXIT) procedure with immediate epicardial pacing has been reported.[32] In the single case, the decision to perform the EXIT procedure was based on that center's historical experience of two newborns dying with pulseless electrical activity within 30 minutes after delivery due to fetal compromise and persistent acidosis despite resuscitation and pacing.

Of note is that neonates with AV block and heart rates of >55 bpm, no congenital heart disease, and good heart function do not typically require immediate intervention in the delivery room though the presence of a neonatologist to initiate resuscitation is suggested in the event of unexpected neonatal compromise.

Postnatal Management

Even if the postnatal baseline heart rate is >55 bpm, it is suggested that neonates with AV block be monitored in an intensive care unit[16] in the first 1 to 2 days, given that occult acidosis may develop from low cardiac output. In the presence of associated congenital heart disease, a higher heart rate is required to maintain cardiac output.

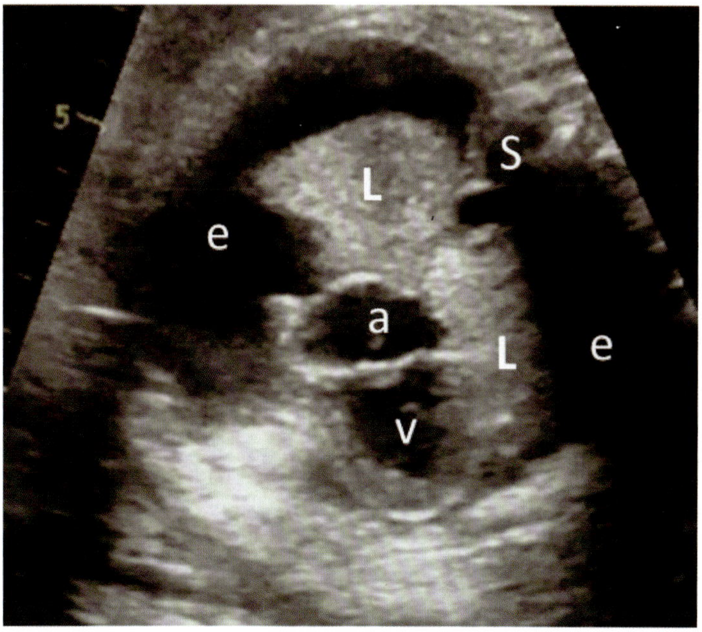

FIGURE 5.3.9 Fetal echocardiogram showing complex single ventricle with a spongy myocardium consistent with left atrial isomerism. Even at 24 weeks, there are large bilateral pleural effusions. A, common atrium; V, single ventricle; L, lung; e, pleural effusions; S, spine.

Early pacing of high-risk neonates with AV block may reduce the adverse consequences of bradycardia in the milieu of increasing metabolic demands after delivery. In one series, transcutaneous pacing was used in five newborns with 3° AV block that required pacing within hours of birth.[12] In another report,[18] 13 patients (9 with maternal anti-Ro/SSA antibodies and 4 with structural cardiac defects) were paced successfully in the first 24 hours of life. Eleven had temporary epicardial pacemakers, thus eliminating the immediate need to perform a larger-scale operation on a tenuous newborn. Two received permanent pacemakers as the initial intervention. A trend toward better outcome was seen in patients whose diagnosis was made before birth and in those in whom pacing was done in a planned manner immediately after birth based on prenatal findings.[18] Of the eight patients who were treated with a planned approach of fetal surveillance, scheduled delivery, and immediate placement of temporary pacing wires, only two deaths occurred in association with congenital heart disease. All patients with structurally normal hearts survived to permanent pacing and hospital discharge.

Fetal findings suggesting that pacing will be necessary in the first 24 to 48 hours of life include hydrops, fetal growth restriction, ventricular dysfunction, and very low FHRs with evidence of ventricular decompensation. Indications for pacing are discussed in Part 4, Chapter 2.

Fetuses With Known or Suspected Channelopathies

Most reports on delivery room management of the fetus with channelopathy relate to patients with known or suspected LQTS. The delivery room management is

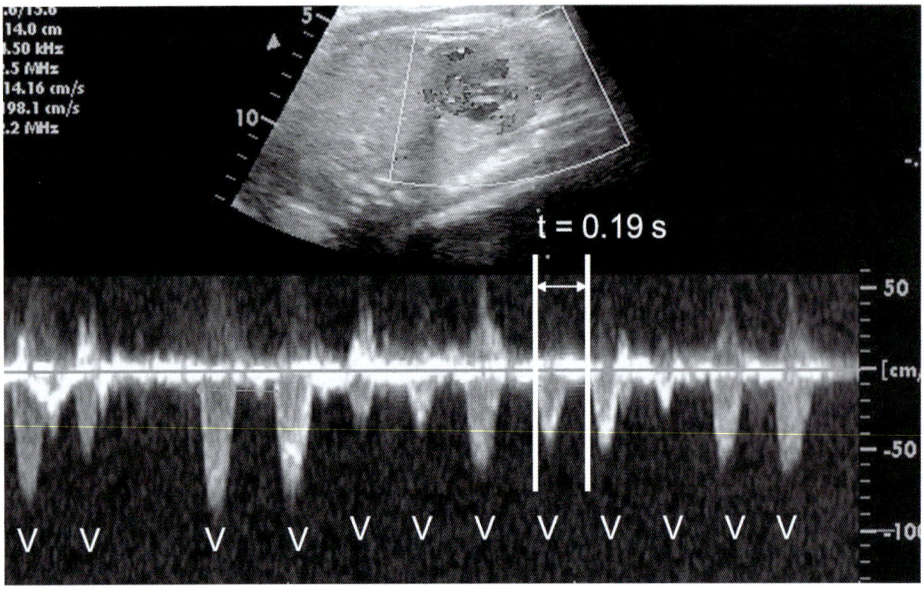

FIGURE 5.3.10 Fetus with long QT syndrome and ventricular tachycardia. Doppler tracing across aortic valve reveals a tachycardia (cycle length [CL] = 190 ms; heart rate = 315 bpm). Ventricular beats (v) have different velocities. This tracing is suggestive of torsades de pointes.

similar for infants with other channelopathies; however, most will not be symptomatic at birth. For fetuses suspected or known to have LQTS because of a low FHR or a family history who manifest only sinus bradycardia, medications that prolong the QT interval should be avoided or, in the case of oxytocin, used carefully and with fetal monitoring. A list of QT-prolonging medications can be found on the sudden arrhythmic death syndrome (SADS) website.[33] If functional 2° AV block or ventricular tachycardia (FIGS. 5.3.10 and 5.3.11) occurs in the setting of LQTS, in utero monitoring and coordination of delivery room care to include pediatric electrophysiologists may improve the likelihood of neonatal survival. The ventricular arrhythmia torsades de pointes that occurs with LQTS has been successfully treated before and after birth[34-36] (FIG. 5.3.12). The channelopathies are discussed in more detail in other chapters.

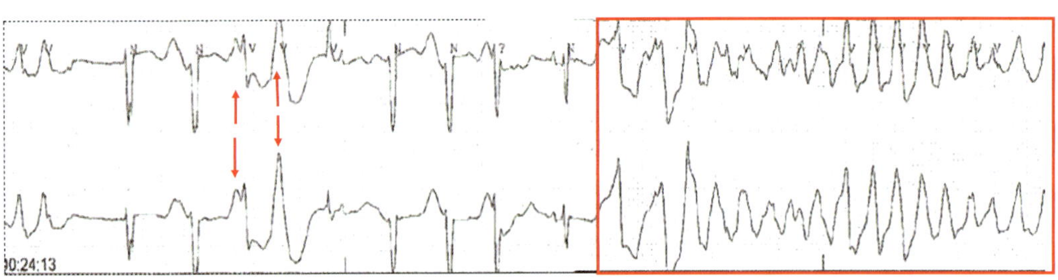

FIGURE 5.3.11 Postnatal rhythm strip in the delivery room showing premature ventricular contractions (red arrows, PVCs) and torsades de pointes in a newborn with no family history of long QT syndrome (LQTS).

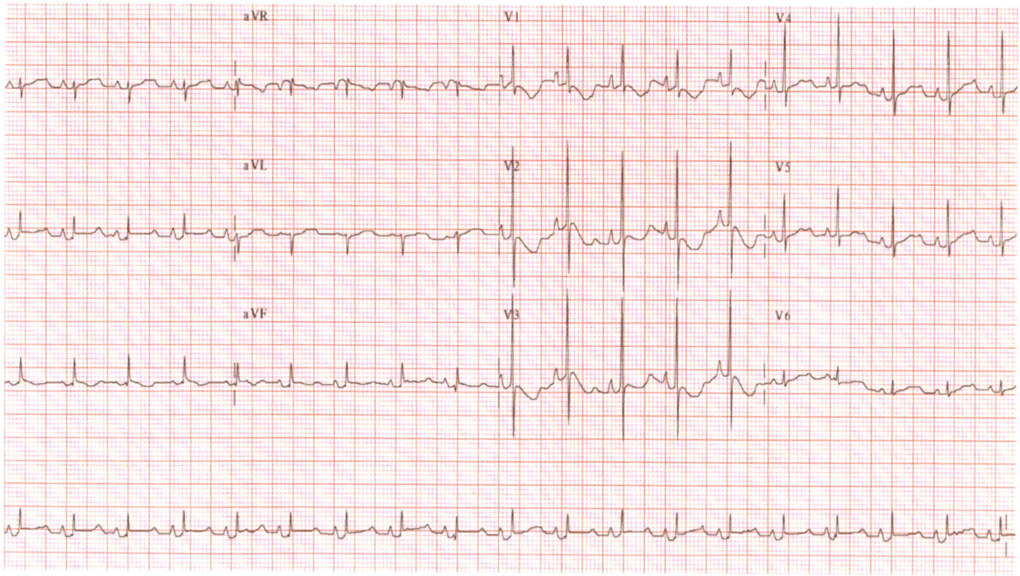

FIGURE 5.3.12 12-Lead ECG of the newborn after successful treatment with intravenous lidocaine, magnesium, and esmolol in the delivery room. The heart rate is 114 bpm, QT is 400 ms, and QTc is 536 ms. The infant had a de novo SCN5A R1623Q pathogenic variant.

SUMMARY

The main goal for the fetus with a clinically significant arrhythmia is a term delivery in sinus rhythm. If this goal is not achievable, the desired outcome is a successful transition of the fetus with arrhythmia to postnatal life. To maximize the likelihood of this outcome, in utero and delivery room care should be coordinated among specialists including obstetricians, maternal-fetal medicine specialists, neonatal and cardiology services, and other specialty teams. Care of the newborn infant should be planned and coordinated for immediate intervention post delivery to treat the arrhythmia and stabilize the circulation, with the overarching goal to minimize hemodynamic compromise and improve outcome.

References

1. Young PC, Glasgow TS, Li X, Guest-Warnick G, Stoddard G. Mortality of late-preterm (near-term) newborns in Utah. *Pediatrics*. 2007;119:e659-e665.
2. Bastek JA, Sammel MD, Paré E, Srinivas SK, Posencheg MA, Elovitz MA. Adverse neonatal outcomes: examining the risks between preterm, late preterm, and term infants. *Am J Obstet Gynecol.* 2008;199:367.e1-367.e8.
3. Cheng YW, Nicholson JM, Nakagawa S, Bruckner TA, Washington AE, Caughey AB. Perinatal outcomes in low-risk term pregnancies: do they differ by week of gestation? *Am J Obstet Gynecol.* 2008;199:370.e1-370.e7.
4. Chiossi G, Lai Y, Landon MB, et al. Timing of delivery and adverse outcomes in term singleton repeat cesarean deliveries. *Obstet Gynecol.* 2013;121:561-569.
5. Costello JM, Pasquali SK, Jacobs JP, et al. Gestational age at birth and outcomes after neonatal cardiac surgery: an analysis of the Society of Thoracic Surgeons Congenital Heart Surgery Database. *Circulation.* 2014;129(24):2511-2517.

6. Bentley JP, Roberts CL, Bowen JR, Martin AJ, Morris JM, Nassar N. Planned birth before 39 weeks and child development: a population-based study. *Pediatrics.* 2016;138(6):e20162002.
7. Maxwell DJ, Crawford DC, Curry PV, Tynan MJ, Allan LD. Obstetric importance, diagnosis, and management of fetal tachycardias. *BMJ.* 1988;297:107-110.
8. Hofstaetter C, Hansmann M, Eik-Nes SH, Huhta JC, Luther SL. A cardiovascular profile score in the surveillance of fetal hydrops. *J Matern Fetal Neonatal Med.* 2006;19(7):407-413.
9. American College of Obstetricians and Gynecologists. ACOG Practice Bulletin No. 106: Intrapartum fetal heart rate monitoring: nomenclature, interpretation, and general management principles. *Obstet Gynecol.* 2009;114(1):192-202
10. Jones NW, Raine-Fenning NJ, Jayaprakasan K, Mousa HA, Taggart MJ, Bugg GJ. Changes in myometrial 'perfusion' during normal labor as visualized by three-dimensional power Doppler angiography. *Ultrasound Obstet Gynecol.* 2009;33:307-312.
11. Jowett VC, Sankaran S, Rollings SL, Hall R, Kyle PM, Sharland GK. Foetal congenital heart disease: obstetric management and time to first cardiac intervention in babies delivered at a tertiary centre. *Cardiol Young.* 2014;24:494-502.
12. Mirlesse V, Cruz A, Le Bidois J, et al. Perinatal management of fetal cardiac anomalies in a specialized obstetric-pediatrics center. *Am J Perinatol.* 2001;18:363-371.
13. Ueda K, Maeno Y, Miyoshi T, et al. The impact of intrauterine treatment on fetal tachycardia: a nationwide survey in Japan. *J Matern Fetal Neonatal Med.* 2018;31(19):2605-2610.
14. Donofrio MT, Moon-Grady AJ, Hornberger LK, et al. Diagnosis and treatment of fetal cardiac disease: a scientific statement from the American Heart Association. *Circulation.* 2014;129:2183-2242.
15. Donofrio MT. Predicting the future: delivery room planning of congenital heart disease diagnosed by fetal echocardiography. *Am J Perinatol.* 2018;35(6):549-552.
16. Wacker-Gussmann A, Wakai RT, Strasburger JF. Importance of fetal arrhythmias to the neonatologist and pediatrician. *Neoreviews.* 2016;17:e568.
17. Cuneo BF, Lee M, Roberson D, et al. A management strategy for fetal atrioventricular block. *J Matern Fetal Neonatal Med.* 2010;23(12):1400-1405.
18. Glatz AC, Gaynor JW, Rhodes LA, et al. Outcome of high-risk neonates with congenital complete heart block paced in the first 24 hours after birth. *J Thorac Cardiovasc Surg.* 2008;136:767-773.
19. Donofrio MT, Gullquist SD, Mehta ID, Moskowitz WB. Congenital complete heart block: fetal management protocol, review of the literature, and report of the smallest successful pacemaker implantation. *J Perinatol.* 2004;24:112-117.
20. ACOG Practice Bulletin. Clinical guidelines for management for obstetrician- gynecologists. #116. 2010.
21. de Caen AR, Berg MD, Chameides L, et al. Part 12: pediatric advanced life Support. 2015 American Heart Association guidelines update for cardiopulmonary resuscitation and emergency cardiovascular care. *Circulation.* 2015;132:S526.
22. Johnson BA, Ades A. Delivery room and early postnatal management of neonates who have prenatally diagnosed congenital heart disease. *Clin Perinatol.* 2005;32:921-946.
23. Wacker-Gussmann A, Strasburger JF, Srinivasan S, Cuneo BF, Lutter W, Wakai RT. Fetal atrial flutter: electrophysiology and associations with rhythms involving an accessory pathway. *J Am Heart Assoc.* 2016;5(6):e003673.
24. Naheed ZJ, Strasburger JF, Deal BJ, Benson DW Jr, Gidding SS. Fetal tachycardia: mechanisms and predictors of hydrops fetalis. *J Am Coll Cardiol.* 1996;27(7):1736-1740.
25. Dubin AM, Triedman JK. Management of supraventricular tachycardia in children. In: Armsby C, ed. *Rapid Interpretation of EKGs.* https://www.uptodate.com/contents/management-of-supraventricular-tachycardia-in-children. Up to Date. 2018.
26. Cuneo BF, Zales VR, Blahunka PC, Benson DW. Pharmacodynamics and pharmacokinetics of esmolol, a short-acting beta-blocking agent, in children. *Pediatr Cardiol.* 1994;15(6):296-301.
27. Jaeggi ET, Hornberger LK, Smallhorn JF, Fouron JC. Prenatal diagnosis of complete atrioventricular block associated with structural heart disease: combined experience of two tertiary care centers and review of the literature. *Ultrasound Obstet Gynecol.* 2005;26:16-21.
28. Schmidt KG, Ulmer HE, Silverman NH, Kleinman CS, Copel JA. Perinatal outcome of fetal complete atrioventricular block: a multicenter experience. *J Am Coll Cardiol.* 1991;17:1360-1366.
29. Minassian VA, Jazayeri A. Favorable outcome in a pregnancy with complete fetal heart block and severe bradycardia. *Obstet Gynecol.* 2002;100:1087-1089.
30. Groves AM, Allan LD, Rosenthal E. Outcome of isolated congenital complete heart block diagnosed in utero. *Heart.* 1996;75:190-194.

31. Eronen M, Siren MK, Ekblad H, et al. Short- and long-term outcome of children with congenital complete heart block diagnosed in utero or as a newborn. *Pediatrics.* 2000;106:86-91.
32. Cuneo BF, Mitchell MB, Marwan AI, et al. Ex utero intrapartum treatment to ventricular pacing: a novel delivery strategy for complete atrioventricular block with severe bradycardia. *Fetal Diagn Ther.* 2017;42(4):311-314.
33. SADs Website for Credible meds.Com.
34. Cuneo BF, Ovadia M, Strasburger JF, et al. Prenatal diagnosis and in utero treatment of torsades de pointes associated with congenital long QT syndrome. *Am J Cardiol.* 2003;91(11):1395-1398.
35. Crimmins S, Vashit S, Doyle L, Harman C, Turan O, Turan S. A multidisciplinary approach to prenatal treatment of congenital long QT syndrome. *J Clin Ultrasound.* 2017;45(3):168-170.
36. Greene EA, Berul CI, Donofrio MT. Prenatal diagnosis of long QT syndrome: implications for delivery room and neonatal management. *Cardiol Young.* 2013;23(1):141-145.

PART

6

Fetal Arrhythmias: Future Directions

The Elusive Fetal Electrocardiogram

Helena M. Gardiner

INTRODUCTION

The major adverse pregnancy outcomes include intrapartum mortality at 0.35 per 1000 births; stillbirth affecting 4.1 per 1000 births a year; birth asphyxia occurring in about 2% of all deliveries contributing to cerebral palsy and lifelong handicap with high litigation costs per damaged child; and prematurity affecting about 5% of all pregnancies, and these adverse outcomes have changed little over the past 20 years.[1] In addition, insecurity of continuous fetal heart rate (FHR) monitoring during labor contributes to an increasing caesarean delivery rate, which is above 30% in many developed countries.

A reliable recording of fetal cardiac activity, the fetal electrocardiogram (fECG), could bring important advances into clinical practice, including noninvasive continuous monitoring of FHR; FHR variability and a reliable indication of hypoxemia during labor; long-duration monitoring "at home" during normal and pathological pregnancies (to provide greater insight into the mechanisms leading to growth restriction and stillbirth); and more accurate diagnosis of fetal arrhythmias to allow administration of the most effective drugs. These fundamental clinical issues remain challenging in the current era and continue to stimulate research to develop better technologies to solve them. As the heart's electrical signal is produced by events occurring at cellular level, it could provide information on mechanisms controlling cardiovascular responses and their neural interaction in the developing fetus, in both normal and pathological pregnancies. The current challenge is to detect the electrical signals produced by the developing fetus consistently and over long enough periods to gain a better understanding of the maturational processes occurring in normal pregnancy. Understanding these responses is the cornerstone to more sophisticated prediction of health and disease in the developing fetus. Furthermore, knowledge of the antecedents of stillbirth and birth asphyxia would increase our understanding of the potential for programming of the neuroendocrine systems that drive later responses and in turn may have important implications for personalized medicine in future years. However, there are major challenges, not yet completely resolved, that provide barriers to fECG acquisition and its implementation as an "at-home" monitoring system and as an improvement on the Doppler cardiotocogram (CTG) in pregnancy and during labor.

CLINICAL APPLICATION OF FETAL ECG

The important clinical parameters that can be recorded from the fetal heart's electrical signals include the basal FHR, its accelerations and decelerations, and heart rate variability. These parameters provide information about fetal well-being during pregnancy and labor. If the fECG morphology can be captured during pregnancy, its time intervals can be measured including atrial and ventricular rates; the P-, QRS-, and T-wave durations; and PR, QRS, and QT time intervals. These could provide information on physiological developmental changes, as well as fetal distress and, in cases of arrhythmias, more accurate assessment leading to improved treatment.

Current Methods of Fetal Heart Monitoring

The current methods of fetal heart monitoring include Doppler, electrocardiographic, and magnetocardiographic methods. Magnetocardiography, cooled by liquid helium, was developed during the 1990s to record and separate the small signals produced by the fetus from its environment, including the mother.[2] Developments in this tool will be discussed fully in Part 2, Chapter 3, while this chapter will discuss the Doppler and fetal ECG methods of monitoring and diagnosis.

DOPPLER METHODS OF FETAL HEART MONITORING

The most commonly used clinical method of FHR monitoring during pregnancy and in labor uses the Doppler principle to produce a semicontinuous recording of fetal cardiac activity, the CTG.[3,4] This method uses transducers mounted on an abdominal belt that emit a weakly focused ultrasound beam of about 1.5 MHz frequency directed toward the fetal thorax with the reflected ultrasound detected within the same transducer. The received signal is complex, including signals from the fetal heart walls and valves. This is demodulated and produces an audio signal, ranging from 200 to 1500 Hz, which the FHR algorithms process to assess periodicity (**FIG. 6.1.1A**). In order to avoid missing or creating heart beats, the algorithms set maximum and minimum heart rates to produce an averaged FHR. The processing is effectively similar to setting a low-pass filter.

Advantages and Limitations of Doppler Methods of Fetal Heart Monitoring

Although this is an inexpensive, portable technique and has been in use for decades, there are important practical drawbacks. The equipment uses belts that are cumbersome, and so the fetal heart trace is easily lost. Monitoring multifetal pregnancies is particularly complicated. Furthermore, the algorithms used in this Doppler technique produce an averaged FHR, and the resultant trace shows no beat-to-beat variability and has limited ability to assess accelerations and decelerations, an important parameter of fetal well-being. Additionally, the Doppler method cannot function reliably if there

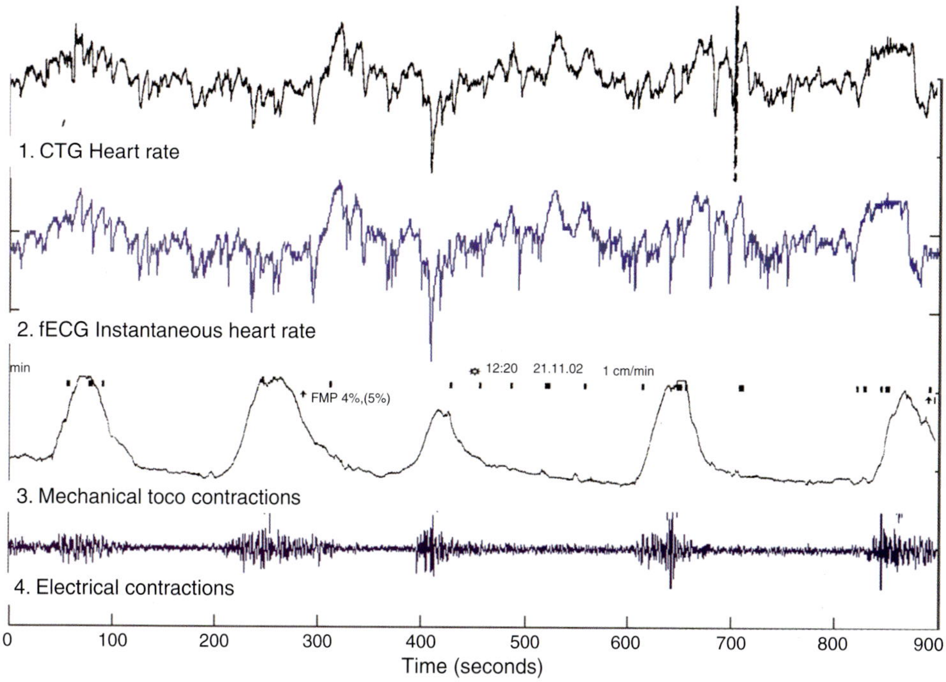

A.

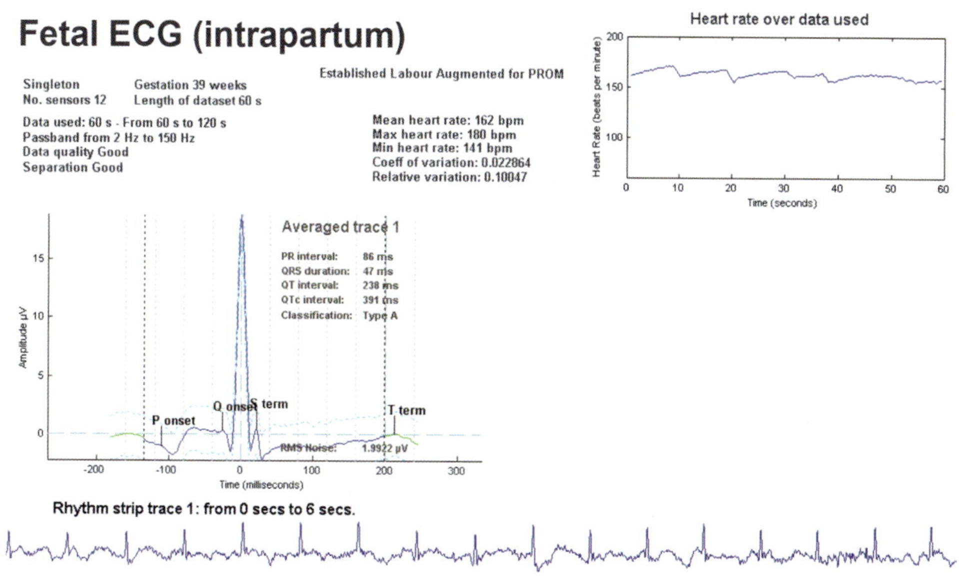

B.

FIGURE 6.1.1 **A:** A composite figure recorded during labor of a fetus at 39 weeks' gestation, comparing the cardiotocographic (CTG) signals with those of 12 maternal abdominal electrodes. The top line shows the averaged fetal heart rate (FHR) recorded by the CTG and the second line, the instantaneous FHR recorded by fECG. The third line shows the mechanical tocograph of uterine contractions and the electronic uterine signals in the fourth line. **B:** Fetal ECG recorded from the same 39-week fetus during labor showing instantaneous FHR, a 6-second strip of the rhythm and the averaged time intervals measured from a coherently averaged signal.

is more than one strong fetal signal as it may produce a doubled FHR or semblance of fetal tachycardia. These factors contribute to the difficulty in interpretation of the CTG, and experienced personnel are required to read the tracings and make clinical decisions affecting management of the pregnancy. Adverse pregnancy outcomes are frequently attributed to suboptimal monitoring and interpretation of fetal heart traces. Computerized CTG systems attempt to improve the interpretation of traces and provide guidance but cannot alter the deficiencies of the underlying Doppler technique.

ST Analysis Method of Fetal Heart Monitoring

A single scalp electrode inserted into the fetal scalp in labor has been shown capable of recording the fetal ECG. Components of the ECG trace are influenced by ion shifts, some of which are oxygen dependent, and alteration of the morphology of the ECG occurs in response to physiological stimuli such as hypoxemia.

There are several practical restrictions: this technique is invasive and only suitable for in-labor monitoring once the membranes have ruptured; the fetus must be in a cephalic presentation to allow access to the fetal scalp; and maternal movements are restricted because of the electrode. The development of this method is based on animal experiments that demonstrated that a reduction in oxygen led to an increase in adrenaline to induce glycogenolysis, which is accompanied by a potassium shift into the fetal myocardial cells. This was shown to alter their relaxation phase resulting in increased T-wave amplitude. ST analysis (STAN) has been assessed in combination with CTG monitoring to determine whether a change in fetal electrical signals can provide additional information to the CTG traces and improve assessment of fetal well-being. While the initial randomized controlled trial reported the combination of STAN and CTG resulted in a reduction in operative delivery and incidence of metabolic acidosis, the results could not be reproduced in other studies. There are several technical issues that contribute to the lack of reproducibility among which the one-dimensional presentation of the cardiac electrical activity and influence of fetal lie are the most important. In the 1960s, Larks described the normal fetal cardiac axis to lie between 100° and 160°, with a mean of 134° at term. The importance of fetal lie in assessing the electrical cardiac axis may be illustrated by the alteration of calculated axis in different fetal presentations. This report assumed the fetal presentation was cephalic and frontal, whereas the mean axis could be calculated to lie closer to 90° in the sagittal plane and a negative axis between 180° and 0° in a breech presentation.[5]

In the STAN technology, an event signaling possible fetal distress occurs if there is an alteration in the ratio of the baseline T-wave size relative to the QRS-wave (the T/QRS ratio) produced by potassium shifts at the cellular level. However, recognition and interpretation of such events are challenging: the propagation in the contraction (QRS) phase differs from that in the relaxation (T) phase, and the magnitude of alteration of the T/QRS ratio depends on the orientation of the electrical heart axis with reference to the fetal scalp electrode. If the fetal scalp lead is perpendicular to the fetal cardiac axis, the T-wave is of small amplitude producing low T/QRS values at baseline. However, if the fetal scalp lead is parallel to the fetal cardiac axis, the T-wave will be larger and produce higher T/QRS ratios at baseline. Thus for a similar fetal response to hypoxemia, the resultant potassium shift could produce very little change in the T/QRS axis if the scalp electrode is perpendicular to the cardiac axis, yet trigger many events if they are parallel to each other.[6] The disadvantage of a single-axis recording system to detect the fECG is clear from its use during in-labor monitoring, but assessment of the signal still proves challenging, even using multichannel recorders.

METHODS OF SIGNAL ACQUISITION OF FETAL ECG

Historical Review of ECG Acquisition

TABLE 6.1.1 details the chronology of acquisition of the electrocardiogram.[7] The first human electrocardiogram recording from the body surface was by Augustus Desire Waller in 1887.[8] He also demonstrated that the electrical signals preceded muscular contraction, and that it was not essential for the electrodes to be applied to the subject's chest, but the ECG could be obtained from two peripheries (hands or feet) immersed in saline. Willem Einthoven developed these techniques further in 1902 using the string galvanometer to enable recognizable recordings of the P, QRS, and T components of the modern ECG waveform from a surface electrode.[9]

The first fetal ECG recording was made in 1906 by Cremer from various maternal sites including a combination of vaginal and abdominal electrodes, as well as from large esophageal leads.[10] However, it was not until the 1950s that reports of human fetal ECG acquisition became more frequent: Smyth developed a silver wire electrode that could be attached directly to the fetus after membrane rupture in 1953,[11] and a year later, Davis and Meares reported successful fECG recording using a Grass Electroencephalograph in a 19-week fetus. They used a multilead system combining abdominal and vaginal electrodes.[12] In 1957, Southern published fECG time intervals recorded from maternal abdominal electrodes. He correlated P and PR time intervals with fetal oxygen saturation and bradycardic episodes and made observations on the ST segment.[13]

TABLE 6.1.1 SUMMARY OF ELECTROCARDIOGRAPHY MILESTONES

1887	First human ECG	A.D. Waller
1902	Surface lead ECG	W. Einthoven
1906	Esophageal ECG	M. Cremer
1933	Unipolar chest wall leads	F.N. Wilson
1936	Vector electrocardiography	F. Schellong
1938	Small triangle F (RA, LA, RL)	W. Nehb
1942	Unipolar amplified extremity leads	E. Goldberger
1956	Corrected orthogonal lead systems	E. Frank
1960	Intracardial leads	G. Giraud and P. Puech
1969	His bundle ECG	B.J. Scherlag

Adapted from Lewalter T, Lüderitz B. Historical milestones of electrical signal recording and analysis. In: Gussak I, Antzelevitch C, Hammill SC, Shen WK, Bjerregaard P, eds. *Cardiac Repolarization. Contemporary Cardiology*.Totowa, NJ: Humana Press;2003.

However, the intense filtering required to separate the fECG from maternal signals used at that time is likely to have reduced the quality of the fECG morphology. Concurrently, intrapartum recordings were also made by placing electrodes within the uterine cavity following rupture of the membranes.[14,15] During the 1960s and 1970s, attempts were made to obtain fECG from maternally sited abdominal electrodes. However, intensive high-pass filtering of the mixed maternal and fetal signal from abdominal electrodes usually led to loss of P- and T-waves from the fECG, as noted previously by Smyth. The desire to monitor the fetal heart in early labor has resulted in a pragmatic approach: use of the averaged R-R interval acquired by Doppler in FHR monitoring that persists until the present day.

Hon reported on the use of the fetal scalp electrode in 1962 and worked on improving the signal-to-noise ratio, describing peaked biphasic P-waves and shortened PR intervals in cases of human fetal hypoxemia.[16] However, small sample size, the use of anencephalic fetuses, and inadequate computing power and filtering methods resulted in major difficulties with signal separation and a concern that responses of anencephalic fetuses to hypoxemia may not be the same as normal fetuses. The chances of detecting P- and T-waves within the fECG were first improved by using a bandwidth of 0.1 to 100 Hz to filter the abdominal signals.[17] However, research still failed to report the anticipated fECG changes (lengthening of PR or QR intervals and ST segment depression or T-wave inversion) in hypoxic subjects.[18,19] Continuing technical challenges into the 1970s resulted in conflicting data from animal studies, particularly in interpretation of the ST segment: some data finding the response to hypoxemia were an elevation of the ST segment and augmented T-waves[20,21]; the latter study corroborated the fECG findings with postmortem studies showing reduced neonatal myocardial glycogen and creatinine phosphate. Other researchers reported the response to hypoxemia manifests as ST segment depression and reversal of the T-waves and also demonstrating an elevated T/QRS ratio on postnatal ECG.[22,23] Only one human study during this era correlated fetal scalp electrode recordings with scalp blood and cord acid-base status after delivery, reporting lengthening of the corrected QT interval and T-wave inversion with fetal acidosis.[24]

As signal processing and computer power increased in the 1980s, large studies were performed in Gothenburg, Sweden, and in Nottingham and Plymouth in the United Kingdom. The changing relationship between FHR (R-R interval) and recorded PR interval in hypoxemia was described: the usual negative relationship in the healthy fetus became a positive one in the setting of fetal acidosis.[25] Building on these findings, the relationship between PR interval and FHR was explored further and termed the conduction index (CI). This manipulation of the data permitted adjustments to long-term fECG recordings during labor to allow for short-term fluctuations, such as blood sampling or catecholamine surges, and enabled more robust interpretation of the data. Improved filtering allowed more reliable separation of the maternal and fECG signals, while subsequent averaging of the fetal waveform allowed the full fECG signature to be demonstrated and time intervals measured off-line. A relationship between the QRS duration and growth restriction was first reported by Brambati and Pardi.[26] Continuing developments in computer power permitted automated analysis of signals, rather than measurement by human investigators and led to computerized measurement of the coherent averaged signal.[27]

Data produced from a range of studies were used to inform the T/QRS ratio, thus providing the platform for the later development of STAN analysis and underpinning studies comparing it with CTG.[28-30]

Current State of Fetal ECG Development

Methods of Signal Separation

There are a variety of fetal ECG extraction algorithms including matched filtering,[31] adaptive filtering and wavelet analysis,[32-34] blind source (signal) separation (BSS),[35,36] independent component analysis (ICA),[37] singular value decomposition,[38] and methods based on neural networks.[39] Adaptive filtering is a simple and fast method of fECG extraction but is affected by maternal ECG and general interference. Wavelet-based methods have shown promise, but appropriate selection of the maternal wavelet is essential to recognize the fetal and maternal ECGs. Traditional BSS methods only deal with steady non-Gaussian signals, and their robustness is limited in the presence of noise.[25] ICA is a newer BSS method with higher convergence and robustness and has been widely used in biomedical signal processing. The most frequently used linear ICA method is the FastICA algorithm, and it assumes that the source signals are statistically independent of each other. It is based on approximate negentropy and Newton iteration that reduces computation, but because the channels containing the separated source components are not fixed, it may require additional algorithms, such as sample entropy. Neural networks is a fast-developing field which holds future promise.

Publicly Available Datasets and Development of Algorithms

Successful filtering depends on many different factors: electrode number and their placement, fetal position, gestation age, and maternal factors. Therefore, there is a need to automate the filter optimization process, and many researchers use an automated generator producing standardized fECG signals to test the range of optimization processes.[33]

One research initiative, the PhysioNet/Computing in Cardiology Challenge 2013 made available three public noninvasive fECG databases and invited researchers to propose various signal processing techniques.[40]

Details of these databases are as follows:

1. The Daisy database constituted of eight channels (four abdominal and three thoracic) and the abdominal ECG lasting for 10 seconds and using a sampling frequency of 250 Hz.
2. The Non-Invasive Fetal Electrocardiogram Database, available on PhysioNet,[41] had a sampling frequency of 1 kHz from 55 multichannel abdominal ECG recordings taken from a single subject between 21 and 40 weeks of gestation, without reference annotations.
3. Abdominal and Direct Fetal Electrocardiogram Database, available on PhysioNet, sampling frequency of 250 Hz with 5 minutes of recordings from four abdominal channels in five women in labor (38-41 weeks of gestation) and a scalp fECG with sampling frequency of 1 Hz for reference.

Such initiatives have resulted in a series of publications reporting the ability of newer algorithms to separate the full fECG; however, in contrast, there are relatively few studies using human or animal experimental data.

Current Clinical Machines and Limitations

The coverage of signal detection, usually achieved by a large number and broad placement of electrodes over the maternal abdomen, is pivotal to the quality and success of fECG **(FIG. 6.1.2)**. Technical issues include the requirement for arrays of multiple sensors to extract the weak fetal cardiac signal of about 10 microVolts from the maternal ECG of about 100 μV. However, these array inputs are of overlapping frequency and require separation from interference in both the temporal and frequency domains, as well as separation from maternal physiological signals, such as ECG, electromyography (EMG), and respiration **(FIG. 6.1.1A)**. In addition, fetal motion during the signal recording period, morphological similarity between the maternal and fetal ECG (for example, during fetal bradycardia), and external noise all present challenges. Whole-body sensors have been proposed and are likely to provide high-quality recordings in the research setting.[42] However, most clinical fECG research has focused on the development of a tool that can be used for long-term monitoring throughout pregnancy as well as during labor **(FIG. 6.1.1)**. Commercial solutions report the use of three-lead fECG collector systems using five electrodes.

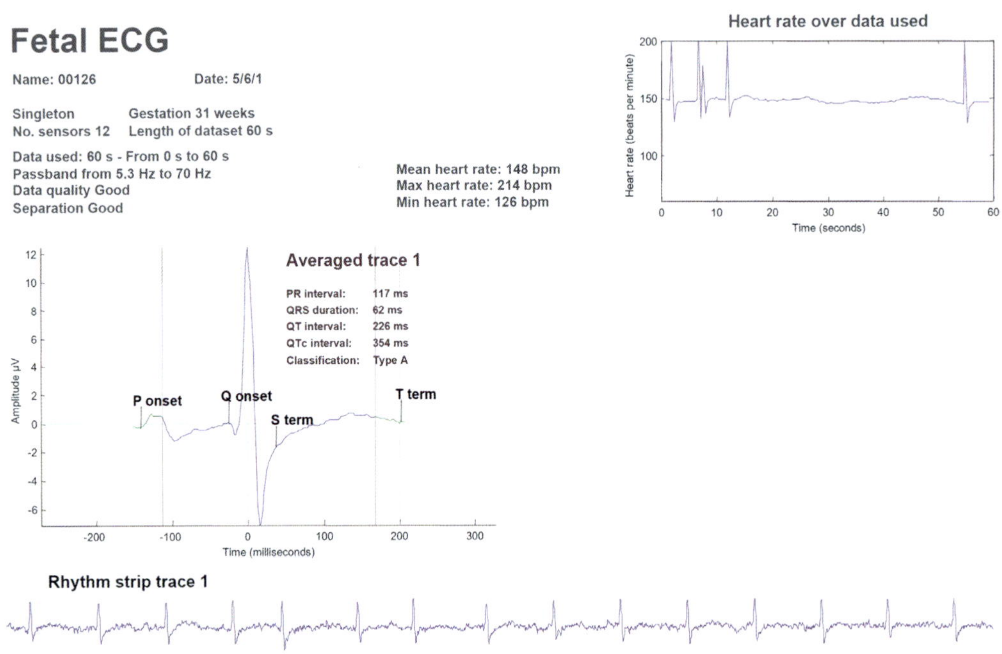

FIGURE 6.1.2 Fetal ECG recorded from 12 maternal abdominal electrodes in a 31-week fetus separated using blind source (signal) separation (BSS). This demonstrates instantaneous fetal heart rate over the recording, a 6-second rhythm strip extracted from the 60-second recording, and the averaged time intervals measured from a coherently averaged signal.

However, despite improved filtering techniques and computing power, this array is often inadequate to confidently detect P-waves and the ST segment because of a high noise-to-signal ratio. The most successful commercial product, the Monica AN24 Wireless Fetal Monitoring System, is an evolution of the Care 2000 system originating from Nottingham University.[27,43] It is based around five electrodes and an ambulatory signal recorder, allowing for the real-time separation of fECG for the determination of instantaneous heart rate. It has evolved as a mobile system that could be worn by women during their pregnancy. Many small studies of this device have shown it to be acceptable and feasible, but major drawbacks included loss of fetal signal, sometimes for 40% of the time worn, as well as reduced reliability in detection of the P- and T-waves.[44,45] The quality of recording was found better during nocturnal recordings when the mothers were still, as well as at later gestational ages. A recent study monitoring small-for-gestational-age fetuses confirmed these findings: overall success rate of FHR signals was only 48.6% and increased to 68.8% beyond 34 weeks' gestation, and success was greater at night.[46] Further developments have enabled this device to monitor the FHR in real time and display to the device via Bluetooth. However, the number of electrodes results in several intrinsic problems with signal acquisition that have resulted in display of the FHR but not the fECG waveform. The FEMO device[47] was also based around three electrodes, a reference, ground, and single channel. Skin preparation is required through the use of abrading tape and alcohol wipe to realize electrode impedance below 5 kΩ. The system is capable of real-time signal extraction with a delay of 0.06 seconds. The basis of the signal processing approach, like the Monica Healthcare system, is the subtraction of the maternal ECG component using double computation to reduce detection errors, particularly the elimination of fECG complexes coincident with subtracted maternal complexes, and to minimize the influence of baseline drift.

The Nemo prototype system for extracting the fECG (NEMO Healthcare BV, the Netherlands) uses eight electrodes on the maternal abdomen, placed in a fixed configuration. A ground and reference electrode are placed near the abdomen, and the six recording electrodes give bipolar signals containing a mix of signals. The fECG signals are digitized and stored, then processed off-line by PC-based dedicated signal processing techniques to retrieve the fECG. Future research aims to normalize the fECG for fetal orientation (based on a simultaneously performed ultrasound assessment of the fetal presentation) by calculating the vectorcardiogram (VCG) of the fetus. The VCG is a three-dimensional representation of the fetal electrical cardiac activity and can be used to calculate standardized fECG leads. Subsequent signal averaging of the fECG waveform allows semiautomatic detection of fECG segments and time intervals. Although a proposal to perform this research was published 3 years ago, no updates are available at this time.[48]

Home-based Monitoring

Smartphones are an ideal platform for home-based monitoring. Researchers have used simulated signals to test the ability of algorithms to extract the fECG for near-real-time monitoring of FHR using a smartphone and cloud-based databases. In one recent paper, a smartphone app was provided with a prerecorded three-channel abdominal ECG signal and the FastICA algorithm was used to separate the source components. The entropy of each sample was used as a measure of the strength of the fECG signal. The sampling frequency was 250 Hz, and the fECG extraction algorithm took approximately 1.5 seconds to process a batch of 400 data points, resulting in a lag of about 1.5 seconds to display the FHR on a smartphone interface. The software is capable of analyzing the heart rate for abnormalities, generating a warning and automatically uploading them to a cloud platform for clinical diagnosis.[49]

Another team has reported on the use of data from public databases widely used by the signal processing community known as the SISTA/DAISY dataset to test transmission of fECG signals via Bluetooth to a smartphone that would then upload the signals to a base station.[50] However, it is important to note that only FHR was extracted in these studies and not the full fECG waveform. Real-time monitoring of the morphological waveform of the fECG has not yet been demonstrated using these simulations, and no clinical studies using cloud-based analysis of fECG have yet been reported.

Current Commercially Available Products

To date, only two noninvasive fetal ECG devices have obtained FDA clearance and have published papers: the Monica AN24 monitor (Monica Healthcare, Nottingham, UK) and the MERIDIAN monitor from MindChild Medical (North Andover, MA). The Monica AN24 uses recordings from three electrodes and produces the FHR, albeit without detailed morphological information of the fECG to date and reports the best results during nighttime recordings when noise from maternal musculature is least. The MERIDIAN M110 monitor was designed for use in term labor and records FHR, uterine contraction, and maternal heart rate data.[51,52] One advantage is that it uses a range of electrodes, applied in strips that require no skin preparation; however, although it produces a reliable FHR derived from the R-R interval, no information on fECG morphology is produced. The technological limitations of current equipment limit the clinical information produced and present important barriers to their clinical utility. Recent innovations in connectivity potentially enable improved use of separated signals, but the essential major challenges remain: the small electrical fetal cardiac signals generated in a noisy environment and their propagation to sensors on the surface are uncertain and variable. Thus essential issues such as signal separation and the identification of an isoelectric line (from which to ascertain ST segment changes) remain challenging, and it is worthwhile comparing information from more recent clinical reports with those produced by research equipment and algorithms during the early 2000s, including the collaboration between a group of signal experts at QinetiQ and a fetal center team who published several fECG studies,[53-56] where the fECG signals were initially analyzed off-line and later in near real time. In 2003, the group described gestational age changes in time intervals from coherently averaged fECG signals in singleton pregnancies and signal separation in multifetal pregnancies (**FIGS. 6.1.3** and **6.1.4**). They described reduced performance during the 27- to 32-week gestational period with only 66% of traces successfully extracted, probably corresponding

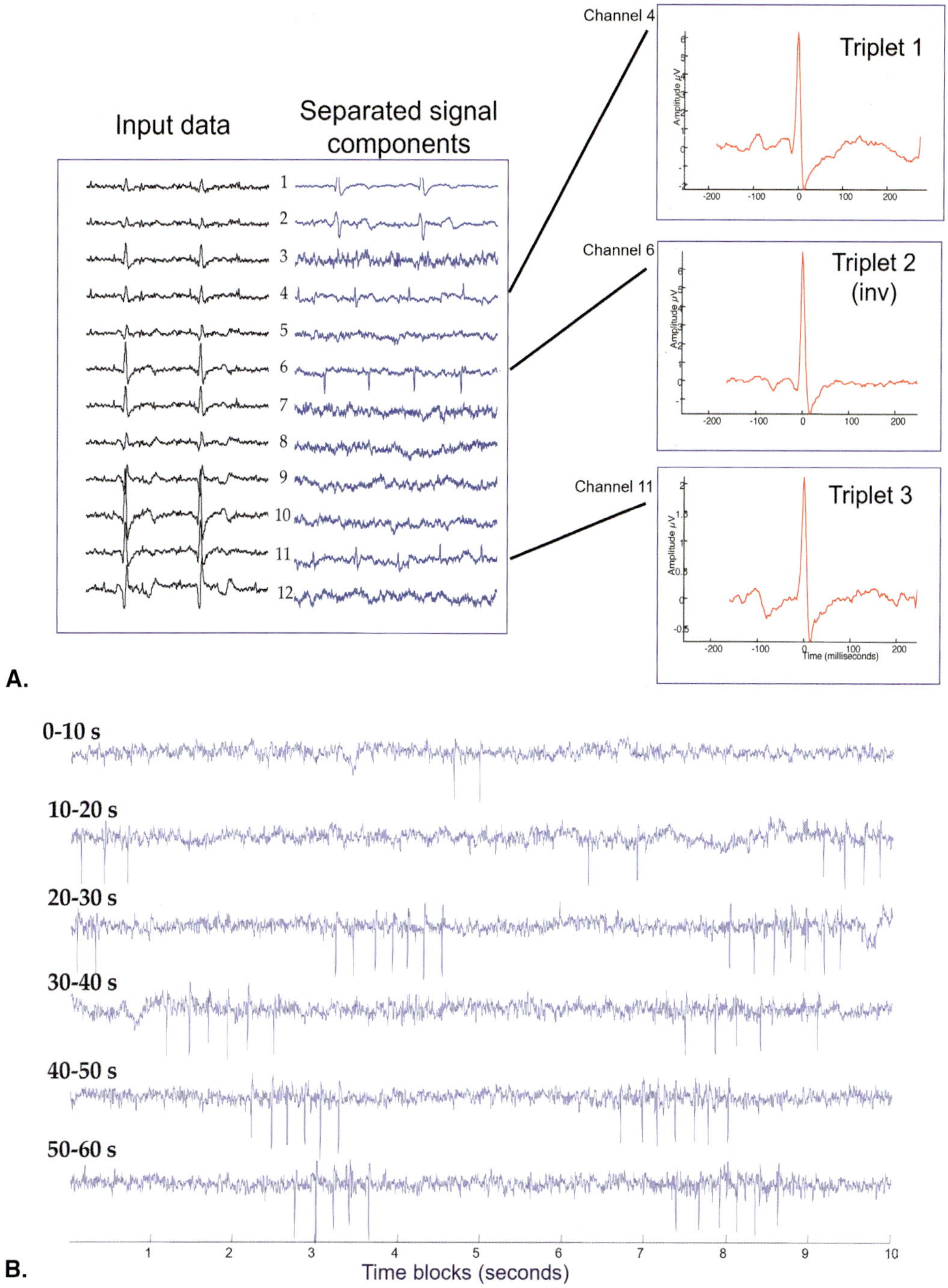

FIGURE 6.1.3 **A:** Fetal ECG demonstrating signal separation in a triplet pregnancy from 12 maternal abdominal electrodes. The input data from the electrodes are shown in the first panel and the extracted fetal signals in the second panel. The coherent averaged signal of the three fetuses shows differing fetal heart rates and axes. **B:** The rhythm strip of the very growth-restricted fetus shows a terminal heart rate pattern recorded shortly before demise.

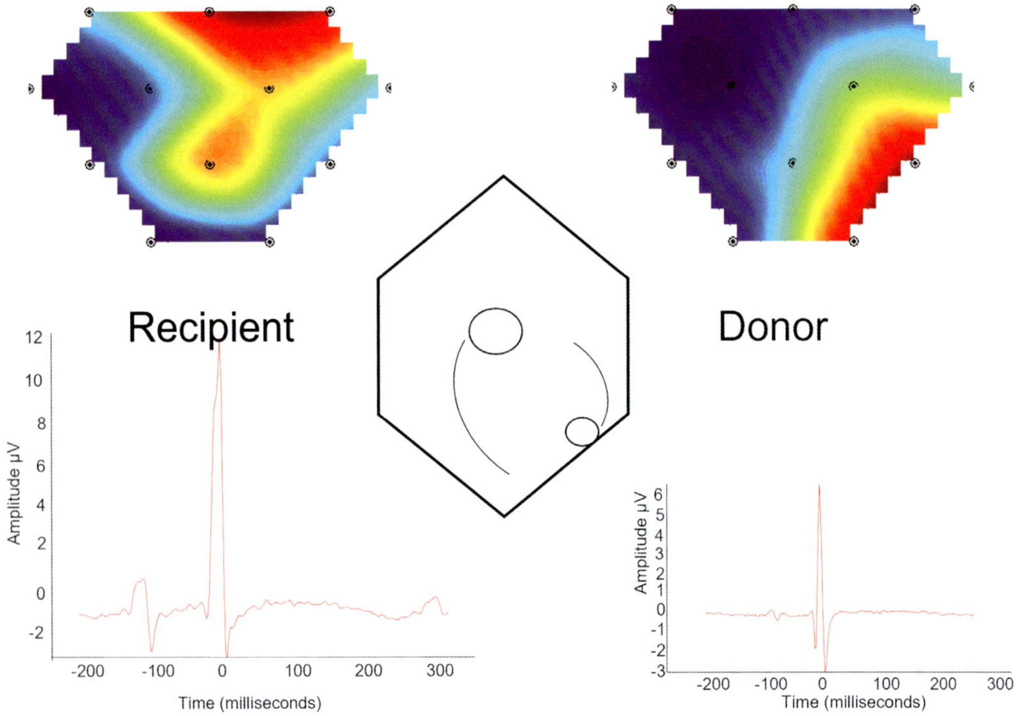

FIGURE 6.1.4 Energy map of monochorionic diamniotic twins with twin-to-twin transfusion syndrome, demonstrating the differing size of the fetal ECG signals in the twins with selective growth restriction.

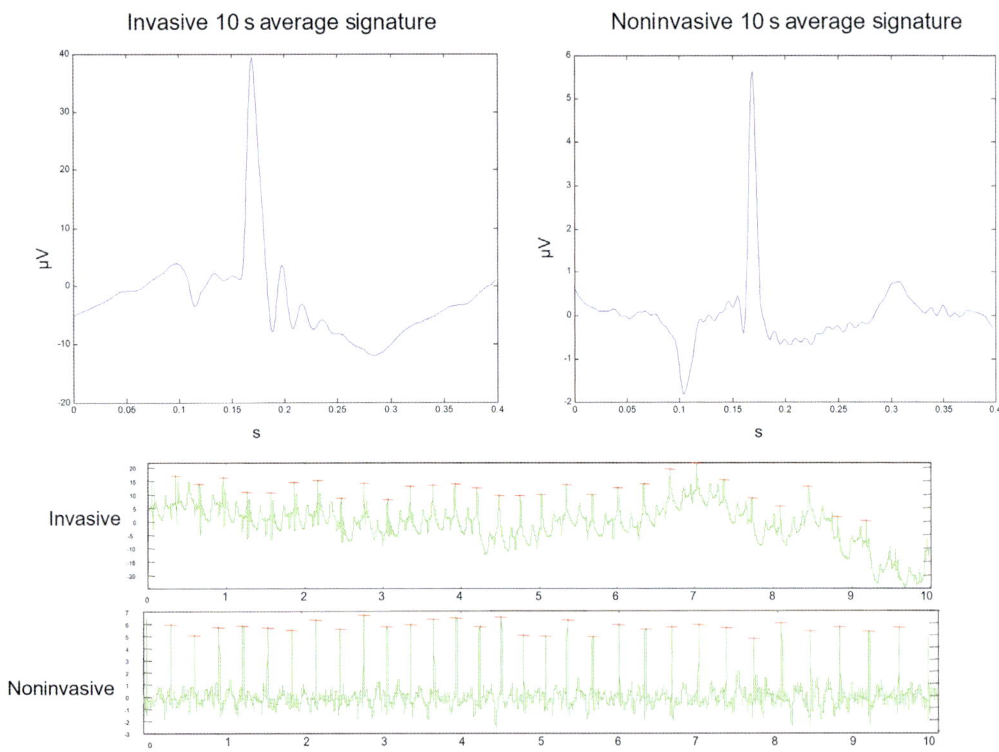

FIGURE 6.1.5 Comparison of traces obtained in an instrumented fetal lamb from both noninvasive abdominally recorded traces and an invasive, direct recording from the fetal chest electrodes. Intermittent cord occlusion produced similar responses using both methods.

with the formation of vernix, an insulating layer surrounding the fetus. It is likely this performance can be improved with higher resolution hardware and reduced noise levels to enable the detection of submicrovolt fECG signals.[53] The group subsequently recorded fECG and maternal contraction patterns in a small sample of laboring women[54] (FIG. 6.1.1). The ability of the equipment to demonstrate ST segment and FHR changes in response to fetal hypoxemia was demonstrated in a study of instrumented fetal lambs undergoing repetitive cord occlusion[55] (FIG. 6.1.5). This method was compared with Doppler in measuring PR intervals in anti-Ro–positive women and a comparison of electrical and Doppler measurements made simultaneously reported.[56] Obtaining a good P-wave signal enables characterization of fetal tachycardia as shown in an fECG at 31 weeks and resurgence of the short RP tachycardia 3 days after delivery at term (FIG. 6.1.6). Thus, many of the desirable features of fECG have been demonstrated already, albeit not providing real-time analysis.

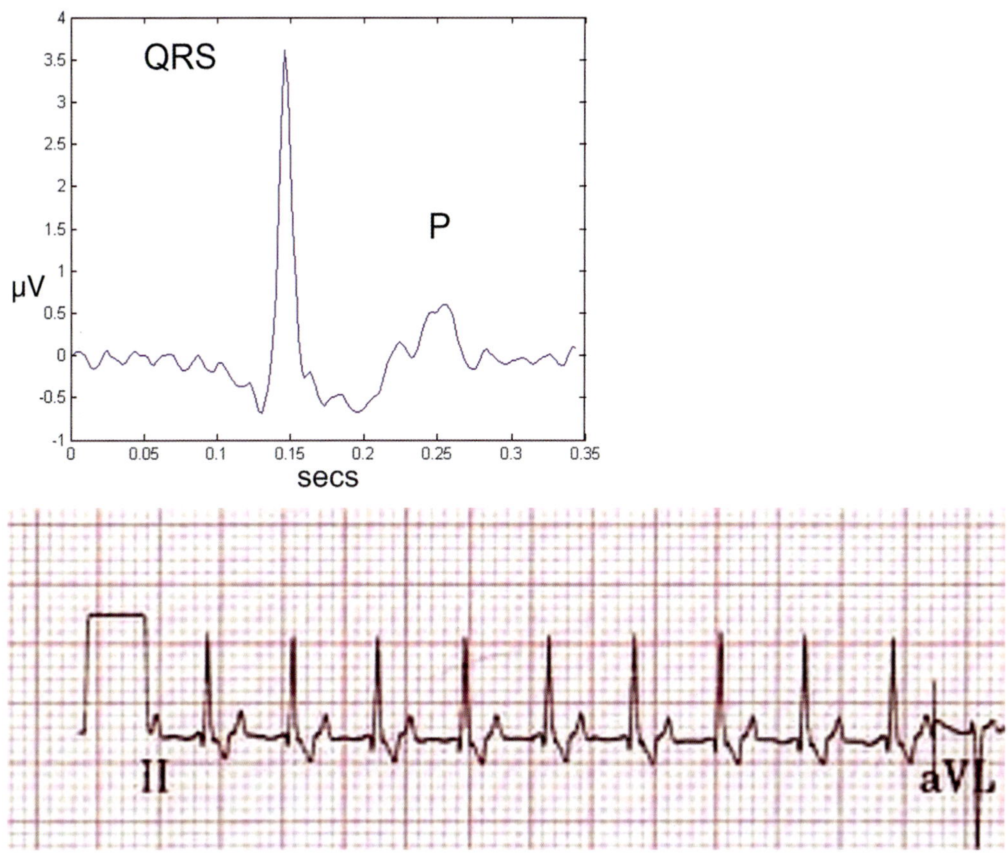

FIGURE 6.1.6 Fetus diagnosed with atrial tachycardia at 31 gestational weeks. The fetal ECG rhythm strip showed P-waves after the QRS complex and synchronous with the T-wave. Coherent signal averaging confirmed it was short RP tachycardia. The arrhythmia resolved with maternal oral Digoxin therapy within 4 days but reoccurred 3 days after birth and is demonstrated on lead 2 in the postnatal rhythm strip.

SUMMARY

In this world of increasing computing power and continual developments in wearable technology, neural networks, smartphones, and cloud-based platforms, is the fetal ECG still elusive? The short answer is yes, but one can imagine developments in computing power will facilitate real-time signal separation and efficient data processing, while sensor arrays will permit more reliable detection of fetal signals during daily activity, so that the fetus can be monitored earlier and for longer periods during pregnancy. The data collected and stored in cloud-based platforms can provide timely feedback to mothers and physicians, either to reassure or warn of potential problems. These data may also feed into repositories of personalized physiological information that may be used to optimize an individual's future medical treatment. Studying the responses of the developing fetus to its environment in greater detail may unlock underlying and treatable mechanisms responsible for intrauterine growth restriction, stillbirth, and cerebral palsy within the coming decades.

References

1. Draper ES, Gallimore ID, Kurinczuk JJ, et al. *MBRRACE-UK Perinatal Mortality Surveillance Report, UK Perinatal Deaths for Births from January to December 2016*. Leicester: The Infant Mortality and Morbidity Studies, Department of Health Sciences, University of Leicester; 2018.
2. Peters MJ, Stinstra JG, van den Broek SP, et al. On the fetal magnetocardiogram. *Bioelectrochem Bioenerg*. 1998;47:273.
3. Peters M, Crowe J, Pieri JF, et al. Monitoring the fetal heart noninvasively: a review of methods. *J Perinat Med*. 2001;29:408-416.
4. Alfirevic Z, Devane D, Gyte GM. Continuous cardiotocography (CTG) as a form of electronic fetal monitoring (EFM) for fetal assessment during labour. *Cochrane Database Syst Rev*. 2013;(5):CD006066.
5. Larks SD. Estimation of the electrical axis of the fetal heart. *Am J Obstet Gynecol*. 1965;91:46-55.
6. Vullings R, Verdurmen KMJ, Hulsenboom ADJ, et al. The electrical heart axis and ST events in fetal monitoring: a post-hoc analysis following a multicentre randomised controlled trial. *PLoS ONE* 2017;12(4):e0175823.
7. Lewalter T, Lüderitz B. Historical Milestones of electrical signal recording and analysis. In: Gussak I, Antzelevitch C, Hammill SC, Shen WK, Bjerregaard P, eds. *Cardiac Repolarization. Contemporary Cardiology*. Totowa, NJ: Humana Press; 2003
8. Waller AG. A demonstration on man of electromotive changes accompanying the heart's beat. *J Physiol*. 1887;8:229-234.
9. Einthoven W. Ein neues galvanometer. *Ann Phys*. 1903;12:1059-1071.
10. Cremer M. Över die direkte Ableitung der Aktionsstrome des menschlichen Herzens vom Oesophagus und tiber das Elektrokardiogramm des Fotus. *Munch Med Wschr*. 1906;53:811-813.
11. Smyth CN. Experimental electrocardiography of the foetus. *Lancet*. 1953;1(6771):1124-1126.
12. Davis J, Meares SD. Preliminary report on an investigation of foetal electrocardiography and foetal stethography. *Med J Aust*. 1954;2(13):501-504.
13. Southern EM. Fetal anoxia and its possible relation to changes in the prenatal fetal electrocardiogram. *Am J Obstet Gynecol*. 1957;73(2):233-247.
14. Sureau C. Fetal electrocardiographic research during pregnancy and labor; first results of a new technic of registration by intrauterine electrodes. *Gynecol Obstet (Paris)*. 1956;55(1):21-33.
15. Kaplan S, Toyama S. Fetal electrocardiography; utilizing abdominal and intrauterine leads. *Obstet Gynecol*. 1958;11(4):391-397.
16. Hon EH, Lee ST. Noise reduction in fetal electrocardiography. II. Averaging techniques. *Am J Obstet Gynecol*. 1963;87:1086-1096.
17. Larks SD, Larks GG. Components of the fetal electrocardiogram and intrauterine electrical axis: quantitative data. *Biol Neonat*. 1966;10(3):140-152.
18. Gennser G, Johansson BW, Kullander S. Electrocardiographic and tissue lactate changes in the hypoxic human fetus in mid-pregnancy. *J Obstet Gynaecol Br Commonw*. 1968;75(9):941-948.

19. Gelli MG, Gyulai F. Effect of glucose infusion in the mother before delivery on the ECG of rabbit foetuses under anoxia. *Acta Obstet Gynecol Scand.* 1969;48(1):56-63.
20. Pardi G, Tucci E, Uderzo A, Zanini D. Fetal electrocardiogram changes in relation to fetal heart rate patterns during labor. *Am J Obstet Gynecol.* 1974;118(2):243-250.
21. Rosén KG, Kjellmer I. Changes in the fetal heart rate and ECG during hypoxia. *Acta Physiol Scand.* 1975;93(1):59-66.
22. Symonds EM. Vectorcardiography and acid-base balance in the human fetus. *J Obstet Gynaecol Br Commonw.* 1972;79(5):416-423.
23. Hökegård KH, Karlsson K, Lilja H, Rosén KG. Neonatal electrocardiographic changes in relation to cardiotocographic changes. *Br J Obstet Gynaecol.* 1978;85(3):165-171.
24. Symonds EM. Configuration of the fetal electrocardiogram in relation to fetal acid-base balance and plasma electrolytes. *J Obstet Gynaecol Br Commonw.* 1971;78(11):957-970.
25. Murray HG. The fetal electrocardiogram: current clinical developments in Nottingham. *J Perinat Med.* 1986;14(6):399-404.
26. Brambati B, Pardi G. The intraventricular conduction time of fetal heart in uncomplicated pregnancies. *Br J Obstet Gynaecol.* 1980;87(11):941-948.
27. Crowe JA, Woolfson MS, Hayes-Gill BR, et al. Antenatal assessment using the FECG obtained via abdominal electrodes. *J Perinat Med.* 1996;24:43.
28. Greene KR, Dawes GS, Lilja H, Rosen KG. Changes in the ST waveform of the fetal lamb electrocardiogram with hypoxemia. *Am J Obstet Gynecol.* 1982;144:950-958.
29. Widmark C, Lindecrantz K, Murray H, Rosen KG. Changes in the PR, RR intervals and ST waveform of the fetal lamb electrocardiogram with acute hypoxemia. *J Dev Physiol.* 1992;18:99-103.
30. Westgate JA, Bennet L, Brabyn C, Williams CE, Gunn AJ. ST waveform changes during repeated umbilical cord occlusions in near-term fetal sheep. *Am J Obstet Gynecol.* 2001;184:743-751.
31. Dessì A, Pani D, Raffo L. An advanced algorithm for fetal heart rate estimation from non-invasive low electrode density recordings. *Physiol Meas.* 2014;35:1621-1636.
32. Behar J, Johnson A, Clifford GD, Oster J. A Comparison of single channel fetal ECG extraction methods. *Ann Biomed Eng.* 2014;42:1340-1353.
33. Martinek R, Kahankova R, Nazeran H, et al. Non-invasive fetal monitoring: a maternal surface ECG electrode placement-based novel approach for optimization of adaptive filter control parameters using the LMS and RLS algorithms. *Sensors.* 2017;17:1154.
34. Wu S, Shen Y, Zhou Z, Lin L, Zeng Y, Gao X. Research of fetal ECG extraction using wavelet analysis and adaptive filtering. *Comput Biol Med.* 2013;43:1622-1627.
35. Sato M, Kimura Y, Chida S, et al. A novel extraction method of fetal electrocardiogram from the composite abdominal signal. *IEEE Trans Biomed Eng.* 2006;54:49-58.
36. Li Y, Yi Z. An algorithm for extracting fetal electrocardiogram. *Neurocomputing.* 2008;71:1538-1542.
37. Liu G, Luan Y. An adaptive integrated algorithm for noninvasive fetal ECG separation and noise reduction based on ICA-EEMD-WS. *Med Biol Eng Comput.* 2015;53:1113-1127.
38. Zhang NN, Zhang JY, Li H, et al. A novel technique for fetal ECG extraction using single-channel abdominal recording. *Sensors.* 2017;17:457.
39. Ma YP, Xiao YG, Wei G, Sun JW. A multichannel nonlinear adaptive noise canceller based on generalized FLANN for fetal ECG extraction. *Meas Sci Technol.* 2016;27:015703.
40. Clifford GD, Silva I, Behar J, Moody GB. Noninvasive fetal ECG analysis. *Physiol Meas.* 2014;35(8):1521-1536.
41. Goldberger AL, Amaral LAN, Glass L, et al. PhysioBank, PhysioToolkit, and PhysioNet: components of a new research resource for complex physiologic signals. *Circulation.* 2000;101(23):e215-e220.
42. Lew S, Hämäläinen MS, Okada Y. Toward noninvasive monitoring of ongoing electrical activity of human uterus and fetal heart and brain. *Clin Neurophysiol* 2017;128:2470-2481.
43. Crawford A, Anyadi P, Stephens L, et al. A mixed-methods evaluation of continuous electronic fetal monitoring for an extended period. *Acta Obstet Gynecol Scand.* 2018;97:1515-1523.
44. Graatsma E, Jacod B, van Egmond L, Mulder E, Visser G. Fetal electrocardiography: feasibility of long-term fetal heart rate recordings. *Br J Obstet Gynaecol.* 2009;116:334-338.
45. Graatsma E, Mulder EJH, Vasak B, et al. Average acceleration and deceleration capacity of fetal heart rate in normal pregnancy and in pregnancies complicated by fetal growth restriction. *J Matern Fetal Neonatal Med.* 2012;25(12):2517-2522.
46. Kapaya H, Dimelow ER, Anumba D. Is portable foetal electrocardiogram monitor feasible for foetal heart rate monitoring of small for gestational age foetuses in the home environment. *J Obstet Gynaecol.* 2019;39(8):1081-1086.
47. Chia EL, Ho TF, Rauff M, Yip WC. Cardiac time intervals of normal fetuses using noninvasive fetal electrocardiography. *Prenat Diagn.* 2005;25(7):546-552.

48. Verdurmen KMJ, Lempersz C, Vullings R, et al. Normal ranges for fetal electrocardiogram values for the healthy fetus of 18-24 weeks of gestation: a prospective cohort study. *BMC Pregnancy Childbirth* 2016;16:227.
49. Yuan L, Yuan Y, Zhou Z, Bai Y, Wu S. A fetal ECG monitoring system based on the android smartphone. *Sensors* 2019, 19, 446.
50. Ali MAS. Continuously monitoring foetal ECG using mobile telemedicine sensor network. *Engineering*. 2013;5:63-66.
51. Clifford G, Sameni R, Ward J, Robinson J, Wolfberg AJ. Clinically accurate fetal ECG parameters acquired from maternal abdominal sensors. *Am J Obstet Gynecol.* 2011;205(1):47.e1-47.e5.
52. Behar J, Andreotti F, Zaunseder S, Li Q, Oster J, Clifford GD. An ECG simulator for generating maternal-foetal activity mixtures on abdominal ECG recordings. *Physiol Meas.* 2014;35(8):1537-1550.
53. Taylor MJ, Smith MJ, Thomas M, et al. Non-invasive fetal electrocardiography in singleton and multiple pregnancies. *Br J Obstet Gynaecol.* 2003;110(7):668-678.
54. Taylor MJ, Thomas MJ, Smith MJ, et al. Non-invasive intrapartum fetal ECG: preliminary report. *Br J Obstet Gynaecol.* 2005;112(8):1016-1021.
55. Cleal JK, Thomas M, Hanson MA, Paterson-Brown S, Gardiner HM, Green LR. Noninvasive fetal electrocardiography following intermittent umbilical cord occlusion in the preterm ovine fetus. *Br J Obstet Gynaecol.* 2010;117(4):438-444.
56. Gardiner HM, Belmar C, Pasquini L, et al. Fetal ECG: a novel predictor of atrioventricular block in anti-Ro positive pregnancies. *Heart.* 2007;93:1454-1460.

Magnetocardiography for the Fetus at Risk for Stillbirth

Janette F. Strasburger

INTRODUCTION

For half a century, the superb diagnostic capabilities of ultrasound and echocardiography have been the primary tools for fetal cardiac rhythm diagnosis. However, fetal magnetocardiography (fMCG) (Part 2, Chapter 3) has taken our understanding to a new level by allowing us to delve into the electrophysiology of these rhythms. With these advances, it should be possible to explore the hypothesis that fMCG may uncover electrophysiologic findings that predispose to the risk of stillbirth. This possibility has been largely unexplored in the field of fetal medicine. Such an approach would be facilitated by 25 years of experience in the Biomagnetism Laboratory at the University of Wisconsin-Madison, where medical physicists and fetal cardiologists have developed normal values for fetal cardiac intervals and repolarization characteristics over a wide range of gestational ages.[1-3] These studies have diagnosed repolarization abnormalities in fetuses with atrioventricular (AV) block, long QT syndrome (LQTS), and congenital heart disease.[4-9] Serial studies of 132 ostensibly normal pregnancies where fMCG-detected QRS-T discordance and ST depression or elevation suggest underlying abnormalities in fetuses thought to be normal by traditional obstetrical parameters.[10] In addition, these studies have shown that treatment can positively effect the electrophysiology of fetuses with conduction system and structural heart disease. This chapter will summarize current information about stillbirth and describe a new study utilizing fMCG. This study proposes to evaluate electrophysiologic findings in fetuses at risk for stillbirth to find markers predicting in utero demise. It is currently evaluating five at-risk groups: mono-dichorionic twins, fetuses with gastroschisis or congenital heart disease, and mothers with a prior history of stillbirth, or those with fetal hydrops.

FETAL MAGNETOCARDIOGRAPHY (fMCG)

FMCG has been described in Part 2, Chapter 3. As previously discussed, fMCG produces no magnetism or energy and is a completely safe passive receiver for cardiac electric and magnetic signals. Currently, fMCG is limited to medical physics laboratories rather than labor and delivery wards. Though approved by the Food and

Drug Administration (FDA) for the indication of fetal cardiac recording with a Class IIa indication for fetal arrhythmia, superconducting quantum interference device (SQUID) magnetometers are extremely expensive to operate. The expense is due to the need to cool the SQUIDs with liquid helium as described in Part 2, Chapter 3. Newer sensors are being developed that use optically pumped magnetometers rather than cryogenics; this change is expected to significantly reduce cost. Optically pumped magnetometers are not yet approved for use in the fetus, but in the Biomagnetism Laboratory at University of Wisconsin-Madison, over 50 pregnant women have undergone this procedure without incident. The quality of the data is equal to that obtained using the SQUID.[11]

STILLBIRTH

Stillbirth is defined as the unexpected in utero death of the fetus at a gestational age (GA) of ≥20 weeks. Almost 25,000 stillbirths occur each year in the United States, more than seven times the frequency of sudden infant death syndrome (SIDS). Worldwide, an estimated 2.5 million stillbirths occur each year. Stillbirth peaks in late gestation[12-14] and has a lifetime impact on the mother and other family members. The cause of at least 30% of stillbirths is unknown. Over 200 risk factors have been associated with stillbirth, such as placenta, cord and membrane complications, and fetal anomalies (FIG. 6.2.1A). Stillbirth also has acute and chronic, intrinsic, and extrinsic triggers.[12,13,15-17] Non-Hispanic black women have almost double the stillbirth rates of other races; Native Americans and Pacific Islanders also are at high risk (FIG. 6.2.1B). The reasons for these disparities are unclear, but epigenetic risk is proposed. Common genetic polymorphisms may also increase this risk.

While the rate of stillbirth has declined over decades, the decreasing rate has not kept pace with the decline of neonatal and infant deaths (FIG. 6.2.2A). This is especially true of stillbirths at 20 to 28 weeks GA (FIG. 6.2.2B). Even if the pregnancy is at increased risk of stillbirth, the timing of delivery to avert such a death is imperfectly predicted, and the obstetrician often chooses between delivering a live baby prematurely and risking a stillbirth.

Little is known of the mechanisms of stillbirth, and tools to identify and monitor the at-risk fetus are limited. Thus, the presence of electrophysiologic abnormalities such as conduction or repolarization prior to stillbirth is unknown. What is needed is a more sensitive monitoring tool to identify the cardiac sequelae of hypoxia and acidosis. To date, monitoring capabilites of fMCG can provide these data.

Known Maternal and Fetal Risk Factors for Stillbirth

Stillbirth is seen in 2% to 30% of major congenital heart defects (especially when chromosomal abnormalities or extracardiac defects are present),[18] in 30% of fetal hydrops cases,[19-21] and in 5% of subsequent pregnancies in women who have had a prior unexplained fetal demise.[14,22,23] Monochorionic twins have a 0.5% to 15% mortality,[24-26] and gastroschisis has a 4.8% to 10% fetal mortality.[27-29] The only obstetrical disease with an increased stillbirth associated with fetal conduction system disease

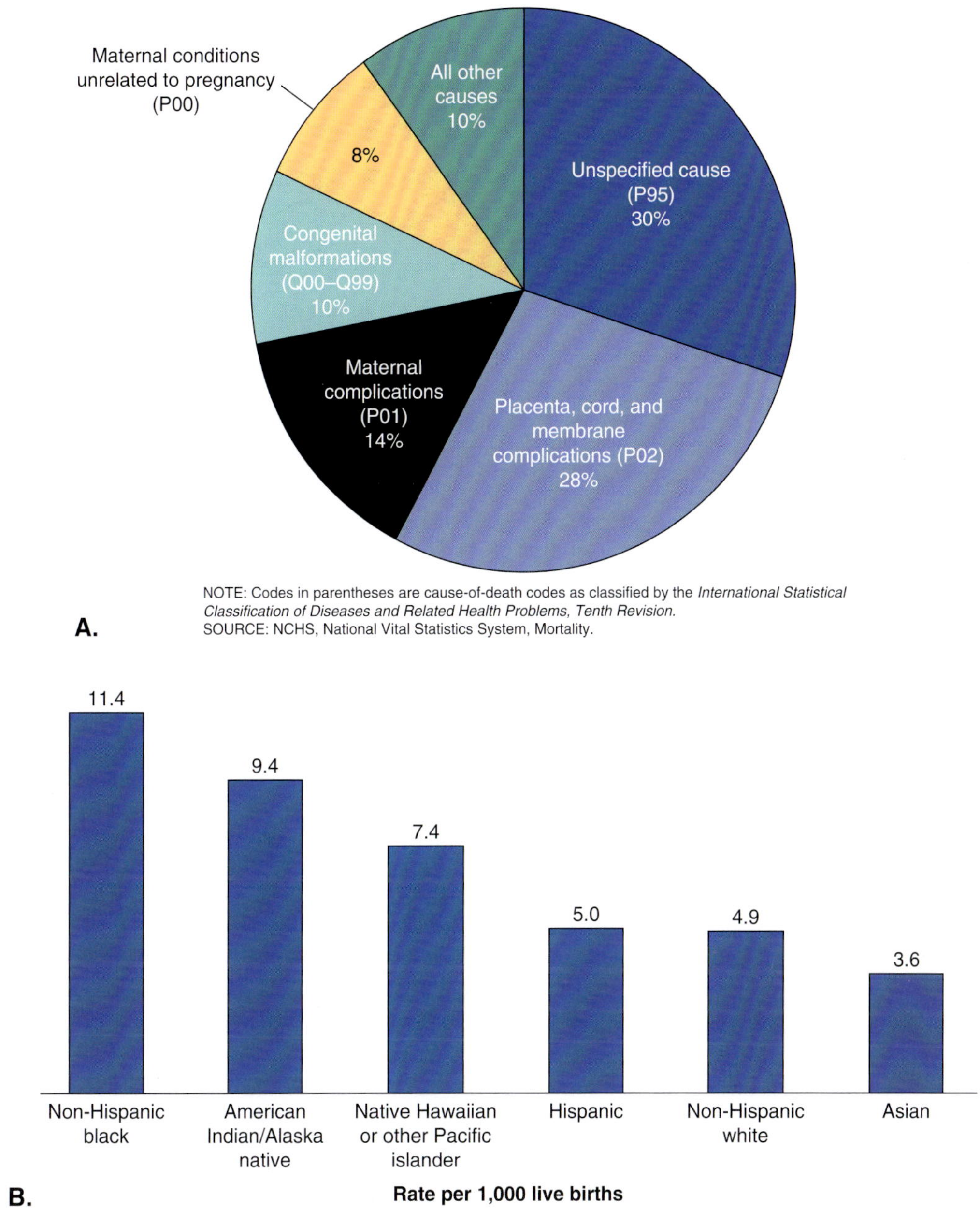

FIGURE 6.2.1 Stillbirth statistics. **A:** Breakdown of the six most common reasons for fetal demise. Note that the largest category is unexplained. **B:** Fetal demise rates among various racial and ethnic groups. Note that non-Hispanic black, and Native American and Native Hawaiian persons have higher rates of fetal demise. (A, Reprinted from Hoyert DL, Gregory ECW. Cause of fetal death: Data From the Fetal Death Report, 2014. *Natl Vital Stat Rep*. 2016;65(7). https://www.cdc.gov/nchs/data/nvsr/nvsr65/nvsr65_07.pdf. B: Reprinted from Centers for Disease Control and Prevention. Infant Mortality. https://www.cdc.gov/reproductivehealth/maternalinfanthealth/infantmortality.htm. Published March 27, 2019.)

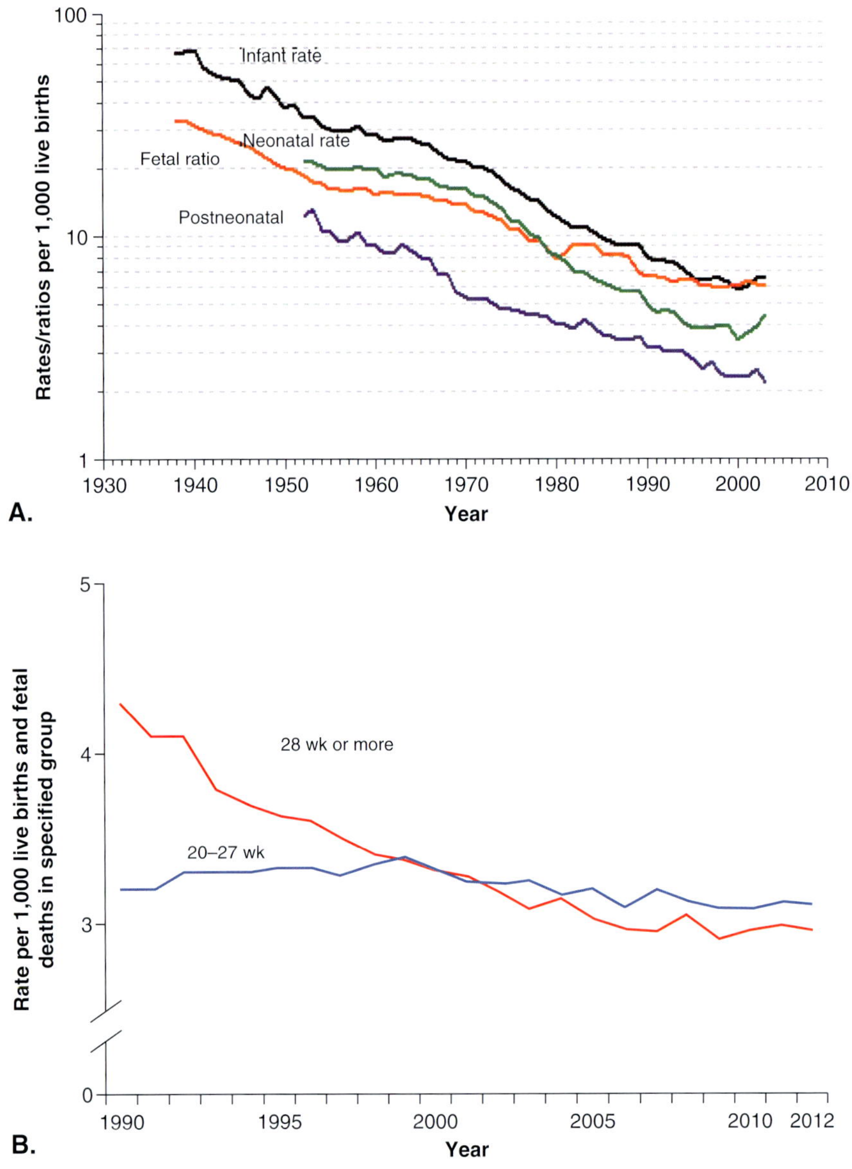

FIGURE 6.2.2 Changes in fetal, neonatal, postneonatal, and infant death ratios over time. **A:** Graph from the Centers for Disease Control and Prevention (CDC) showing the decline in fetal death ratios (stillbirths/1000 live births plus fetal deaths) compared with all postnatal deaths between 1930 and 2004. **B:** CDC/National Vital Statistics graph from 1990 to 2012 showing that while fetal deaths after 28 weeks have declined, deaths between 20 and 28 weeks have not. (Reprinted from CDC/NCHS, National Vital Statistics System)

is intrahepatic cholestasis (IHC). It is known that bile acids have an arrhythmogenic effect, and in a case series, the fetuses of pregnant women with IHC had significantly longer PR intervals than controls.[30] In a case report, treatment of IHC with ursodeoxycholic acid reduced the mother's symptoms and shortened the fetal AV interval from 163 to 143 ms.[31]

Speculations on the Mechanism and Harbingers of Stillbirth

Few studies have documented brain death in the fetus or the heart rate and rhythm patterns that are present prior to fetal demise.[32] In those that have made such observations, the fetus is flaccid, without breathing movements, with flat heart rate pattern absent variability, and sometimes with tachycardia or ectopy. Usually, cardiac function is abnormal. Hydramnios can occur due to lack of fetal swallowing. In one observed case, contraction of only the atrium without contraction of the ventricles immediately prior to stillbirth was seen. Using fMCG, ST depression, marked QT interval prolongation, QRS discordance, T-wave alternans, and torsades de pointes ventricular tachycardia have been seen in the hours and days prior to death. These findings were seen in fetuses with structural heart disease, cardiomyopathy, ion channelopathies, or severe growth restriction (**FIGS. 6.2.3-6.2.6**). FMCG has also shown that treatment can positively affect the electrophysiology of fetuses at risk for stillbirth, specifically those with conduction system disease and structural heart disease (**FIGS. 6.2.7** and **6.2.8**).

However, there may be other harbingers of stillbirth. In the fetus with severe QTc prolongation, a pattern of progressive bursts of ventricular tachycardia has been seen to develop; this may be the mechanism of death. FMCG has identified rhythms that

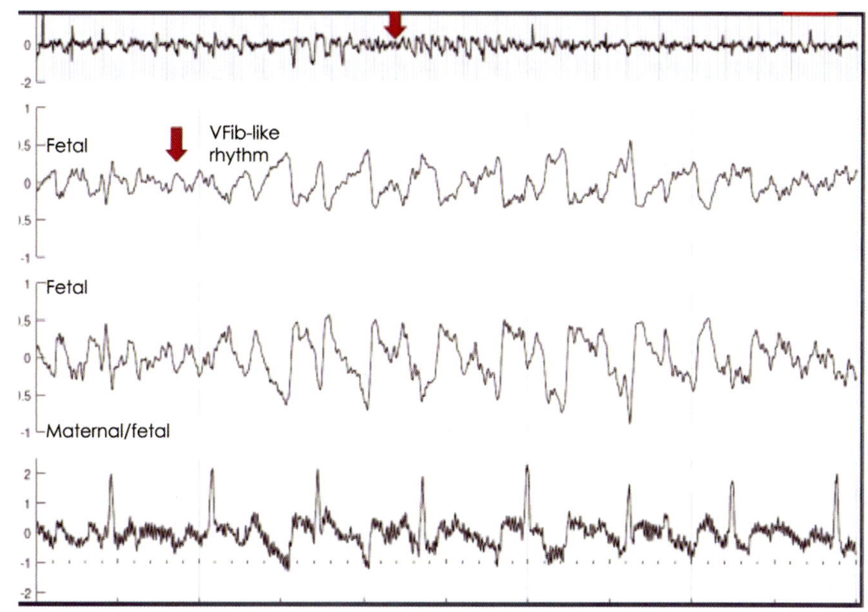

FIGURE 6.2.3 Torsades de pointes in a 33-week fetus with known long QT syndrome (LQTS). The inset at the top is a longer tracing of this segment, and along the bottom, the maternal/fetal channel. At times, the rhythm appeared to be disorganized, as in ventricular fibrillation, and at other times, it was more organized. This fetus died in utero at approximately 34-weeks gestational age; genetic testing results are pending. In over 30 cases of LQTS, fetuses with de novo pathogenic variants have a 44% mortality, whereas familial (inherited) fetuses have about a 14% mortality. The timelines are 0.5 seconds.

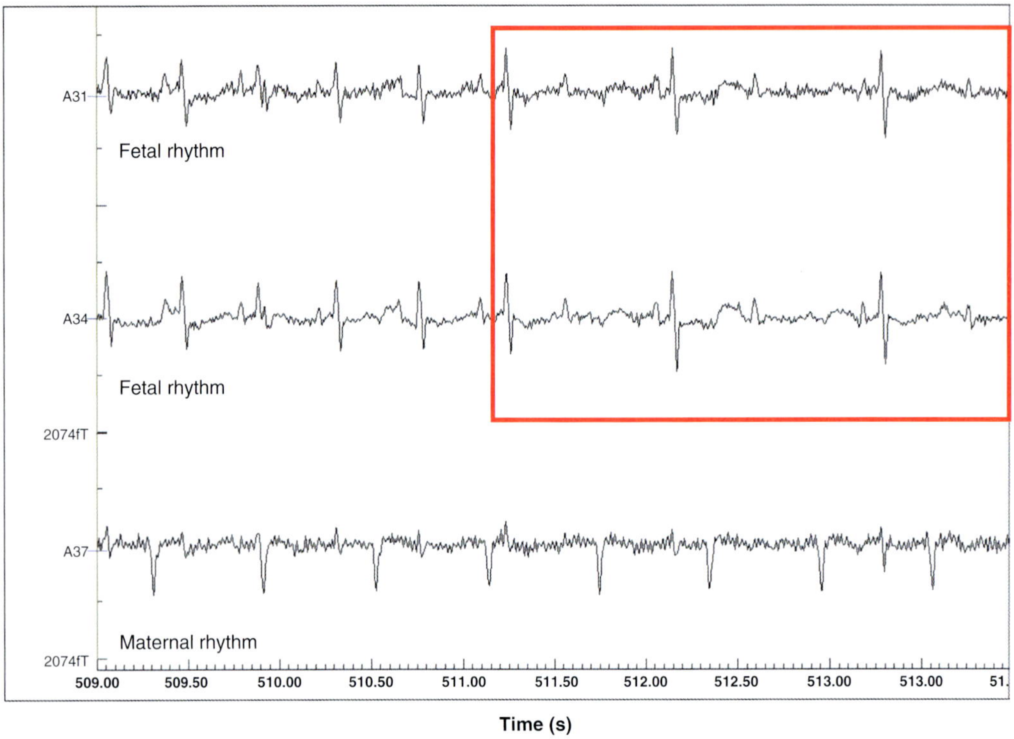

FIGURE 6.2.4 Fetal magnetocardiography (fMCG) rhythm tracings of a 34-week fetus with critical aortic stenosis and tricuspid valve dysplasia with severe tricuspid insufficiency. The top two tracings are of the fetus (the maternal signal has been moved) and the bottom tracing is from the mother. The red square shows a period of 2° AV block, which occurred numerous times during the fMCG but had not been detected on numerous prior fetal echocardiograms. Fetal heart rate variability was reduced. The fetus died within a week.

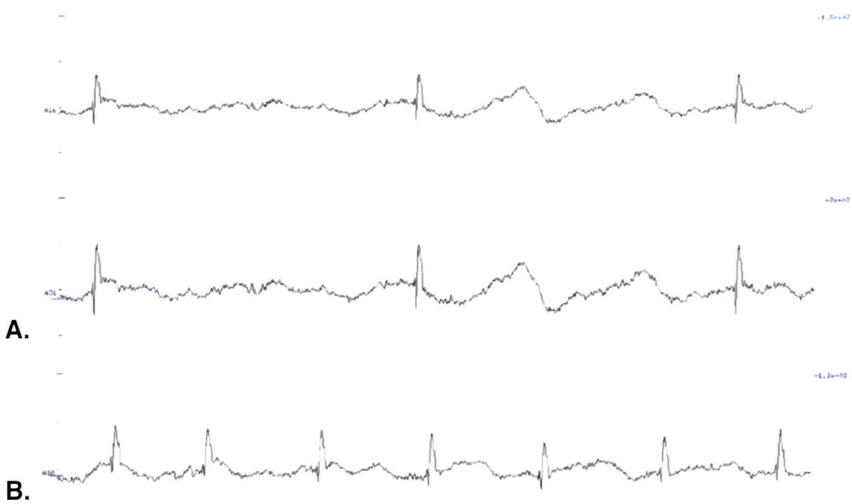

FIGURE 6.2.5 Fetal magnetocardiography (fMCG) rhythm tracings from a 23-week fetus with dilated cardiomyopathy. **A:** ST segment elevation seen in the first QRS complex suggestive of ischemia, which occurs before a significant deceleration. **B:** T-wave alternans later in the fMCG of the same fetus. The fetus died several days later. (Reprinted from Cuneo BF, Strasburger JF, Wakai RT. Magnetocardiography in the evaluation of fetuses at risk for sudden cardiac death before birth. *J Electrocardiol.* 2008;41(2):116.e1-116.e6.)

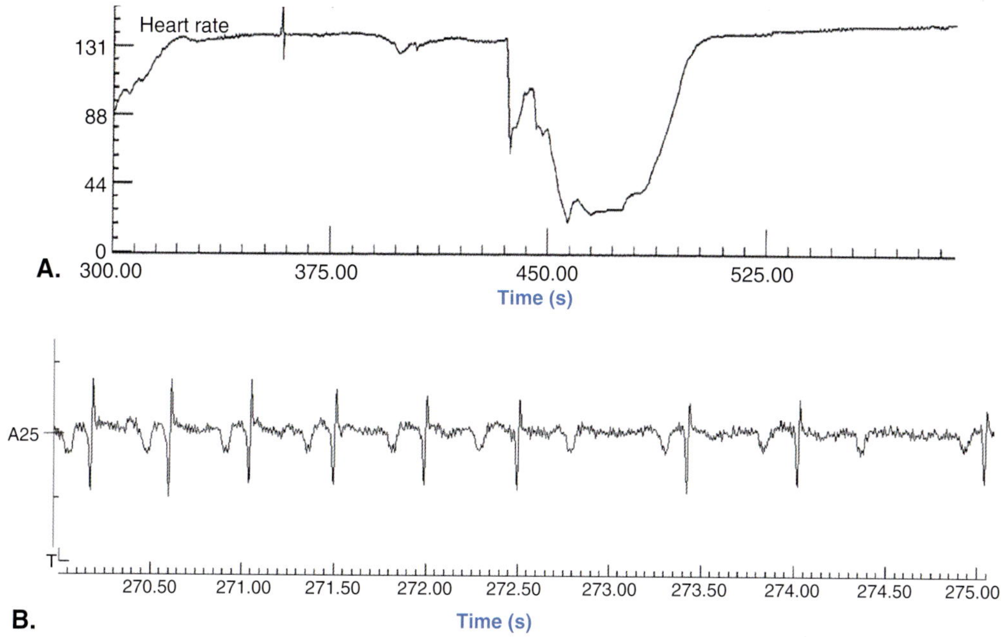

FIGURE 6.2.6 A 32-week fetus with severe Ebstein anomaly of the tricuspid valve. **A:** Fetal heart rate tracing over time showing a deep and prolonged deceleration. **B:** The fetal magnetocardiography (fMCG) rhythm tracing showed not sinus bradycardia, but 2° AV block was the rhythm during the deceleration. (Reprinted from Cuneo BF, Strasburger JF, Wakai RT. Magnetocardiography in the evaluation of fetuses at risk for sudden cardiac death before birth. *J Electrocardiol*. 2008;41(2):116.e1-116.e6.)

mimic ventricular fibrillation though without immediate death (FIG. 6.2.3). For fetuses manifesting less significant electrophysiologic abnormalities, it is possible that QT lengthening reduces the reserve of the fetus to withstand bouts of acidosis. This could result in electromechanical dissociation or ventricular fibrillation causing death.[6] Still other cardiac findings reported to be prognosticators of poor outcome in adults have been also seen in fetuses, but whether the significance is the same at both time periods is not known (FIG. 6.2.9).

Underappreciated Maternal and Fetal Risk Factors for Stillbirth

Certain pregnancies have unrecognized or underappreciated risk factors. Mothers with hypokalemia, hypomagnesemia, hypocalcemia, or chronic vitamin D deficiency[5] may be asymptomatic, yet these deficiencies may affect fetal cardiac repolarization (FIG. 6.2.10). Over 165 medications prolong maternal QT interval and, after crossing the placenta, may prolong the fetal QT interval. Several medications commonly prescribed in obstetrics,[33] for example, oxytocin (Pitocin), ondansetron (Zofran), antacids, antidepressants, and antihistamines effect maternal and fetal QT interval. Multiple QT-prolonging drugs may be given to mothers with opioid use disease (OUD) in pregnancy. Recently, a case series comparing eight mothers with OUD treated with buprenorphine with eight controls found that the mean (range) of QTc in the treatment group was 505 (396-642) ms compared to controls 383

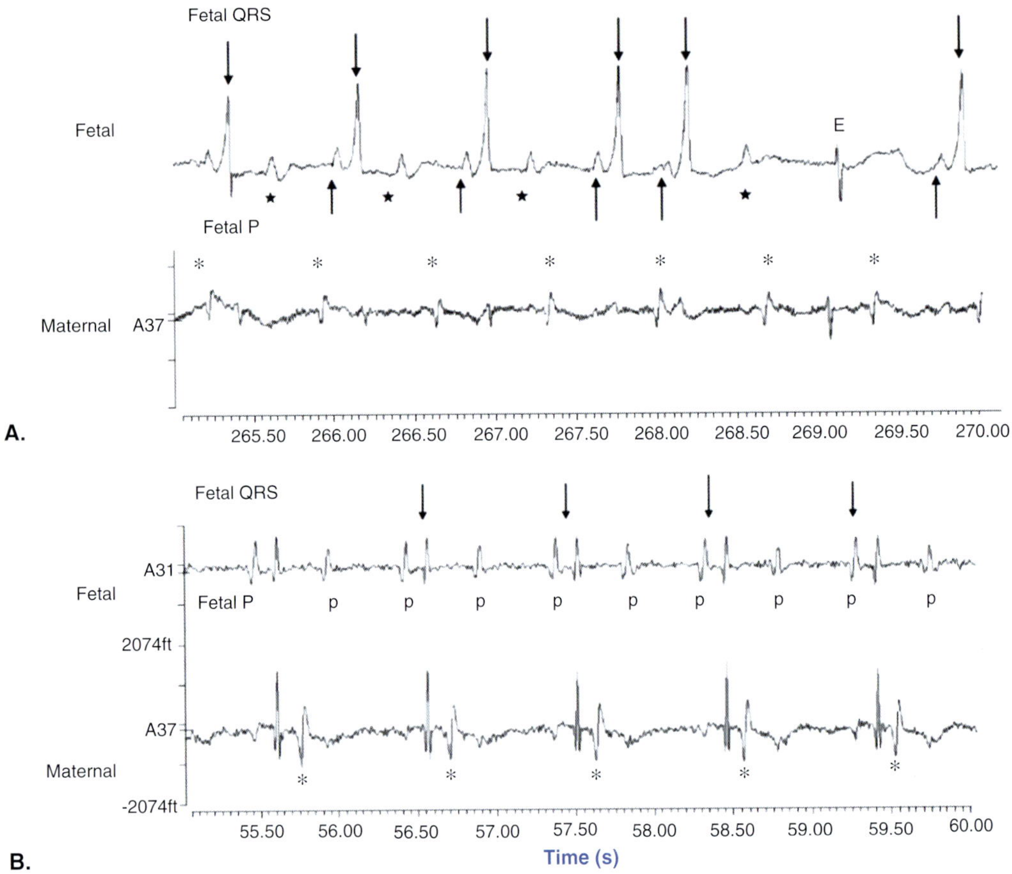

FIGURE 6.2.7 A 32-week fetus with maternal anti-Ro/SSA antibodies who presented with an irregular rhythm. **A:** The fetal rhythm (top tracing) shows 3:2 and 2:1 conduction across an accessary connection. No atrioventricular (AV) node conduction was seen. (Bottom tracing is maternal/fetal rhythm.) **B:** After 1 week of dexamethasone treatment, intermittent conduction (2° AV block) is restored across the AV node (fetal: top tracing). Stars represent P-waves in fetal tracings and fetal QRS complexes in maternal/fetal tracings. (Reprinted from Cuneo BF, Strasburger JF, Wakai RT, Ovadia M. Conduction system disease in fetuses evaluated for irregular cardiac rhythm. *Fetal Diagn Ther*. 2006;21(3):307-313.)

(280-477 ms, $P = .02$).[34] There has been personal experience with the fetus of a treated mother with mild bradycardia. The infant's postnatal QTc was 500 ms (B. Cuneo, personal communication).

FMCG Assessment of Pregnancies at Risk for Stillbirth

An NIH-funded prospective 5-year observational study is currently being conducted to evaluate the fMCG recorded from an FDA-approved SQUID Biomagnetometer in pregnancies at risk for stillbirth. Women at 20 to 27 weeks' gestation are being recruited from Maternal-Fetal Medicine (MFM) specialty clinics. The protocol includes an initial fMCG at 20 to 27 weeks followed by a repeat fMCG at 30 to

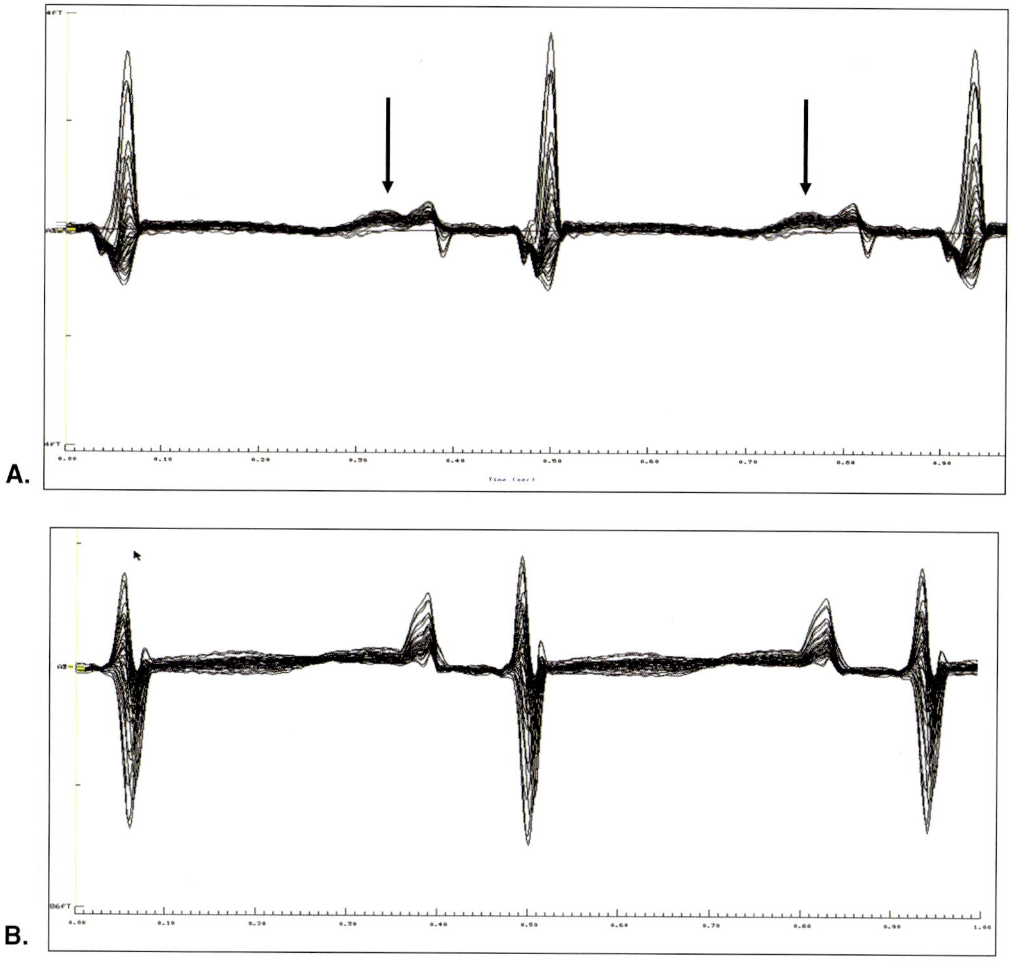

FIGURE 6.2.8 Signal-averaged rhythm tracing of a 28-week fetus with critical aortic stenosis. **A:** Before in utero balloon valvuloplasty. **B:** After in utero balloon valvuloplasty. T-wave alternans were present both before and after the procedure (not shown). The P-wave morphology changed from bifid to single, and the QT interval shortened after in utero valvuloplasty.

37 weeks of gestation. The purpose of the second fMCG is to detect abnormalities that might not have been present at initial visit. The study will determine how the fetal beat-to-beat heart rate variability and cardiac intervals (RR, P duration, PR, QRS, QT, QTc, QTUc, and ST segment changes) compare with gestation-matched control data. The purpose, first, is to determine whether unique "signature" electrophysiological abnormalities are present and, second, to define at what trimester these signature findings are first seen. Finally, the study plans to correlate fMCG findings with pregnancy outcomes.

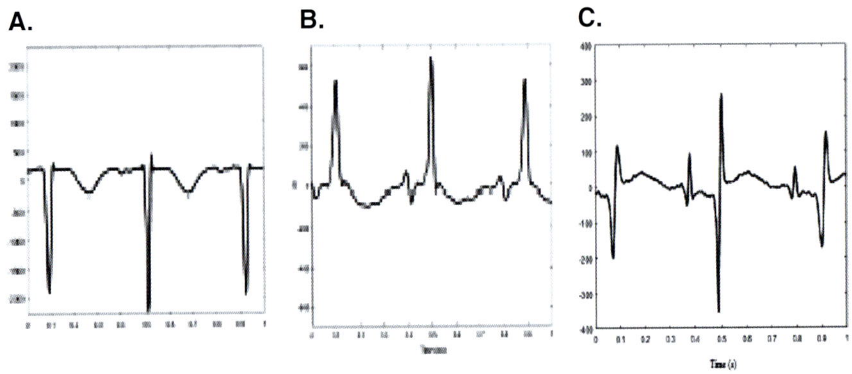

FIGURE 6.2.9 QRS- and T-wave concordance and discordance. **A:** Tracings from fetus at 38 5/7 weeks' gestational age. Note the T-wave and QRS are concordant (both downward). **B:** A second fetus at 21 weeks with QRS-T discordance (up-down). A J-wave hump is noted at the end of the QRS complex, which is of unknown significance but, in adults, is linked to risk of sudden death. **C:** Fetus at 21 4/7 weeks with ST "depression" (because the QRS is inverted, the ST segment is upright and elevated). The significance of the ST-T wave changes and QRS-T discordance is not known in the fetus. Although such findings are abnormal in postnatal life, they may be variants of normal before birth.

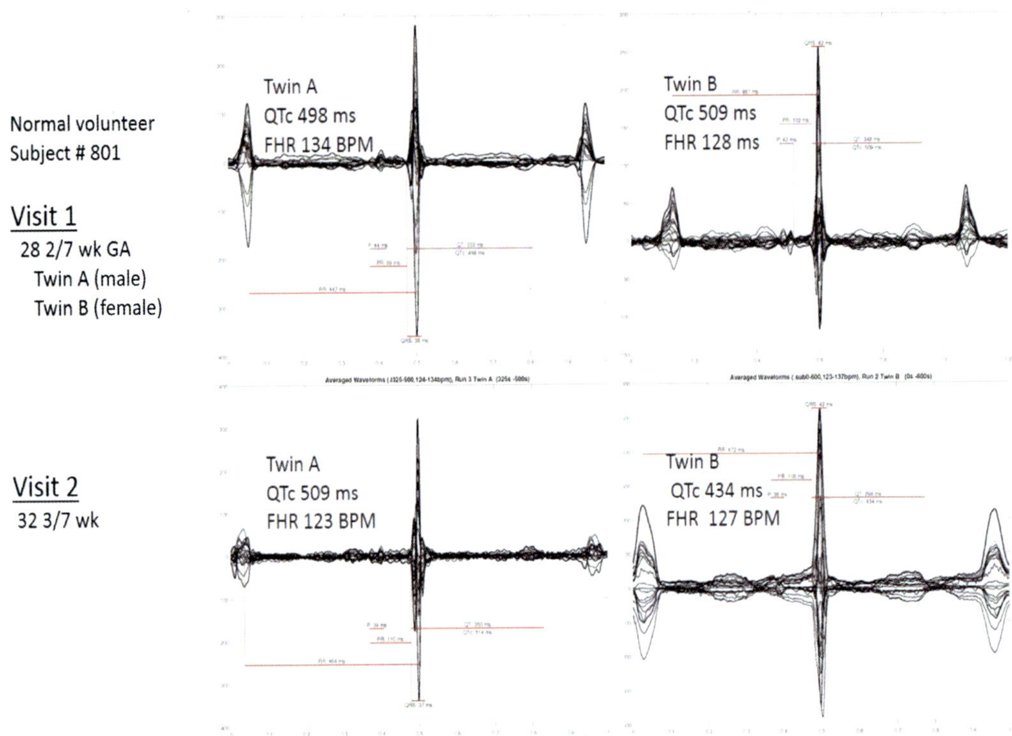

FIGURE 6.2.10 In this normal volunteer with twin fetuses, abnormal QTc values (498 and 509 ms) were present in both twins at visit 1, 28 2/7 weeks' gestational age (GA). The maternal magnesium level was 1.3 mEq/L (nl > 1.6) with normal albumin, and she was placed on oral magnesium oxide 200 mg/d. In F/U 1 month later, 32 3/7 weeks' GA, twin B showed resolution of QTc prolongation (434 ms); however, QTc remained significantly prolonged in twin A (509 ms). Both twins have borderline low fetal heart rates (FHRs) for gestation. Measurements on postnatal ECGs were within normal limits.

SUMMARY

We speculate that undetected electrophysiologic abnormalities such as conduction system disorders and repolarization anomalies may herald the risk of stillbirth. If data-support this speculation, routine use of fMCG may become standard of care for at-risk pregnancies and provides guidelines for prenatal care and delivery. In the American Heart Association's 2014 Scientific Statement of Fetal Diagnosis and Treatment, fMCG received a Class IIa indication for fetal arrhythmias suggesting that the majority of physicians find it valuable, with a benefit >> risk ratio.[35] By expanding the use of fMCG to the fetus with no apparent cardiac pathology but at risk for stillbirth, we will be able to detect repolarization and conduction system abnormalities invisible to traditional obstetric monitoring. By providing a more complete cardiac assessment of the fetus, we hope to identify the harbingers of stillbirth.

References

1. Horigome H, Takahashi MI, Asaka M, Shigemitsu S, Kandori A, Tsukada K. Magnetocardiographic determination of the developmental changes in PQ, QRS and QT intervals in the foetus. *Acta Paediatr.* 2000;89(1):64-67.
2. Horigome H, Ogata K, Kandori A, et al. Standardization of the PQRST waveform and analysis of arrhythmias in the fetus using vector magnetocardiography. *Pediatr Res.* 2006;59(1):121-125.
3. Leuthold A, Wakai RT, Martin CB. Noninvasive in utero assessment of PR and QRS intervals from the fetal magnetocardiogram. *Early Hum Dev.* 1999;54(3):235-243.
4. Cuneo BF, Ovadia M, Strasburger JF, et al. Prenatal diagnosis and in utero treatment of torsades de pointes associated with congenital long QT syndrome. *Am J Cardiol.* 2003;91(11):1395-1398.
5. Cuneo BF, Strasburger JF, Wakai RT. Magnetocardiography in the evaluation of fetuses at risk for sudden cardiac death before birth. *J Electrocardiol.* 2008;41(2):116.e1-116.e6.
6. Cuneo BF, Strasburger JF, Yu SH, et al. In utero diagnosis of long QT syndrome by magnetocardiography. *Circulation.* 2013;128(20):2183-2191.
7. Strasburger JF, Wakai RT. Fetal cardiac arrhythmia detection and in utero therapy. *Nat Rev Cardiol.* 2010;7(5):277-290.
8. Zhao H, Cuneo BF, Strasburger JF, Huhta JC, Gotteiner NL, Wakai RT. Electrophysiological characteristics of fetal atrioventricular block. *J Am Coll Cardiol.* 2008;51(1):77-84.
9. Cuneo BF, Strasburger JF, Wakai RT, Ovadia M. Conduction system disease in fetuses evaluated for irregular rhythm. *Fetal Diagn Ther.* 2006;21:307-313.
10. Strand SA, Strasburger JF, Wakai RT. Fetal magnetocardiogram waveform characteristics. *Physiol Meas.* 2019;40(3):035002.
11. Strand S, Lutter W, Strasburger JF, Shah V, Baffa O, Wakai RT. Low-cost fetal magnetocardiography: a comparison of SQUID and optically-pumped magnetometers. *J Am Heart Assoc.* 2019;8(16):e013436..
12. Reddy UM, Goldenberg R, Silver R, et al. Stillbirth classification–developing an international consensus for research: executive summary of a National Institute of Child Health and Human Development workshop. *Obstet Gynecol.* 2009;114(4):901-914.
13. Silver RM, Varner MW, Reddy U, et al. Work-up of stillbirth: a review of the evidence. *Am J Obstet Gynecol.* 2007;196(5):433-444.
14. Silver RM. Previous stillbirth, late preterm, and early-term birth. *Semin Perinatol.* 2011;35(5):302-308.
15. Lawn JE, Blencowe H, Pattinson R, et al. Stillbirths: where? When? Why? How to make the data count? *Lancet.* 2011;377(9775):1448-1463.
16. de Bernis L, Kinney MV, Stones W, et al. Stillbirths: ending preventable deaths by 2030. *Lancet.* 2016;387(10019):703-716.
17. Lawn JE, Blencowe H, Waiswa P, et al. Stillbirths: rates, risk factors, and acceleration towards 2030. *Lancet.* 2016;387(10018):587-603.
18. Divanovic A, Bowers K, Michelfelder E, et al. Intrauterine fetal demise after prenatal diagnosis of congenital heart disease: assessment of risk. *Prenat Diagn.* 2016;36(2):142-147.

19. Berg C, Geipel A, Kamil D, et al. The syndrome of left isomerism: sonographic findings and outcome in prenatally diagnosed cases. *J Ultrasound Med.* 2005;24(7):921-931.
20. Bellini C, Donarini G, Paladini D, et al. Etiology of non-immune hydrops fetalis: an update. *Am J Med Genet A.* 2015;167A(5):1082-1088.
21. Huhta JC. Diagnosis and treatment of foetal heart failure: foetal echocardiography and foetal hydrops. *Cardiol Young.* 2015;25(suppl 2):100-106.
22. Bukowski R, Hansen NI, Pinar H, et al. Altered fetal growth, placental abnormalities, and stillbirth. *Plos One.* 2017;12(8):e0182874.
23. Page JM, Christiansen-Lindquist L, Thorsten V, et al. Diagnostic tests for evaluation of stillbirth: results from the stillbirth collaborative research network. *Obstet Gynecol.* 2017;129(4):699-706.
24. Fong F, Thangaratinam S, Zamora J. Increased stillbirth in uncomplicated monochorionic twin pregnancies: a systematic review and meta-analysis. *Obstet Gynecol.* 2013;122(6):1302.
25. McPherson JA, Odibo AO, Shanks AL, Roehl KA, Macones GA, Cahill AG. Impact of chorionicity on risk and timing of intrauterine fetal demise in twin pregnancies. *Am J Obstet Gynecol.* 2012;207(3):190.e1-190.e6.
26. Danon D, Sekar R, Hack KE, Fisk NM. Increased stillbirth in uncomplicated monochorionic twin pregnancies: a systematic review and meta-analysis. *Obstet Gynecol.* 2013;121(6):1318-1326.
27. Meyer MR, Shaffer BL, Doss AE, Cahill AG, Snowden JM, Caughey AB. Prospective risk of fetal death with gastroschisis. *J Matern Fetal Neonatal Med.* 2015;28(17):2126-2129.
28. Sparks TN, Shaffer BL, Page J, Caughey AB. Gastroschisis: mortality risks with each additional week of expectant management. *Am J Obstet Gynecol.* 2017;216(1):66.e1-66.e7.
29. Landisch RM, Yin Z, Christensen M, Szabo A, Wagner AJ. Outcomes of gastroschisis early delivery: a systematic review and meta-analysis. *J Pediatr Surg.* 2017;52(12);1962-1971.
30. Rodríguez M, Moreno J, Márquez R, et al. Increased PR interval in fetuses of patients with intrahepatic cholestasis of pregnancy. *Fetal Diagn Ther.* 2016;40(4):298-302.
31. Rodríguez M, Sprohnle A, Muñoz J, Cadena C, Corvalán R, Sepúlveda-Martínez A. Treatment of intrahepatic cholestasis of pregnancy with ursodeoxycholic acid associated with improvement of fetal first-degree atrioventricular block. *Ultrasound Obstet Gynecol.* 2018;52(6):801-802.
32. Pacora P, Romero R, Jaiman S, et al. Mechanisms of death in structurally normal stillbirths. *J Perinat Med.* 2019;47(2):222-240.
33. Viskin S, Justo D, Halkin A, Zeltser D. Long QT syndrome caused by noncardiac drugs. *Prog Cardiovasc Dis.* 2003;45(5):415-427.
34. Bolin EH, Escalona-Vargas D, Daily JA, et al. Magnetocardiographic identification of prolonged fetal corrected QT interval in women receiving treatment for opioid use disorder. *J Obstet Gynaecol Res.* 2019;45(10);1989-1996.
35. Donofrio MT, Moon-Grady AJ, Hornberger LK, et al. Diagnosis and treatment of fetal cardiac disease: a scientific statement from the American Heart Association. *Circulation.* 2014;129(21):2183-2242.
36. Dutton PJ, Warrander LK, Roberts SA, et al. Predictors of poor perinatal outcome following maternal perception of reduced fetal movements--a prospective cohort study. *Plos One.* 2012;7(7):e39784.

The Fetal Pacemaker

Yaniv Bar-Cohen • Gerald E. Loeb • Michael J. Silka • Jay D. Pruetz • Ramen H. Chmait

INTRODUCTION

Severe bradycardia, particularly when there is a sustained fetal heart rate (FHR) < 50 beats per minute (bpm), is infrequent but carries a high mortality and is usually associated with hydrops fetalis due to the development of heart failure.[1] There are several reasons for the poor outcome of these fetuses. First, functional elements to increase cardiac output are limited in the fetal heart. Cardiac myocytes lack well-developed sarcoplasmic reticulum, sympathetic innervation, and beta-adrenergic receptors.[2-4] Beyond 19 weeks of gestation, the fetal heart is operating near the top of the Frank-Starling curve[5]; that is, both ventricles have a diminished capacity to increase stroke volume from increased preload.[5,6] With reduced contractility and a limited ability to increase stroke volume, fetal cardiac output is largely FHR dependent. Second, medical therapy with chronotropic agents such as terbutaline may increase FHR for a time, but tachyphylaxis develops, and maternal side effects are often not tolerated.[7,8] After birth, several reliable options are available for cardiac pacing in the neonate, child, and adult.[9] However, in utero pacing to resolve hydrops and prolong the pregnancy to a mature gestation is a tremendous challenge. Currently, there are no proven methods available for successful fetal pacing.

Etiologies of Bradycardia

There are multiple etiologies for bradycardia, but not all are severe. The bradycardias with a 1:1 atrioventricular (AV) relationship result from sinus node (SAN) abnormalities associated with heterotaxy, usually left atrial isomerism in which the SAN is frequently absent. Although mutations of ion channel coding genes such as SCN5[10] and HCN4[11] and genes involved in SAN development[12-14] have been identified as a cause of bradycardia during postnatal life, these appear to be rare in the fetus. Lastly, the SAN can be damaged by inflammation leading to fibrosis from viruses and maternal anti-Ro/SSA antibodies.[15,16] In some cases, the entire atrium can be rendered electrically inert secondary to maternal antibodies.[17]

The bradycardias without a 1:1 relationship include AV block associated with maternal anti-Ro/SSA antibodies, structural cardiac anomalies, or functional AV block in long QT syndrome (LQTS).[18] Regardless of etiology, fetuses with AV block are at high risk for severe bradycardia. It is this population that may benefit most from fetal cardiac pacing.

The development of hydrops fetalis due to congestive heart failure is seen in a quarter of pregnancies complicated by anti-Ro/SSA antibody–mediated AV block.[1,19] The risk is higher in those with structural heart anomalies and AV block but unknown in fetuses with LQTS and functional AV block. Once hydrops fetalis occurs, if the fetus cannot be delivered due to prematurity or other clinical concerns, fetal demise is nearly inevitable.[1,19] Although the degree of myocardial dysfunction is variable, successful pacing of a fetus with AV block and hydrops fetalis could theoretically allow resolution of hydrops over several weeks and permit and conclude in a term gestation. As a result, the specific group of patients with AV block and hydrops fetalis has historically been a target for fetal pacing despite the untested and invasive procedures. Unfortunately, to date, all attempts at pacing human fetuses have invariably failed with no survivors.

To address the challenge of fetal pacing, investigators at Children's Hospital Los Angeles and the University of Southern California have developed a novel pacing system specifically designed for minimally invasive implantation in a human fetus. This chapter will discuss the challenges of fetal pacing, describe a number of historical attempts at fetal pacing, and outline the indications for and strategy behind a proposed fetal micropacemaker.

HISTORY OF FETAL PACING

In the setting of a fetus with severe bradycardia, the development of hydrops fetalis carries an extremely poor prognosis. During the past three decades, there have been several reports attempting fetal pacing. Indications in all cases have been severe bradycardia, hydrops fetalis, and AV block. These cases are described below.

In 1986, Carpenter et al first reported an attempt at fetal pacing[20] in a fetus with maternal anti-Ro/SSA–mediated AV block and an FHR of 44 bpm at 27 1/2 weeks of gestation. A 17-gauge needle was advanced though the uterine cavity and fetal thorax and into the right ventricular cavity. A bipolar pigtail pacing catheter was placed through this needle into the fetal right ventricle, and the needle was subsequently removed. The pacing wire was attached to an external pacing system, and pacing was initiated at 120 bpm. Initially, the capture threshold (the minimum amount of energy required to a cause cardiac contraction) was 1.5 mA, and the heart was paced at 6 mA. After 4 hours and 15 minutes, intermittent heart tones were heard, and the output was increased to 20 mA without improvement. Five minutes later, heart sounds were absent, and an ultrasound confirmed asystole, despite the pacing catheter having remained in the right ventricle with no evidence for hematoma, thrombi, or pericardial effusions. At postmortem examination, a serosanguinous pericardial effusion was present, but the cause of loss of pacing capture was not clear. Although the cause of death was not known, the authors describe the pacing lead as being only moderately flexible with the possibility of dislodgement or injury with vigorous fetal movement.

A second fetal pacing attempt was made on a 24-week fetus of an anti-Ro/SSA–positive pregnancy who also had hydrops and AV block but had not survived.[21] The fetal umbilical vein was punctured using a 20-gauge needle, and a Teflon-coated pacing lead (0.009 in) was placed into the inferior vena cava just below the diaphragm and advanced through the right atrium into the right ventricle. Extra loops of wire were positioned in the fetal abdomen and in the amniotic fluid, and the pacing wire was connected to a Legend II pacemaker (Medtronic Inc., Minneapolis, MN) which was implanted subcutaneously in the maternal abdominal wall. Pacing at 140 bpm was initiated (at 5 V with a 0.5 ms pulse width—capture threshold was 0.5 V), and the heart rate was 140 bpm 8 hours later. Soon thereafter, however, a return to a slow heart rate was seen, which was presumed to be due to lead displacement. Five days later, an attempt at placing a larger pacing wire along the complete length of the umbilical cord was made in an attempt to reduce the risk for dislodgement. The placental cord was directly punctured, and an 18-gauge needle was used. However, just after the umbilical vein was punctured, the heart rate fell further and asystole followed. An autopsy did not show hemorrhage or tamponade of the cord, but a bright yellow spot was visible at the right ventricular apex, the presumed initial site of pacing.

In 1998, the next report of an attempt at fetal pacing for severe bradycardia and immune-mediated AV block was via an open fetal surgery (maternal laparotomy and hysterotomy) and fetal thoracotomy for direct epicardial pacemaker placement. Unfortunately, the fetus did not survive the procedure.[22]

The first reported pacing attempt in a fetus with complex congenital heart disease and AV block was described by Assad et al in 2003.[23] The fetus was at 24-week gestation at the time of the procedure and had complete AV block, severe bradycardia, marked hydrops, and left atrial isomerism with an atrioventricular septal defect. The novel lead was T-shaped and was introduced through an 18-gauge needle directly into the fetal myocardium (FIG. 6.3.1). A second lead was placed in the thoracic wall for bipolar stimulation, and both leads were connected to a pacemaker (Biotronik ERA 300; Berlin, Germany) implanted in the maternal abdominal wall. Pacing at 140 bpm was initiated, but cardiac tamponade was apparent during the procedure and managed with pericardiocentesis. By the first postoperative day, myocardial function had recovered with a mild pericardial effusion present. After 36 hours of pacing, however, asystole was noticed by ultrasound, and the pericardial effusion appeared significant. Fetal autopsy suggested that a moderate bloody effusion in the pericardial sac was the probable cause of death; the leads were in the left ventricle muscle and thoracic wall as expected.

Another attempt at open fetal pacing was described in 2011 by Eghtesady et al[24] who reported on a 32-year-old mother with a 29-week gestation with immune-mediated AV block, hydrops fetalis, and heart rates in the mid-40s bpm. Open fetal surgery was

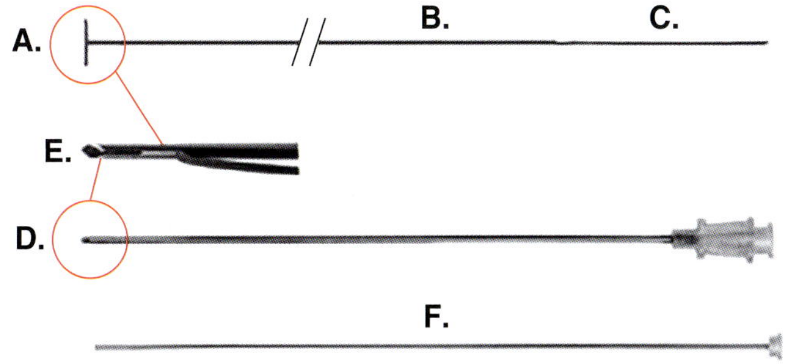

FIGURE 6.3.1 An introducer needle with a novel T-bar lead. **A:** Stainless steel bar; **B:** pacing wire; **C:** straight needle; **D:** 18-gauge introducer needle with a beveled tip fashioned with a 7-mm longitudinal side slot cut from the heel of the bevel (**E**); **F:** needle stylet. (Reprinted from Assad RS, Zielinsky P, Kalil R, et al. New lead for in utero pacing for fetal congenital heart block. *J Thorac Cardiovasc Surg*. 2003;126:300-302.)

performed to implant the small Microny pacemaker (St. Jude Medical Inc., St. Paul, MN). On the first postoperative day, mild oligohydramnios was present, but cardiac output had appeared to be 150% of the prepacing cardiac output assessment. The next day, an attempt was made to increase the pacing rate due to persistent oligohydramnios; however, communication with the device to alter the pacing parameters was not successful despite repositioning attempts. Fetal demise was seen 5 days after the procedure and was attributed to chronic multiorgan failure based on the autopsy findings.

A final description of pacing for anti-Ro/SSA–mediated AV block fetal was recently described via *ex utero* intrapartum treatment (EXIT) procedure in a 21-year-old mother at 36 weeks of gestation with severe bradycardia and cardiac dysfunction.[25] Rather than prolonging the gestation, this procedure had the goal of improving the transition to extrauterine life. The fetal head, chest, and upper extremities were delivered through a low transverse uterine incision. A temporary right ventricular lead was placed by a subxyphoid incision, and pacing was initiated at 70 bpm. The infant was delivered 55 minutes after the fetus was exteriorized, and a permanent pacemaker was ultimately implanted at 3 days of age.

Although never used in a human fetus, a novel pacing technique with potential for human fetal pacing was tested in a rat model by Dell'orfano et al.[26] In this procedure, the diaphragm was exposed via a subcostal incision, and a J-wire was advanced to the thorax. A custom-made 6 Fr pacing lead with a pigtail shape, a single central lumen, and a single electrode at the distal end was then advanced over the J-wire and positioned as close as possible to the mediastinum. The pacing lead was then connected to a Medtronic 5320 external pacemaker (Medtronic 5320, Medtronic Inc, Minneapolis, MN), and pacing was successful in 10 of the 11 rats. Despite being developed for use in humans, no human fetal pacing attempts using this system have been subsequently described.

Although there are many reasons these early attempts at in utero pacing failed, these experiences were helpful in developing a novel fetal pacemaker. Due to the risk to the fetus, potential risk to the mother,[27,28] and failure of sustained fetal pacing with open surgery, the team wanted to develop a less invasive method. Since the last report on fetal pacing, several novel techniques were developed for placing a pacing lead without open fetal surgery. However, the general paradigm of placing a pacing lead on the fetal heart and connecting that lead to an extracorporeal pacemaker (either an external pacemaker or a pacemaker implanted in the maternal abdomen) poses a significant theoretical challenge that occurs because the fetus is moving in the amniotic space and is tethered to the mother by both the umbilical cord and the pacing lead (which may be more prone to dislodge). Although dislodgement was not the etiology of failure in every case reported, ensuring adequate contact of the pacing electrode in the setting of fetal movement is of vital importance.

DEVELOPMENT OF A FETAL MICROPACEMAKER

In order to find a potential solution to the conundrum of fetal pacing, a system was needed that would address the two major challenges of fetal pacing: avoiding open fetal surgery and avoiding exteriorized fetal pacing leads. To accomplish this, the study team fabricated a micropacemaker that could be contained entirely within the fetus and be implanted percutaneously without the need for open fetal surgery. The fetal pacemaker was designed as a small cylindrical device that could be implanted through a cannula, and the study team ensured that the entire system (electrode, lead, and pacemaker) could be implanted through that same single long cannula. To maximize the chance for survival from the procedure, the delivery system was fabricated to be able to use fetal procedural equipment already in use with demonstrated safety.[29]

The pacing system and implantation equipment are shown in **FIG. 6.3.2.**[30] Under ultrasound guidance, the cannula and obturator are advanced through the uterus and fetal chest wall and toward the cardiac ventricles. By definition, the hydropic fetus undergoing micropacemaker implantation would have a pericardial effusion that could be exploited to facilitate surgical access to the ventricles. Once ultrasound imaging suggests that the cannula is near the heart, the obturator is removed, and the pacemaker implantation system is advanced through the cannula so that the distal electrode screw is in direct contact with the epicardium. The system is then rotated clockwise, allowing the pacing electrode screw to be advanced into the myocardium. The entire device is then released by slowly withdrawing the cannula while keeping the device in place with a pushrod. The pacing electrode would therefore remain attached to the myocardium, and the cylindrical pacing device would reside in the fetal chest (likely within a pleural effusion) with a flexible connecting lead absorbing any relative motion during each heartbeat **(FIGS. 6.3.3.** and **6.3.4)**

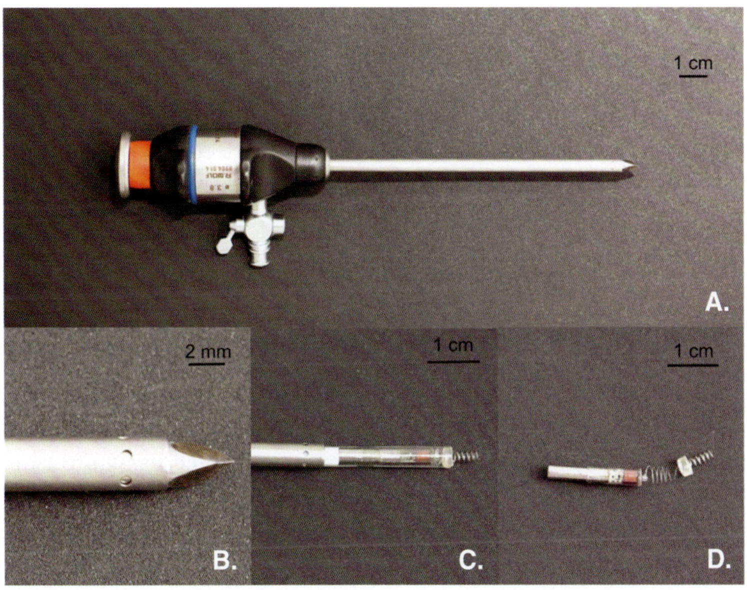

FIGURE 6.3.2 The fetal micropacemaker implantation equipment is shown. **A:** The implantation cannula with an obturator inside. **B:** The sharp tip of the obturator protrudes from the end of the cannula when inserted into the body. **C:** The micropacemaker is shown inside its implantation sheath protruding through the cannula. **D:** The micropacemaker device (micropacemaker [3.475 mm diameter, 18 mm long]) is connected to the distal electrode screw via a coiled flexible lead. (Reprinted from Bar-Cohen Y, Loeb GE, Pruetz J, et al. Preclinical testing and optimization of a novel fetal micropacemaker. *Heart Rhythm*. 2015;12:1683-1690.)

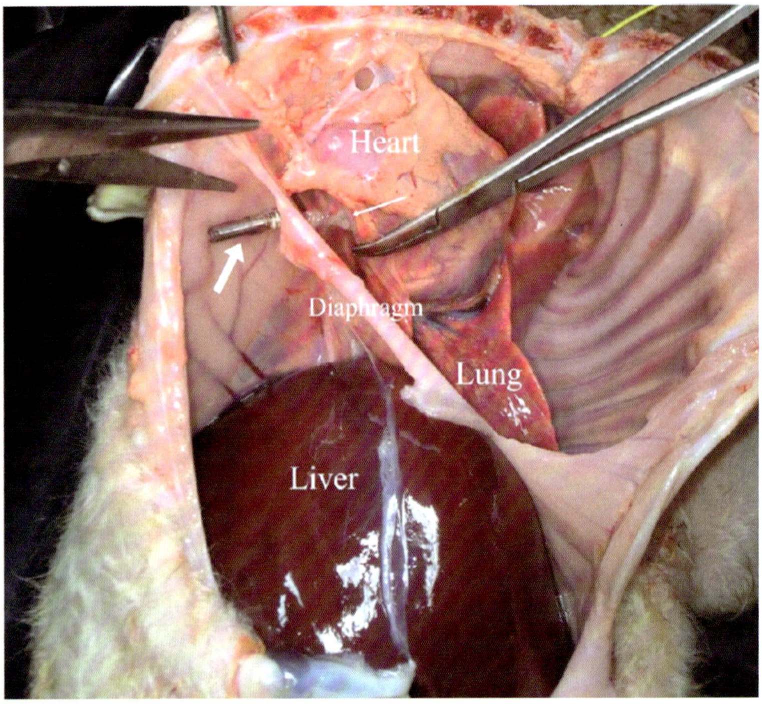

FIGURE 6.3.3 Necropsy specimen of fetal sheep. The micropacemaker is seen passing through the diaphragm (large arrow). The electrode (small arrow) penetrates the left ventricular wall. (Reprinted from Bar-Cohen Y, Loeb GE, Pruetz J, et al. Preclinical testing and optimization of a novel fetal micropacemaker. *Heart Rhythm.* 2015;12:1683-1690.)

The initial experiments focused on the pacing properties of the electrode screw and were open-chest experiments in rabbits to test the electrode—myocardial properties.[31] Thereafter, a nonfunctional, but similarly shaped, device was implanted into an anesthetized adult rabbit through a subxyphoid approach.[31] These early experiments allowed the study team to optimize the pacing properties of the pacemaker and validated the implantation model. Further optimization included the incorporation of a rechargeable battery and a system for wireless recharging of the pacemaker from outside the maternal body.[32]

After these modification, more recent experiments were in a fetal sheep model and allowed further optimization of the pacing system.[30] In a series of seven fetal sheep experiments, micropacemaker devices were implanted using ultrasound guidance, and a series of alterations were made to the system through the iterative process: electrode design changes, circuit board alterations, and refinements to the procedure itself. Several limitations of the fetal sheep model are noteworthy and made the implantation procedures more difficult than anticipated in a human fetus with severe bradycardia. First, the fetal sheep had normal hearts without bradycardia. In order to demonstrate that pacing was successful in a fetus without bradycardia, the experiments required implantation of electrodes on the fetuses' skin for ECG assessment. Although this allowed appropriate assessment of pacing,[30] it required a far more invasive procedure and a uterine incision for the skin electrode implantation. In addition,

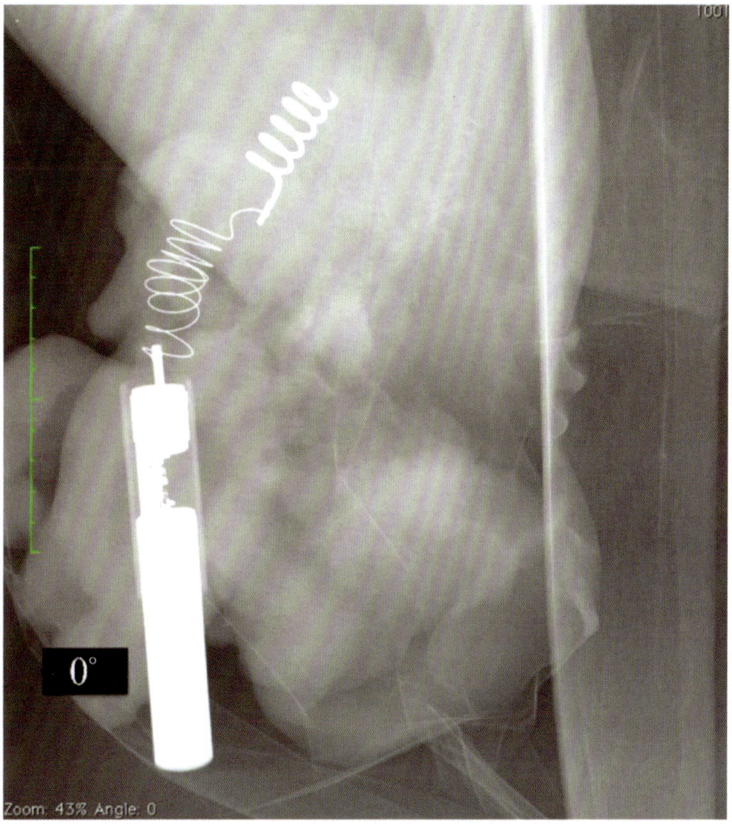

FIGURE 6.3.4 Radiograph of a fetal sheep heart specimen. The electrode is connected to the micropacemaker via a flexible lead. (Reprinted from Bar-Cohen Y, Loeb GE, Pruetz J, et al. Preclinical testing and optimization of a novel fetal micropacemaker. *Heart Rhythm*. 2015;12:1683-1690.)

the fetal sheep did not have hydrops fetalis and therefore did not have a pericardial effusion. The fetal pacemaker was developed for implantation in a fetus with hydrops fetalis in which the implantation scheme would be greatly facilitated by the presence of a pericardial effusion and free space in which to place the cannula tip against the epicardial surface of the heart. The study attempted to accommodate for the intrinsic lack of pericardial effusion in later experiments by infusing saline into the pericardial space. By doing so, it created a pericardial effusion in the final four animals. However, in addition to the further risk of this additional technical step, only a small amount of fluid could be infused into the pericardium without significant risk for tamponade and cardiac compromise. Ultimately, successful capture of the myocardium was demonstrated in five of the seven fetal sheep, but the limitations of the fetal sheep model made conclusions regarding safety and longer term efficacy of the fetal micropacemaker difficult to discern. These experiments, however, did provide support for and demonstrate the necessity of a clinical trial to confirm the viability of the fetal micropacemaker for treating the hydropic fetus with 3° AV block. Histologic data (FIG. 6.3.5) and evidence of increasing capture thresholds over time also provided important data on the inflammatory reaction present at the electrode-myocardial interface

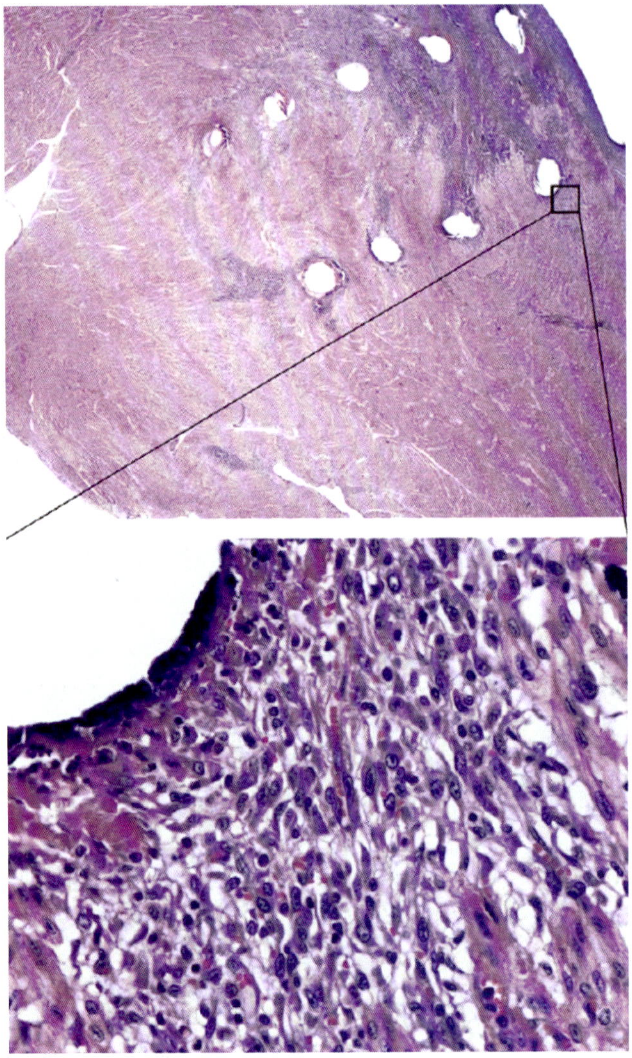

FIGURE 6.3.5 Histology at the implantation site. Histology demonstrates the path of the electrode (seen as round voids) as it tunneled into the myocardium. There is moderate myocardial degeneration and necrosis with a mixed inflammatory reaction including macrophages, lymphocytes, and neutrophils. (Reprinted from Bar-Cohen Y, Loeb GE, Pruetz J, et al. Preclinical testing and optimization of a novel fetal micropacemaker. *Heart Rhythm*. 2015;12:1683-1690.)

in the fetus. Because the literature suggests that fetuses demonstrate less fibrosis than seen in children and adults,[33] the degree of inflammation and subsequent increases in threshold were difficult to predict. However, based on the fetal sheep results, the study team has concluded that inflammation of the fetal epicardium should be viewed as similar to that seen after birth and that the addition of a steroid-eluding plug near the electrode tip may be beneficial to modulate the consequences of inflammation on pacing threshold.[34,35]

THE FETAL MICROPACEMAKER: CURRENT STATUS

The fetal micropacemaker is currently untested in humans, and much clinical work will be required before the device is ultimately approved for use in the human fetus. The fetal micropacemaker has received a humanitarian use device (HUD) designation from the Food and Drug Administration (FDA) due to the small number of patients who would ultimately require its use. This HUD designation does allow for a shorter path to approval, but the rarity of cases when the fetal micropacemaker would be indicated still portends a long course to ultimate FDA approval and commercialization.

At this time, the only indications for fetal pacing using the micropacemaker are fetuses with anti-Ro/SSA–mediated AV block, severe bradycardia, and hydrops fetalis. Due to the invasive nature of any procedure performed on a fetus, a high expected mortality (if untreated) would be required for a patient to be considered a candidate. In addition, the initial target population includes only those fetuses with 3° AV block and hydrops fetalis without other significant heart disease. The lack of previous pacing successes in the hydropic fetus makes it difficult to predict the expected improvement in fetal health after successful pacing. However, the study team has been working under the assumption that successful pacing and treatment of bradycardia may reverse or even cure the hydrops within several weeks as seen in other hydropic conditions.[36]

While hydrops fetalis due to 3° AV block can manifest in a number of ways in the human fetus, a pericardial effusion is required as an inclusion criterion for pacing at this point in the work. As described above, a major challenge of the fetal sheep model was accurately placing the cannula tip within the pericardium space and directly against the epicardial surface. Advancing the cannula through the pericardium without injuring the underlying epicardium (separated normally by only a potential space) proved difficult, while the presence of a pericardial effusion would both help visibility and greatly facilitate positioning of the cannula correctly in that space.

Although the appropriate gestational age for implanting the device is not yet clear, a gestational age of 18 to 32 weeks has been considered as a reasonable window to consider for implantation of the micropacemaker device because viability of a hydropic fetus less than 34 weeks' gestation is poor.[37] The very small chest size at smaller gestational ages than 18 weeks makes that a relative lower limit for age. At the same time, gestational ages significantly above 32 weeks, gestation should trigger a decision for delivery in the near future as opposed to an experimental and untested procedure. Recognition of the potential harm from the procedure to the fetus and the mother makes the presence of multiple gestations a contraindication for the pacemaker at this time. In addition, other medical problems that would portend a poor outcome for the infant (in addition to other heart disease) may be a contraindication to pacing depending on the condition.

The study team anticipates that a neonate with AV block will require lifelong cardiac pacing. The fetal micropacemaker is not designed for such prolonged use, and its fragile flexible lead may not survive long after chest expansion at birth. In addition, although the fetal micropacemaker is intended to be recharged throughout the gestation, each charge lasts less than 1 week, which makes the device impractical for prolonged use after birth. At present, infants needing permanent cardiac pacing require open-chest surgery to implant an epicardial lead connected to a conventional pacemaker in the abdomen. Using many of the concepts from the development of the fetal micropacemaker, efforts are underway to develop a minimally invasive technology to implant a larger version of the micropacemaker that would reside entirely within the pericardial space.[38]

SUMMARY

Although pacing the child or adult with bradycardia is now considered straightforward and routine, successfully pacing a fetus has remained a significant challenge. Pacing a fetus with severe bradycardia and hydrops fetalis is appealing due to the potential to reverse the hydrops caused by cardiovascular compromise from the bradycardia and potentially allow the pregnancy to continue to term. Nonetheless, the continued challenge of fetal pacing has been clearly demonstrated by the numerous failed attempts over the past 30 years with no survivors to date. A fetal micropacemaker is currently being developed to allow an entire self-contained pacing system to be implanted into a fetus percutaneously without open surgery. While human testing has yet to be performed, the device has been tested in fetal sheep and offers great potential as a viable option for the treatment of this life-threatening condition.

References

1. Eliasson H, Sonesson SE, Sharland G, et al; for the Fetal Working Group of the European Association of Pediatric Cardiology. Isolated atrioventricular block in the fetus: a retrospective, multinational, multicenter study of 175 patients. *Circulation*. 2011;124:1919-1926.
2. Mahony L, Jones LR. Developmental changes in cardiac sarcoplasmic reticulum in sheep. *J Biol Chem*. 1986;261(32):15257-15265.
3. Birk E, Tyndall MR, Erickson LC, Rudolph AM, Roberts JM. Effects of thyroid hormone on myocardial adrenergic beta-receptor responsiveness and function during late gestation. *Pediatr Res*. 1992;31(5):468-473.
4. Lebowitz EA, Novick JS, Rudolph AM. Development of myocardial sympathetic innervation in the fetal lamb. *Pediatr Res*. 1972;6(12):887-893.
5. Thornburg KL, Morton MJ. Filling and arterial pressures as determinants of left ventricular stroke volume in fetal lambs. *Am J Physiol*. 1986;251(5 pt 2):H961-H968.
6. Reller MD, Morton MJ, Reid DL, Thornburg KL. Fetal lamb ventricles respond differently to filling and arterial pressures and to in utero ventilation. *Pediatr Res*. 1987;22(6):621-626.
7. Cuneo BF, Zhao H, Strasburger JF, Ovadia M, Huhta JC, Wakai RT. Atrial and ventricular rate response and patterns of heart rate acceleration during maternal-fetal terbutaline treatment of fetal complete heart block. *Am J Cardiol*. 2007;100(4):661-665.
8. Padovani TR, Guyatt G, Lopes LC. Nifedipine versus terbutaline, tocolytic effectiveness and maternal and neonatal adverse effects: a randomized, controlled pilot trial. *Basic Clin Pharmacol Toxicol*. 2015;116(3):244-250.
9. Ebstein AE, Dimarco JP, Ellenbogen KA, et al. Device-based therapy of cardiac rhythm abnormalities: a report of the American College of Cardiology Foundation/American Heart Association Task Force on practice guidelines and the Heart Rhythm Society ACCF/AHA/HRS focused update incorporated into the ACCF/AHA/HRS 2008 guidelines. *J Am Coll Cardiol*. 2013;61(3):4-75.
10. Benson DW, Wang DW, Dyment M, et al. Congenital sick sinus syndrome caused by recessive mutations in the cardiac sodium channel gene (SCN5A). *J Clin Invest*. 2003;112(7):1019-1028.
11. Milanesi R , Baruscotti M, Gnecchi-Ruscone T, DiFrancesco D. Familial sinus bradycardia associated with a mutation in the cardiac pacemaker channel. *N Engl J Med*. 2006;354(2):151-157.
12. Ye W, Song Y, Huang Z, Zhang Y, Chen Y. Genetic regulation of sinoatrial node development and pacemaker program in the venous Pole. *J Cardiovasc Dev Dis*. 2015;2(4):282-298.

13. Vicente-Steijn R, Kelder TP, Tertoolen LG, et al. RHOA-ROCK signalling is necessary for lateralization and differentiation of the developing sinoatrial node. *Cardiovasc Res.* 2017;113(10):1186-1197.
14. Liu H, Espinoza-Lewis RA, Chen C, Hu X, Zhang Y, Chen Y. The role of Shox2 in SAN development and function. *Pediatr Cardiol.* 2012;33(6):882-889.
15. Chockalingam P, Jaeggi ET, Rammeloo LA, et al. Persistent fetal sinus bradycardia associated with maternal anti-SSA/Ro and anti-SSB/La antibodies. *J Rheumatol.* 2011;38(12):2682-2685.
16. Cuneo BF, Strasburger JF, Niksch A, Ovadia M, Wakai RT. An expanded phenotype of maternal SSA/SSB antibody-associated fetal cardiac disease. *J Matern Fetal Neonatal Med.* 2009;22(3):233.
17. Jaeggi ET, Chitayat D, Taylor G. Atrial standstill associated with loss of atrial myocytes: a rare cause of fetal bradyarrhythmia. *Heart Rhythm.* 2009;6(9):1370-1372.
18. Cuneo BF. Fetal bradycardia. In: Yagel S, Silverman NH, Gembruch U, eds. *Fetal Cardiology*. London: Taylor and Francis, LLC; 2019: 515-529.
19. Lopes LM, Tavares GM, Damiano AP, et al. Perinatal outcome of fetal atrioventricular block: one-hundred-sixteen cases from a single institution. *Circulation.* 2008;118:1268-1275.
20. Carpenter RJ Jr, Strasburger JF, Garson A Jr, Smith RT, Deter RL, Engelhardt HT Jr. Fetal ventricular pacing for hydrops secondary to complete atrioventricular block. *J Am Coll Cardiol.* 1986;8:1434-1436.
21. Walkinshaw SA, Wlech CR, McCormack J, Walsh K. In utero pacing for fetal congenital heart block. *Fetal Diagn Ther.* 1994;9:183-185.
22. Silverman NH, Kohl T, Harrison MR, Hanley FL. Experimental fetal surgery in the animal model and in the human fetus. In: Imai Y, Momma K, eds. *Proceedings of the Second World Congress of Pediatric Cardiology and Cardiac Surgery*. Armonk, NY: Futura Publishing Co; 1998:622-623.
23. Assad RS, Zielinsky P, Kalil R, et al. New lead for in utero pacing for fetal congenital heart block. *J Thorac Cardiovasc Surg.* 2003;126:300-302.
24. Eghtesady P1, Michelfelder EC, Knilans TK, Witte DP, Manning PB, Crombleholme TM. Fetal surgical management of congenital heart block in a hydropic fetus: lessons learned from a clinical experience. *J Thorac Cardiovasc Surg.* 2011;141:835-837.
25. Cuneo BF, Mitchell MB, Marwan AI, et al. Ex utero intrapartum treatment to ventricular pacing: a novel delivery strategy for complete atrioventricular block with severe bradycardia. *Fetal Diagn Ther.* 2017;42(4):311-314.
26. Dell'Orfano J, Chou HA, Park D, et al. The monolithic fetal pacemaker: prototype lead design for closed thorax deployment. *Pacing Clin Electrophysiol.* April 2003;26(4 Pt 1):805-811.
27. Golombeck K, Ball RH, Lee H, et al. Maternal morbidity after maternal-fetal surgery. *Am J Obstet Gynecol.* 2006;194:834-839.
28. Wilson RD, Lemerand K, Johnson MP, et al. Reproductive outcomes in subsequent pregnancies after a pregnancy complicated by open maternal-fetal surgery (1996-2007). *Am J Obstet Gynecol.* 2010;203:209.e1-209.e6.
29. Chmait R, Kontopoulos E, Quintero R. Fetoscopic management of complicated monochorionic twins. *Clin Obstet Gynecol.* 2009;52:647-653.
30. Bar-Cohen Y, Loeb GE, Pruetz J, et al. Preclinical testing and optimization of a novel fetal micropacemaker. *Heart Rhythm.* 2015;12:1683-1690.
31. Loeb GE, Zhou L, Zheng K, et al. Design and testing of a percutaneously implantable fetal pacemaker. *Ann Biomed Eng.* 2013;41(1):17-27.
32. Vest AN, Zhou L, Huang X, et al. Design and testing of a transcutaneous RF recharging system for a fetal micropacemaker. *IEEE Trans Biomed Circuits Syst.* 2017;11(2):336-346.
33. Dang C, Ting K, Soo C, Longaker MT, Lorenz HP. Fetal wound healing current perspectives. *Clin Plast Surg.* 2003;30:13-23.
34. Horenstein MS, Hakimi M, Walters H III, Karpawich PP. Chronic performance of steroid-eluting epicardial leads in a growing pediatric population: a 10-year comparison. *Pacing Clin Electrophysiol.* 2003;26(7 pt 1):1467-1471.
35. Mond HG, Stokes KB. The steroid-eluting electrode: a 10-year experience. *Pacing Clin Electrophysiol.* 1996;19:1016-1020.
36. Macé G, Sauvan M, Castaigne V, et al. Clinical presentation and outcome of 20 fetuses with parvovirus B19 infection complicated by severe anemia and/or fetal hydrops. *Prenat Diagn.* 2014;34(11):1023-1030.
37. Norton ME, Chauhan SP, Dashe JS. Society for maternal-fetal medicine (SMFM) clinical guideline #7: nonimmune hydrops fetalis. *Am J Obstet Gynecol.* 2015;212(2):127-139.
38. Bar-Cohen Y, Silka MJ, Hill AC, et al. Minimally invasive implantation of a micropacemaker into the pericardial space. *Circ Arrhythm Electrophysiol.* 2018;11:e006307.

Diagnosis from a Distance: Telecardiology in the Evaluation of Fetal Arrhythmias

J. Fred Thomas • Christina A. Olson • Gerard Frunzi • Bettina F. Cuneo

INTRODUCTION

There are several reasons that a timely and accurate diagnosis of a fetal arrhythmia is beneficial to the fetus and to the pregnancy. First, diagnosis sets the stage for appropriate care. Second, risk stratifying fetal arrhythmias efficiently utilizes healthcare resources.[1,2] Third, after the diagnosis is made, the parents can consult with the physician to develop a care plan, which can reduce stress and anxiety.[3]

However, fetal arrhythmia expertise is usually concentrated in cardiac centers, often many miles from the pregnant woman's home. In the absence of this expertise, initial triage of fetuses with arrhythmias is performed by obstetricians, family physicians, or mid-wives ("OB providers") in the local community. One solution to expand access to limited but necessary expertise is by partnering OB providers from the local community with fetal cardiologists at a distant cardiac center through a form of telemedicine we call "fetal telecardiology." Fetal telecardiology is the real-time performance of fetal echocardiograms at the local community site with a face-to-face virtual interpretation, diagnosis, and consultation by fetal cardiologists at the distant cardiac center.

Such a partnership between OB providers in the local community and fetal cardiologists at the distant cardiac center is possible due to recent advancements in telecommunication technologies including the digital transmission of objective data blended with video conferencing software. Telemedicine has reduced cost, increased efficiency, improved quality, and expanded patient access to subspecialists in some areas of medicine, including obstetrics.[4-14] Fetal teleECHO for identification of structural heart disease during screening echocardiograms has been described,[15-17] but there are few data on the use of fetal telecardiology in the evaluation and management of fetal arrhythmias.

This chapter will describe the results of one fetal telecardiology program, the necessary resources needed to develop such a program, and the real and potential impact on providers, patients, and the healthcare system.

DEVELOPMENT OF A FETAL TELECARDIOLOGY PROGRAM

Feasibility

The feasibility of a fetal telecardiology program is strongly dependent on several factors. First, OB providers in the community must understand and desire the benefits of such a program for their patients and themselves, the latter in the form of continued education and practice quality improvement. Second, a respectful and collaborative relationship between fetal cardiologists in the distant cardiac center and OB providers in the community needs to be established and nurtured; without this effort, employing fancy technology and equipment has little value. Third, OB sonographers in the community must be comfortable scanning fetal hearts independently with virtual coaching and guidance. Fourth, the fetal cardiologist must be committed to providing care "on demand," outside of regular clinic hours, as some fetal arrhythmias require urgent evaluation. Fifth, telemedicine technical support is necessary at the distant and community sites to prevent interruption of services. Sixth, in many cases, the fetal cardiologist must be comfortable with teaching and supervising OB sonographers rather than pediatric echo technicians. Lastly, the health system administrators, physicians, and providers at both the community and distant cardiac center must be aligned and agree on long-term goals, such as improving fetal cardiology productivity, expanding clinical coverage across the region, and increasing clinical capacity of the cardiac center.

Aims

The key aims of a comprehensive fetal telecardiology program are to:

1. Advance the education and training of local OB sonographers in fetal cardiac imaging and arrhythmia ascertainment.
2. Increase the access, efficiency, and process of care for the patients needing these services.
3. Demonstrate that this new and innovative care model has the same diagnostic quality as face-to-face encounters.
4. Determine that fetal telecardiology is accepted and even preferable by mothers and their OB providers in the community.

Education and Training of Sonographers

Expertise and experience in fetal anatomic surveys provide a good background for training in fetal arrhythmia diagnosis. The training period for OB sonographers already competent in fetal scans is usually 3 to 6 months. Training begins with implementing standard fetal echocardiography protocols under the supervision of experienced fetal echo sonographers and fetal cardiologists at the distant cardiac center. Once protocols are firmly established, the OB sonographers observe images of fetal rhythm abnormalities. Lastly, the sonographer applies the echo protocol to systematically evaluate fetuses with arrhythmias. Most of training occurs at the cardiac center, but skills are reinforced by repetitive in-person instruction by the fetal cardiologist working with the OB sonographers at the community hospital. The importance of in-depth, multisession training cannot be understated, as high-quality rhythm assessment by the sonographer is critical for appropriate diagnosis and treatment.

Ideally, the self-reported confidence, fetal echo skills, and efficiency of the sonographers increase significantly after this educational period. In our experience, the time to complete a teleECHO on a fetus with an arrhythmia decreased from 45 minutes in the first year of the telecardiology program to 25 minutes in the third year.[18] In addition, pathological arrhythmias, such as atrioventricular block and supraventricular tachycardia, were differentiated from benign arrhythmias including premature atrial contractions and sinus tachycardia.

Establishing Clinic Process and Efficiency (Fig. 6.4.1)

Pregnant women with risk factors for fetal arrhythmia[2] can be scheduled once a week in a virtual fetal telecardiology clinic at the community site. If a fetus is recognized to have an arrhythmia outside of the clinic time, the sonographer contacts the fetal cardiologist who makes himself available for a virtual echo review and consultation.

After arriving at the community site, the mother completes the intake form including her medical, family, and obstetrical histories, which is reviewed by the fetal cardiologist. Once the echocardiogram is completed by the local sonographer, the fetal cardiologist is connected to the community site (see below for technical details).

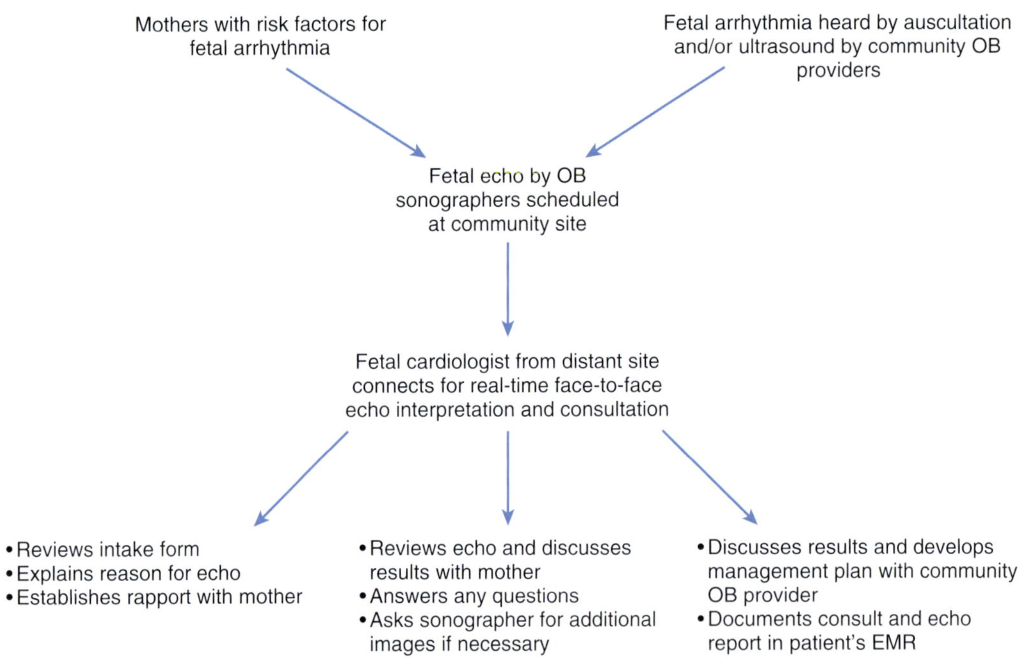

FIGURE 6.4.1 Workflow between the community hospital and providers and fetal cardiologist in the fetal telecardiology model. EMR = electronic medical record.

Through a real-time face-to-face virtual encounter, the fetal cardiologist reviews the fetal echo images captured by the local sonographer. If echo images were unclear or of nondiagnostic quality, the sonographer can rescan the mother while the fetal cardiologist observes. The results of the fetal echo are then discussed with the mother who can ask questions to the fetal cardiologist. The referring OB provider is contacted, and management and follow-up are discussed.

Acceptance of Fetal Telecardiology

One of the critical aspects of evaluating a fetal telecardiology model is satisfaction of both the patient and local OB provider. For the patient, the advantages of local care include convenience and cost savings by avoiding travel to the distant cardiac center without sacrificing quality of care. In our experience, 33 mothers with a fetal arrhythmia saved 46,280 driving miles by staying in their community, and the cost per visit was almost 10 times less ($61.2 vs. $580.5) compared to traveling to the distant cardiac center.[18] For the OB provider, satisfaction is based on developing a plan with the fetal cardiologist that in most instances keeps the patient under his care in the community, while improving his understanding of fetal arrhythmias. Keeping patients local also supports the financial viability of rural hospitals.[19]

A second critical aspect of program evaluation is the accuracy of rhythm diagnosis and risk stratification for postnatal management. In our experience, both have been equal to care provided on site at the cardiac center.[18]

FETAL TELECARDIOLOGY TECHNOLOGY

High bandwidth and internet speed are necessary for successful fetal telecardiology because of the large amount of data transferred during the fetal echocardiogram and the high resolution needed for a diagnostic-quality video stream. The two parts of fetal telecardiology are a bidirectional video conferencing system that allows a virtual face-to-face consultation between the mother and fetal cardiologist and a high-resolution video feed that receives the images from the ultrasound machine at the community site and transmits them real time to the distant cardiac center. These requirements are fulfilled by either a hosted video conference system or a Cloud solution with embedded or separate video conference system (FIGS. 6.4.2 and 6.4.3).

There are several video conference platforms available that support fetal telecardiology (FIG. 6.4.2). Common to all is the ability to receive the video feed (the images) from the ultrasound machine at the community site. The ultrasound images then feed into a video codec which treats the feed as if it were a high-resolution camera input. Ultrasound images from the local codec are transmitted to the codec at the distant cardiac center. The local codec can be switched from the ultrasound video feed (echo images) to video conferencing between the mother and OB sonographer, and the fetal cardiologist.

The video feed and conferencing data can be transferred from the community site to the distant cardiac center and vice versa in several ways (TABLE 6.4.1). The first is via a dedicated point-to-point data circuit such as a T-1 line, which provides excellent

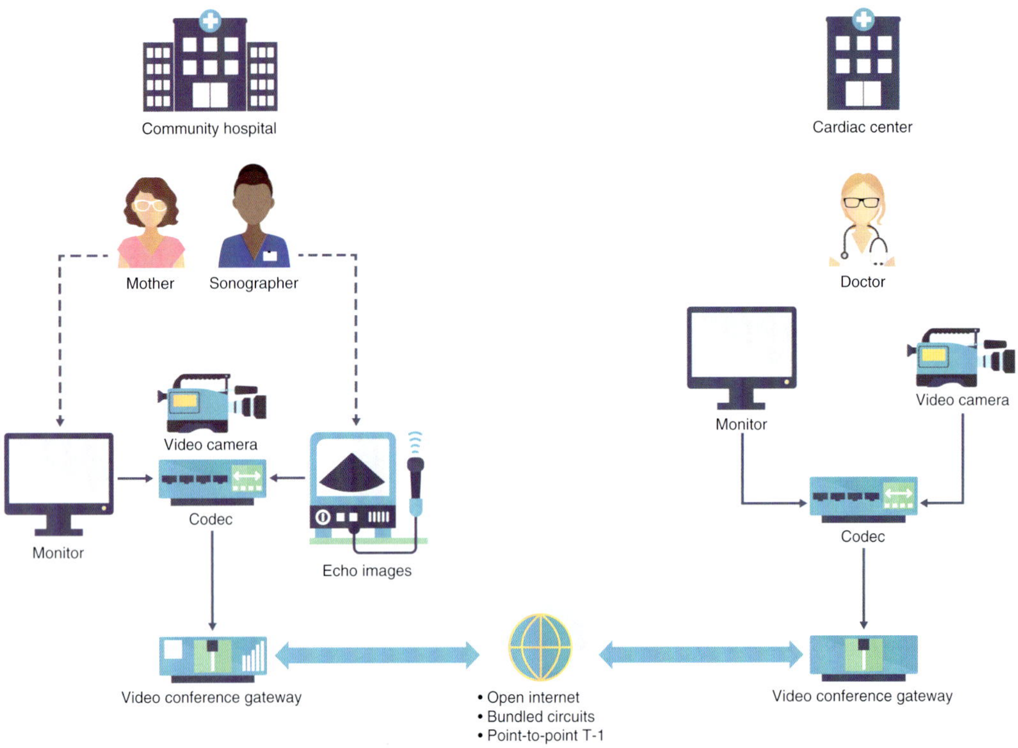

FIGURE 6.4.2 Shared video conference telemedicine solution. Images from the community hospital including fetal echo images, and the sonographer and mother are transmitted to the cardiac center via a video conferencing gateway, which is either a dedicated point-to-point circuit, a bundled circuit, or the open internet. The live and real-time images from the echo are viewed by the fetal cardiologist (doctor); the codec can then be switched for bidirectional video conferencing between the two sites.

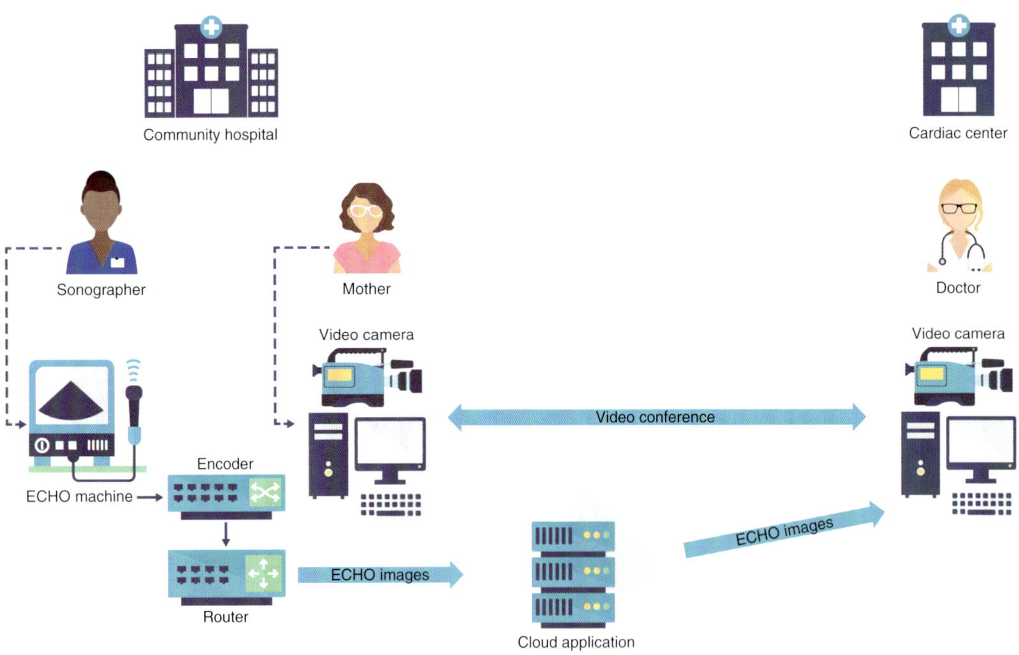

FIGURE 6.4.3 Cloud-based telemedicine solution. Images from the community hospital including fetal echo images, and the sonographer and mother are sent via the encoder and router to the cardiac center. The fetal cardiologist (doctor) reviews the echo images, then speaks to the mother and sonographer through two-way video conferencing.

TABLE 6.4.1 METHODS TO TRANSFER VIDEO FEED AND CONFERENCING FROM COMMUNITY TO DISTANT SITE

Method	Tech Level	Advantages	Disadvantages
Point-to-point data circuit	T1 or multiple DSL lines	Excellent quality at all times	Expensive
Bundled circuit: rented space in telehealth network	DS3 lines	Network is already established, reasonable costs	Data packet loss is high during peak use times and images are not of diagnostic quality
Open internet circuit	Internet	Very inexpensive	Same as for bundled circuit

image quality, but is expensive. The second is data transfer over a "bundled circuit" rented from a public telehealth organization. Not all states have such organizations: for example, Colorado has a telehealth network (using DS3 lines) which connects some but not all the hospitals within the state. Hospitals utilizing the network pay a monthly rental fee to the organization. Lastly, some sites opt to have an open internet circuit large enough to handle the video feed and conference data plus normal organizational operations. The disadvantage of the second and third method is that heavy internet traffic will slow the data transfer speed (also referred to as "packet loss"), resulting in pixilation and small delays in data transfer that render the diagnostic quality of the video feed unacceptable.

The Cloud solution with separate or embedded video conferencing **(FIG. 6.4.3)** leverages the power of the open internet and innovative companies in the telehealth industry. This solution focuses on the need for a high-resolution video stream from the ultrasound feed while allowing for lower speeds in the conferencing between the distant fetal cardiologist and the mother and sonographer in the community.

With the Cloud solution, the local site is provided with an encoder and internet router. The encoder, which replaces the codec used in the video conferencing solution, takes the high-resolution digital outfeed from the ultrasound machine at the local site. The digital outfeed is encrypted and sent through the internet router to a Cloud server. The distant site accesses the Cloud and downloads the ultrasound images to an application or a website. Some vendors include a video product, such as a tablet or cart, that allows conferencing between the community and distant sites. Other vendors separate the conference data from the video digital ultrasound data. Limitations of the Cloud solution include cost (currently they are more expensive than the hosted video conference solution) and lack of regulation and standards within the industry.

Ultrasound companies are developing telehealth options by adding network interface cards to their ultrasound platforms which allow direct transfer of ultrasound images via the internet from the community site to a tablet or computer at the distant site. This eliminates the need for a separate router (used in the Cloud solution) or a high-resolution video codec (used in the hosted video conference). The ultrasound telehealth option will still need a video conferencing system to allow the virtual face-to-face interaction between the mother and fetal cardiologist. In the next few years, telehealth in general and fetal telecardiology specifically, will be much easier and less expensive to perform.

BARRIERS TO FETAL TELECARDIOLOGY SUCCESS

Fetal telecardiology is a novel healthcare delivery system, and it is not surprising that there are both real and imagined barriers to its success. These barriers include the following:

1. Inconsistencies in state and national policies related to the use and reimbursement of telemedicine, as well as regulatory and compliance issues for virtual care which may seem daunting to administrators and physicians.
2. Concerns for cost of the fetal telecardiology enterprise have reduced the enthusiasm in some institutions largely due to misunderstanding about billing. In many states, both the professional component of the echo interpretation and the evaluation and management codes for a face-to-face encounter can be billed by the distant cardiac center.
3. Concerns that the OB providers in the community and/or their patients will not accept virtual care.
4. Satisfaction with the "store and forward" interpretation of fetal echoes in which the echo performed at the community site is transmitted after the fact to the distant site for interpretation. However, store and forward has several disadvantages: the mother may receive the results until days later, causing unnecessary stress and anxiety; she does not have the opportunity to ask questions of the fetal cardiologist; and if the study is incomplete, she must return for further imaging.
5. Difficulty in explaining to administrators and key stake holders the advantages of real-time fetal telecardiology over store and forward, which is less costly and does not need immediate interpretation.

With time, education, and patience, these barriers can be overcome.

SUMMARY

Fetal telecardiology programs are in their infancy, but results to date have been encouraging. A fetal telecardiology program is feasible, has diagnostic accuracy and precise risk stratification. In addition, such a program is well accepted by patients and their OB providers in the local community, offers significant cost savings to the family, and does not sacrifice the integrity of the physician-patient relationship.

References

1. Sanapo L, Pruetz JD, Slodki M, Goens MB, Moon-Grady AJ, Donofrio MT. Fetal echocardiography for planning perinatal and delivery room care of neonates with congenital heart disease. *Echocardiography*. 2017;34(12):1804-1821.
2. Donofrio MT, Moon-Grady AJ, Hornberger LK, et al. Diagnosis and treatment of fetal cardiac disease: a scientific statement from the American Heart Association. *Circulation*. 2014;129(21):2183-2242.
3. Pinto NM, Weng C, Sheng X, et al. Modifiers of stress related to timing of diagnosis in parents of children with complex congenital heart disease. *J Matern Fetal Neonatal Med*. 2016;29(20):3340-3346.
4. Scalvini S, Zanelli E, Conti C, et al. Assessment of prehospital chest pain using telecardiology. *J Telemed Telecare*. 2002;8(4):231-236.
5. Klersy C, de Silvestri A, Gabutti G, et al. A meta-analysis of remote monitoring of heart failure patients. *J Am Coll Cardiol*. 2009;54(18):1683-1694.

6. Inglis SC, Clark RA, McAlister FA, et al. Structured telephone support or telemonitoring programmes for patients with chronic heart failure. *Cochrane Database Syst Rev.* 2010;8:CD007228.
7. Scalvini S, Glisenti F. Centenary of tele-electrocardiography and telephonocardiography — where are we today? *J Telemed Telecare.* 2005;11(7):325-330.
8. Molinari G, Rebo G, Frascio M, et al. The role of telecardiology in supporting the decision-making process of general practitioners during the management of patients with suspected cardiac events. *J Telemed Telecare.* 2002;8(2):97-101.
9. Molinari G, Valbusa A, Terrizzano M, et al. Nine years' experience of telecardiology in primary care. *J Telemed Telecare.* 2004;10(5):249-253.
10. Clark RA, Inglis SC, McAlister FA, et al. Telemonitoring or structured telephone support programmes for patients with chronic heart failure: systematic review and meta-analysis. *Br Med J.* 2007;334(7600):942-945.
11. Maric B, Kaan A, Ignaszewski A, et al. A systematic review of telemonitoring technologies in heart failure. *Eur J Heart Fail.* 2009;11(5):506-517.
12. Lowery C, Bronstein J, McGhee J, et al. ANGELS and University of Arkansas for Medical Sciences paradigm for distant obstetrical care delivery. *Am J Obstet Gynecol.* 2007;196:534.e1-534.e9.
13. Magann EF, McKelvey SS, Hitt WC, Smith MV, Azam GA, Lowery CL. The use of telemedicine in obstetrics: a review of the literature. *Obstet Gynecol Surv.* 2011;66:170-178.
14. Lowery CL, Bronstein JM, Benton TL, Fletcher DA. Distributing medical expertise: the evolution and impact of telemedicine in Arkansas. *Health Aff (Millwood).* 2014;33:235-243.
15. McCrossan BA, Sands AJ, Kileen T, Cardwell CR, Casey F. Fetal diagnosis of congenital heart disease by telemedicine. *Arch Dis Child Fetal Neonatal Ed.* 2011;96:F394-F397.
16. Sharma S, Parness IA, Kamenir SA, et al. Screening fetal echocardiography by telemedicine: efficacy and community acceptance. *J Am Soc Echocardiogr.* 2003;16:202-208.
17. McCrossan BA, Sands AJ, Kileen T, Doherty NW, Casey FA. A fetal telecardiology service: patient preference and socioeconomic factors. *Prenatal Diagn.* 2012;32:883-887.
18. Cuneo BF, Olson C, Haxel C, et al. Risk stratification of fetal cardiac anomalies in an underserved population using telecardiology. *Obstet Gynecol.* 2019;134(5):1096-1103.
19. Albritton JE, Maddox L, Dalto J, Ridout E, Minton S. The effect of a newborn telehealth program on transfers avoided: a multiple-baseline study. *Health Aff.* 2018;37(12):1990-1996.

Note: Page numbers followed by "f" indicate figures and "t" indicate tables.

R

S

T